T0321746

Medical Data Security for Bioengineers

Butta Singh
Guru Nanak Dev University, India

Barjinder Singh Saini
Dr. B. R. Ambedkar National Institute of Technology, India

Dilbag Singh
Dr. B. R. Ambedkar National Institute of Technology, India

Anukul Pandey
Dumka Engineering College, India

A volume in the Advances in Bioinformatics and
Biomedical Engineering (ABBE) Book Series

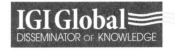

Published in the United States of America by
IGI Global
Medical Information Science Reference (an imprint of IGI Global)
701 E. Chocolate Avenue
Hershey PA, USA 17033
Tel: 717-533-8845
Fax: 717-533-8661
E-mail: cust@igi-global.com
Web site: http://www.igi-global.com

Library of Congress Cataloging-in-Publication Data

Names: Singh, Butta, 1981- editor. | Saini, Barjinder Singh, 1970- editor. |
  Singh, Dilbag, editor. | Pandey, Anukul, editor.
Title: Medical data security for bioengineers / Butta Singh, Barjinder Singh
  Saini, Dilbag Singh, and Anukul Pandey, editors.
Description: Hershey, PA : Medical Information Science Reference, [2019] |
  Includes bibliographical references.
Identifiers: LCCN 2018041395| ISBN 9781522579526 (hardcover) | ISBN
  9781522579533 (ebook)
Subjects: | MESH: Computer Security | Medical Informatics | Confidentiality |
  Signal Processing, Computer-Assisted | Cloud Computing
Classification: LCC R858 | NLM W 26.5 | DDC 610.285--dc23 LC record available at https://lccn.loc.gov/2018041395

This book is published in the IGI Global book series Advances in Bioinformatics and Biomedical Engineering (ABBE) (ISSN: 2327-7033; eISSN: 2327-7041)

British Cataloguing in Publication Data
A Cataloguing in Publication record for this book is available from the British Library.

All work contributed to this book is new, previously-unpublished material. The views expressed in this book are those of the authors, but not necessarily of the publisher.

For electronic access to this publication, please contact: eresources@igi-global.com.

Advances in Bioinformatics and Biomedical Engineering (ABBE) Book Series

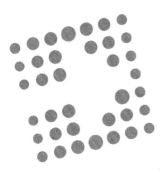

Ahmad Taher Azar
Benha University, Egypt

ISSN:2327-7033
EISSN:2327-7041

MISSION

The fields of biology and medicine are constantly changing as research evolves and novel engineering applications and methods of data analysis are developed. Continued research in the areas of bioinformatics and biomedical engineering is essential to continuing to advance the available knowledge and tools available to medical and healthcare professionals.

The **Advances in Bioinformatics and Biomedical Engineering (ABBE) Book Series** publishes research on all areas of bioinformatics and bioengineering including the development and testing of new computational methods, the management and analysis of biological data, and the implementation of novel engineering applications in all areas of medicine and biology. Through showcasing the latest in bioinformatics and biomedical engineering research, ABBE aims to be an essential resource for healthcare and medical professionals.

COVERAGE

- DNA Structure
- Algorithms
- Biomedical Sensors
- Genetic Engineering
- Structural Biology
- Finite Elements
- Nucleic Acids
- Bayesian methods
- Protein Engineering
- Drug Design

IGI Global is currently accepting manuscripts for publication within this series. To submit a proposal for a volume in this series, please contact our Acquisition Editors at Acquisitions@igi-global.com or visit: http://www.igi-global.com/publish/.

Titles in this Series

For a list of additional titles in this series, please visit: www.igi-global.com/book-series

Expert System Techniques in Biomedical Science Practice
Prasant Kumar Pattnaik (KIIT University, India) Aleena Swetapadma (KIIT University, India) and Jay Sarraf (KIIT University, India)
Medical Information Science Reference • copyright 2018 • 280pp • H/C (ISBN: 9781522551492) • US $205.00 (our price)

Nature-Inspired Intelligent Techniques for Solving Biomedical Engineering Problems
Utku Kose (Suleyman Demirel University, Turkey) Gur Emre Guraksin (Afyon Kocatepe University, Turkey) and Omer Deperlioglu (Afyon Kocatepe University, Turkey)
Medical Information Science Reference • copyright 2018 • 381pp • H/C (ISBN: 9781522547693) • US $255.00 (our price)

Applying Big Data Analytics in Bioinformatics and Medicine
Miltiadis D. Lytras (Deree - The American College of Greece, Greece) and Paraskevi Papadopoulou (Deree - The American College of Greece, Greece)
Medical Information Science Reference • copyright 2018 • 465pp • H/C (ISBN: 9781522526070) • US $245.00 (our price)

Comparative Approaches to Biotechnology Development and Use in Developed and Emerging Nations
Tomas Gabriel Bas (University of Talca, Chile) and Jingyuan Zhao (University of Toronto, Canada)
Medical Information Science Reference • copyright 2017 • 592pp • H/C (ISBN: 9781522510406) • US $205.00 (our price)

Computational Tools and Techniques for Biomedical Signal Processing
Butta Singh (Guru Nanak Dev University, India)
Medical Information Science Reference • copyright 2017 • 415pp • H/C (ISBN: 9781522506607) • US $225.00 (our price)

Handbook of Research on Computational Intelligence Applications in Bioinformatics
Sujata Dash (North Orissa University, India) and Bidyadhar Subudhi (National Institute of Technology, India)
Medical Information Science Reference • copyright 2016 • 514pp • H/C (ISBN: 9781522504276) • US $230.00 (our price)

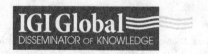

701 East Chocolate Avenue, Hershey, PA 17033, USA
Tel: 717-533-8845 x100 • Fax: 717-533-8661
E-Mail: cust@igi-global.com • www.igi-global.com

Table of Contents

Detailed Table of Contents

Siva Janakiraman, Shanmugha Arts, Science, Technology, and Research Academy (Deemed), India
Sundararaman Rajagopalan, Shanmugha Arts, Science, Technology, and Research Academy (Deemed), India
Rengarajan Amirtharajan, Shanmugha Arts, Science, Technology, and Research Academy (Deemed), India

Images have been widely used in the medical field for various diagnostic purposes. In the field of healthcare IoT, secure communication of a medical image concerned with an individual is a crucial task. Embedding patients' personal information as an invisible watermark in their medical images helps to authenticate the ownership identification process. Reliable communication of medical image can be thereby ensured concerning authentication and integrity. Images in DICOM format with a pixel resolution of 8-bit depth are used for medical diagnostics. This chapter deals about the development of a lightweight algorithm to insert patients' identities as an invisible watermark in random edge pixels of DICOM images. This chapter describes the implementation of the proposed lightweight watermarking algorithm on a RISC microcontroller suitable for healthcare IoT applications. Imperceptibility level of the watermarked medical image was analyzed besides its lightweight performance validation on the constrained IoT platform.

Neetika Soni, Guru Nanak Dev University, India
Indu Saini, Dr. B. R. Ambedkar National Institute of Technology, India
Butta Singh, Guru Nanak Dev University, India

The upsurge in the communication infrastructure and development in internet of things (IoT) has promoted e-healthcare services to provide remote assistance to homebound patients. It, however, increases the demand to protect the confidential information from intentional and unintentional access by unauthorized persons. This chapter is focused on steganography-based data hiding technique for ECG signal in which the selected ECG samples of non-QRS region are explored to embed the secret information. An embedding site selection (ESS) algorithm is designed to find the optimum embedding locations. The performance of the method is evaluated on the basis of statistical parameters and clinically supportive measures. The efficiency is measured in terms of embedding capacity and BER while key space measures its robustness. The implementation has been tested on standard MIT-BIH arrhythmia database of 2 mins and 5 mins duration and found that the proposed technique embarks the proficiency to securely hide the secret information at minimal distortion.

Chapter 3

Charu Bhardwaj, Jaypee University of Information Technology, India
Urvashi Sharma, Jaypee University of Information Technology, India
Shruti Jain, Jaypee University of Information Technology, India
Meenakshi Sood, Jaypee University of Information Technology, India

Compression serves as a significant feature for efficient storage and transmission of medical, satellite, and natural images. Transmission speed is a key challenge in transmitting a large amount of data especially for magnetic resonance imaging and computed tomography scan images. Compressive sensing is an optimization-based option to acquire sparse signal using sub-Nyquist criteria exploiting only the signal of interest. This chapter explores compressive sensing for correct sensing, acquisition, and reconstruction of clinical images. In this chapter, distinctive overall performance metrics like peak signal to noise ratio, root mean square error, structural similarity index, compression ratio, etc. are assessed for medical image evaluation by utilizing best three reconstruction algorithms: basic pursuit, least square, and orthogonal matching pursuit. Basic pursuit establishes a well-renowned reconstruction method among the examined recovery techniques. At distinct measurement samples, on increasing the number of measurement samples, PSNR increases significantly and RMSE decreases.

Chapter 4

Varinder Singh, Guru Nanak Dev University, India
Shikha Dhiman, Panjab University, India

The framers of Indian Constitution were very much cognizant about the significance of human nobility and worthiness and hence they incorporated the "right to life and personal liberty" in the Constitution of India. Right to life is considered as one of the primordial fundamental rights. There is no doubt that Indian Judiciary has lived up to the expectations of the Constitution framers, both in interpreting and implementing Article 21 initially, but there are still a few complications left as to the viability of Article 21 in modern times. Looking at the wider arena of right to life, it can be articulated that broader connotation of "right to life" aims at achieving the norms of "privacy" as well.

    Harminder Kaur, Dr. B. R. Ambedkar National Institute of Technology, India
    Sharvan Kumar Pahuja, Dr. B. R. Ambedkar National Institute of Technology, India

The aging population is vulnerable to various illnesses and health conditions because with increase in age the people suffer from chronic disease. Quite often, they are partially handicapped due to their restricted mobility and their reduced mental abilities. To resolve these problems, health monitoring systems are designed for real-time monitoring of patients. WBAN use medical sensors for acquiring patient physiological data with wireless technologies to send data to healthcare providers. Due to wireless transmission, the chances of attacking and occurring security issues in the data are more. So, the security of the system is the main concern because the system consists of patient privacy concerns. Due to these reasons there is need of designing security algorithms to prevent data from being stolen by attackers. The aim of this chapter is to present a review of different attacks that occurred during transmission of data and security issues related to data. The chapter also describes different algorithms to prevent data from being stolen through various attacks and security issues.

    Anukul Pandey, Dumka Engineering College, India
    Butta Singh, Guru Nanak Dev University, India
    Barjinder Singh Saini, Dr. B. R. Ambedkar National Institute of Technology, India
    Neetu Sood, Dr. B. R. Ambedkar National Institute of Technology, India

The primary objective of this chapter is to analyze the existing tools and techniques for medical data security. Typically, medical data includes either medical signals such as electrocardiogram, electroencephalogram, electromyography, or medical imaging like digital imaging and communications in medicine, joint photographic experts group format. The medical data are sensitive, subject to privacy preservation, and data access rights. Security in e-health field is an integrated concept which includes robust combination of confidentiality, integrity, and availability of medical data. Confidentiality ensures the data is inaccessible to unauthorized access. Integrity restricts the alteration in data by the unauthorized user. Whereas availability provides the readiness of the data when needed by the authorized user. Additionally, confidentiality, integrity and availability, accountability parameter records the back action list which answers the why, when, what, and whom data is accessed. The selected tools and techniques used in medical data security in e-health applications is discussed.

    Atul Kumar Verma, Dr. B. R. Ambedkar National Institute of Technology, India
    Indu Saini, Dr. B. R. Ambedkar National Institute of Technology, India
    Barjinder Singh Saini, Dr. B. R. Ambedkar National Institute of Technology, India

In this chapter, the BAT-optimized fuzzy k-nearest neighbor (FKNN-BAT) algorithm is proposed for discrimination of the electrocardiogram (ECG) beats. The five types of beats (i.e., normal [N], right bundle block branch [RBBB], left bundle block branch [LBBB], atrial premature contraction [APC], and premature ventricular contraction [PVC]) are taken from MIT-BIH arrhythmia database for the experimentation. Thereafter, the features are extracted from five type of beats and fed to the proposed BAT-tuned fuzzy KNN classifier. The proposed classifier achieves the overall accuracy of 99.88%.

Chapter 8

Padmapriya Praveenkumar, Shanmugha Arts, Science, Technology, and Research Academy (Deemed), India

Santhiyadevi R., Shanmugha Arts, Science, Technology, and Research Academy (Deemed), India

Amirtharajan R., Shanmugha Arts, Science, Technology, and Research Academy (Deemed), India

In this internet era, transferring and preservation of medical diagnostic reports and images across the globe have become inevitable for the collaborative tele-diagnosis and tele-surgery. Consequently, it is of prime importance to protect it from unauthorized users and to confirm integrity and privacy of the user. Quantum image processing (QIP) paves a way by integrating security algorithms in protecting and safeguarding medical images. This chapter proposes a quantum-assisted encryption scheme by making use of quantum gates, chaotic maps, and hash function to provide reversibility, ergodicity, and integrity, respectively. The first step in any quantum-related image communication is the representation of the classical image into quantum. It has been carried out using novel enhanced quantum representation (NEQR) format, where it uses two entangled qubit sequences to hoard the location and its pixel values of an image. The second step is performing transformations like confusion, diffusion, and permutation to provide an uncorrelated encrypted image.

Chapter 9

Taranjit Kaur, Indian Institute of Technology Delhi, India

Barjinder Singh Saini, Dr. B. R. Ambedkar National Institute of Technology, India

Savita Gupta, Panjab University, India

Multilevel thresholding is segmenting the image into several distinct regions. Medical data like magnetic resonance images (MRI) contain important clinical information that is crucial for diagnosis. Hence, automatic segregation of tissue constituents is of key interest to clinician. In the chapter, standard entropies (i.e., Kapur and Tsallis) are explored for thresholding of brain MR images. The optimal thresholds are obtained by the maximization of these entropies using the particle swarm optimization (PSO) and the BAT optimization approach. The techniques are implemented for the segregation of various tissue constituents (i.e., cerebral spinal fluid [CSF], white matter [WM], and gray matter [GM]) from simulated images obtained from the brain web database. The efficacy of the thresholding technique is evaluated by the Dice coefficient (Dice). The results demonstrate that Tsallis' entropy is superior to the Kapur's entropy for the segmentation CSF and WM. Moreover, entropy maximization using BAT algorithm attains a higher Dice in contrast to PSO.

The risk of encountering new diseases is on the rise in medical centers globally. By employing advancements in medical sensors technology, new health monitoring programs are being developed for continuous monitoring of physiological parameters in patients. Since the stored medical data is personal health record of an individual, it requires delicate and secure handling. In wireless transmission networks, medical data is disposed of to avoid loss due to alteration, eavesdropping, etc. Hence, privacy and security of the medical data are the major considerations during wireless transfer through Medical Sensor Network of MSNs. This chapter delves upon understanding the working of a secure monitoring system wherein the data could be continuously observed with the support of MSNs. Process of sanctioning secure data to authorized users such as physician, clinician, or patient through the key provided to access the file are also explained. Comparative analysis of the encryption techniques such as paillier, RSA, and ELGamal has been included to make the reader aware in selecting a useful technique for a particular hospital application.

Signal processing technology comprehends fundamental theory and implementations for processing data. The processed data is stored in different formats. The mechanism of electrocardiogram (ECG) steganography hides the secret information in the spatial or transformed domain. Patient information is embedded into the ECG signal without sacrificing the significant ECG signal quality. The chapter contributes to ECG steganography by investigating the Bernoulli's chaotic map for 2D ECG image steganography. The methodology adopted is 1) convert ECG signal into the 2D cover image, 2) the cover image is loaded to steganography encoder, and 3) secret key is shared with the steganography decoder. The proposed ECG steganography technique stores 1.5KB data inside ECG signal of 60 seconds at 360 samples/s, with percentage root mean square difference of less than 1%. This advanced 2D ECG steganography finds applications in real-world use which includes telemedicine or telecardiology.

Chapter 12

Atul Kumar Verma, Dr. B. R. Ambedkar National Institute of Technology, India
Indu Saini, Dr. B. R. Ambedkar National Institute of Technology, India
Barjinder Singh Saini, Dr. B. R. Ambedkar National Institute of Technology, India

In the chapter, dynamic time domain features are extracted in the proposed approach for the accurate classification of electrocardiogram (ECG) heartbeats. The dynamic time-domain information such as RR, pre-RR, post-RR, ratio of pre-post RR, and ratio of post-pre RR intervals to be extracted from the ECG beats in proposed approach for heartbeat classification. These four extracted features are combined and fed to k-nearest neighbor (k-NN) classifier with tenfold cross-validation to classify the six different heartbeats (i.e., normal [N], right bundle branch block [RBBB], left bundle branch block [LBBB], atrial premature beat [APC], paced beat [PB], and premature ventricular contraction[PVC]). The average sensitivity, specificity, positive predictivity along with overall accuracy is obtained as 99.77%, 99.97%, 99.71%, and 99.85%, respectively, for the proposed classification system. The experimental result tells that proposed classification approach has given better performance as compared with other state-of-the-art feature extraction methods for the heartbeat characterization.

Chapter 13

Ramgopal Kashyap, Amity University Chhattisgarh, India
Surendra Rahamatkar, Amity University Chhattisgarh, India

Medical image segmentation is the first venture for abnormal state image analysis, significantly lessening the multifaceted nature of substance investigation of pictures. The local region-based active contour may have a few burdens. Segmentation comes about to intensely rely on the underlying shape choice which is an exceptionally capable errand. In a few circumstances, manual collaborations are infeasible. To defeat these deficiencies, the proposed method for unsupervised segmentation of viewer's consideration object of medical images given the technique with the help of the shading boosting Harris finder and the center saliency map. Investigated distinctive techniques to consider the image data and present a formerly utilized energy-based active contour method dependent on the choice of high certainty forecasts to allocate pseudo-names consequently with the point of diminishing the manual explanations.

Chapter 14

Sundararaman Rajagopalan, Shanmugha Arts, Science, Technology, and Research Academy (Deemed), India
Siva Janakiraman, Shanmugha Arts, Science, Technology, and Research Academy (Deemed), India
Amirtharajan Rengarajan, Shanmugha Arts, Science, Technology, and Research Academy (Deemed), India

The healthcare industry has been facing a lot of challenges in securing electronic health records (EHR). Medical images have found a noteworthy position for diagnosis leading to therapeutic requirements. Millions of medical images of various modalities are generally safeguarded through software-based encryption. DICOM format is a widely used medical image type. In this chapter, DICOM image encryption implemented on cyclone FPGA and ARM microcontroller platforms is discussed. The methodology includes logistic map, DNA coding, and LFSR towards a balanced confusion – diffusion processes for encrypting 8-bit depth 256×256 resolution of DICOM images. For FPGA realization of this algorithm, the concurrency feature has been utilized by simultaneous processing of 128×128 pixel blocks which yielded a throughput of 79.4375 Mbps. Noticeably, the ARM controller which replicated this approach through sequential embedded "C" code took 1248 bytes in flash code memory and Cyclone IV FPGA consumed 21,870 logic elements for implementing the proposed encryption scheme with 50 MHz operating clock.

Preface

Healthcare systems are life-critical, context-aware, and networked systems of medical devices that provide tight integration between the cyber world of computing, communications and the physical world. Recent advances in mobile and wearable healthcare, communication, and Cloud computing technologies are making healthcare systems a promising platform for scientific advancement and development of new tools that may improve patients' health and wellbeing. Coming along with the potential social, economic and personal healthcare benefits are significant security, privacy, and trustworthiness challenges, due to unreliable embedded software controlling medical devices, weak computing and networking capabilities, and adaptive privacy requirements introduced by complicated physiological dynamics of patient bodies.

This edited book should be of interest to a broad spectrum of medical practitioners and bioengineers associated with biomedical data security. Many of the chapters cover topics that can be adequately covered only in a book dedicated solely to these areas. In this sense, every chapter represents a serious compromise with respect to comprehensive coverage of the associated topics. Practicing biomedical engineers, computer scientists, information technologists, medical physicists, and data-processing specialists working in diverse areas of biomedical signal applications, and hospital information systems may find this edited book valuable in their quest to learn advanced techniques for biomedical signal processing.

In Chapter 1, authors provides the development of a algorithm to insert patient's identity as an invisible watermark in random edge pixels of DICOM images. Random positions are identified at edge pixels that can be effectively utilized for the insertion of patient's personal information as an invisible watermark in images used for medical diagnostic applications. This chapter elaborates image security application using a microcontroller which open-up usage of constrained devices like microcontrollers for image-based security implementations on IoT platforms.

Chapter 2 is focussed on steganography based data hiding technique for ECG signal in which the selected ECG samples of non-QRS region are explored to embed the secret information. An embedding site selection (ESS) algorithm is designed to find the optimum embedding locations. The performance of the method is evaluated on the basis of statistical parameters and clinically supportive measures. The efficiency is measured in terms of embedding capacity and BER while key space measures its robustness. The implementation has been tested on standard MIT-BIH Arrhythmia database of 2mins and 5mins duration and found that the proposed technique embarks the proficiency to securely hide the secret information at minimal distortion.

Compression provides a main motive for efficient storage and transmission of medical, satellite and natural images (Chapter 3). Transmission speed is a key challenge in transmitting large amount of data especially for Magnetic Resonance Imaging (MRI) and Computed Tomography (CT) Scan images. Compressive sensing (CS) is an optimization based option to acquire sparse signal using sub-Nyquist criteria exploiting only the signal of interest. This chapter explores a nascent area of CS for correct sensing, acquisition and reconstruction of clinical images. CS performance is estimate for 1D signal and different medical image samples of MRI and CT- Scan. It is observed that the value of samples should be taken in such a way that there is appropriate balance between the recovered image quality and sampling rate. Quality metrics are obtained for L1, L2 and OMP algorithms for different image samples and it is estimated that L1 technique is better than other reconstruction algorithms in terms of PSNR, RMSE, SSIM and CR. Perfect image recovery is possible by L1 technique as it resembles more to the original image in comparison to L2 and OMP reconstruction methods. It is concluded that all quality metrics are better obtained by L1 and this is the best recovery technique among other implemented algorithms.

Privacy and confidentiality of an individual are most significant and influential values which is linked to person's autonomy and is considered to be highly prized in a country like India which has a democratic as well as republican set up. Chapter 4 appriciates shielding the confidentiality, privacy and data security of bio-medical information in India. Right to Life is considered as one of the primordial fundamental rights. There is no doubt that Indian Judiciary has lived up to the expectations of the Constitution framers, both in interpreting and implementing Article 21 initially, but there is still little amount of complication left as to the viability of Article 21 in modern times. Furthuremore, Chapter 5 reviewed security of system as main concern of patient privacy concerns which has been transmitted through wireless channel. Due to these reasons there is need of designing security algorithms to prevent data from attacker. Aim of this chapter is to present review of different attacks which are occurred during transmission of data and security issues related to data. The chapter also described different algorithms to prevent data from various attacks and security issues. the use of the wireless sensor networks in designing healthcare applications and currently available health monitoring systems.

Chapter 6 analyse the existing tools and techniques for medical data security. Typically, medical data includes either medical signals such as Electrocardiogram, Electroencephalogram, Electromyography or medical imaging like Digital Imaging and Communications in Medicine, Joint Photographic Experts Group format. The medical data are sensitive, subject to privacy preservation, and data access rights. Security in e-health field is an integrated concept which includes robust combination of confidentiality, integrity and availability of medical data. Confidentiality ensures the data is inaccessible to unauthorized access. Integrity restricts the alteration in data by the unauthorized user. Whereas availability provides the readiness of the data when needed by the authorized user. Additionally, confidentiality, integrity and availability; accountability parameter records the back action list which answers the why, when, what, and whom data is accessed. The selected tools and techniques used in medical data security in e-health applications is discussed.

Chapter 7 deals with the BAT optimized Fuzzy k-nearest neighbor (FKNN-BAT) algorithm for discrimination of the electrocardiogram (ECG) beats. The five types of beats i.e., Normal (N), Right Bundle Block Branch (RBBB), Left Bundle Block Branch (LBBB), Atrial Premature Contraction (APC), and Premature Ventricular Contraction (PVC) of ECG are taken from MIT-BIH arrhythmia database for the experimentation. The features are extracted from five type of beats and fed to the proposed BAT tuned Fuzzy KNN classifier. The comparative results of the classification accuracy using the existing and the proposed classification approach are presented

Chapter 8 focused in transferring and preservation of medical diagnostic reports and images across the globe in internet era, which become inevitable for the collaborative tele-diagnosis and tele-surgery. Consequently, it is of prime importance to protect it from unauthorized users and to confirm integrity and privacy of the user. Quantum Image Processing (QIP) paves way by integrating security algorithms in protecting and safeguarding medical images. This chapter proposes a Quantum assisted encryption scheme by making use of Quantum gates, chaotic maps and hash function to provide reversibility, ergodicity and integrity respectively. The first step in any quantum related image communication is the representation of the classical image into quantum. It has been carried out using Novel Enhanced Quantum Representation (NEQR) format, where it uses two entangled qubit sequences to hoard the location and its pixel values of an image. Secondly transformations like confusion, diffusion and permutation was carried out to provide an uncorrelated encrypted image.

Chapter 9 presents multilevel thresholding based segmention of the medical data like magnetic resonance images (MRI) into several distinct regions. Standard entropies, i.e., Kapur's and Tsallis are explored for thresholding of brain MRI. The optimal thresholds are obtained by the maximisation of these entropies using the Particle Swarm Optimization (PSO) and the BAT optimization approach. The techniques are implemented for the segregation of various tissue constituents, i.e., cerebral spinal fluid (CSF), white matter (WM) and, gray matter (GM) from simulated images obtained from the brain web database. The efficacy of the thresholding technique is evaluated by the Dice coefficient (Dice).

Chapter 10 covers the risk of encountering new diseases on the rise in medical centres. By employing medical sensors technology, health monitoring are being developed for monitoring physiological parameters of patients. Since the stored medical data is personal health record of an individual, it requires delicate and secure handling. In wireless transmission network, medical data is disposed to infect such as alteration, eavesdropping etc. Hence privacy and security of the medical data are the major considerations during wireless transfer through MSN. This chapter delves upon understanding the working of a secure monitoring system wherein the data could be continuously observed with the support of MSNs. Process of sanctioning secure data to authorised users such as physician, clinician or patient through the, key provided to access the file are also explained.

Chapter 11 describes the mechanism of Electrocardiogram (ECG) steganography in the spatial or transformed domain. Patient information is embedded into the ECG signal without sacrificing the significant ECG signal quality. This present chapter contributes to ECG steganography by investigating the Bernoulli's Chaotic map for 2D ECG Image Steganography. The methodology adopted is 1) Convert ECG signal into the 2D cover image 2) the cover image is loaded to steganography encoder, and 3) Secret key is shared with the steganography decoder. The proposed ECG steganography technique stores 1.5KB data inside ECG signal of 60 seconds at 360 samples/s, with percentage root mean square difference of less than 1%.

Chapter 12 proposes a new dynamic time-domain features are extracted in the proposed approach for the accurate classification of electrocardiogram (ECG) heartbeats. The dynamic time-domain information such as RR, Pre-RR, Post-RR, ratio of Pre-Post RR, and ratio of Post-Pre RR intervals to be extracted from the ECG beats in proposed approach for heartbeat classification. the new feature vector set is fed to the k-NN classifier with tenfold cross-validation scheme to classify the six different beats. The experimental results demonstrate that the proposed classification approach achieves an overall accuracy of 99.85%.

In Chapter 13 medical image segmentation for abnormal state image analysis for lessening the multifaceted nature of substance investigation of pictures has been presented. The local region-based active contour may have a few burdens. Segmentation comes about to intensely rely on upon the underlying shape choice which is an exceptionally capable errand. In a few circumstances, manual collaborations are infeasible. To defeat these deficiencies, the proposes method for unsupervised segmentation of viewer's consideration object of medical images given the technique with the help of the shading boosting Harris finder and the center saliency map.

Chapter 14 dicusses the Healthcare industry challenges in securing Electronic Health Records (EHR). Medical images have found a noteworthy position for diagnosis leading to therapeutic requirements. Millions of medical images of various modalities are generally safeguarded through software based encryption. DICOM format is a widely used medical image type. DICOM image encryption implemented on Cyclone FPGA and ARM microcontroller platforms. The methodology includes logistic map, DNA coding and LFSR towards a balanced confusion – diffusion processes for encrypting 8-bit depth 256 × 256 resolution of DICOM images. On the Microcontroller implementation, 1,248 flash code memory bytes and 65,992 flash data bytes were utilized by taking a computational time of 336.732 ms for encrypting the same size DICOM image with 50 MHz operating frequency.

Butta Singh
Guru Nanak Dev University, India

Barjinder Singh Saini
Dr. B. R. Ambedkar National Institute of Technology, India

Dilbag Singh
Dr. B. R. Ambedkar National Institute of Technology, India

Anukul Pandey
Dumka Engineering College, India

Acknowledgment

We are extremely happy to express our thanks to the Worthy Vice Chancellor, Guru Nanak Dev University, Amritsar, India and Worthy Director, National Institute of Technology, Jalandhar, India for providing the academic environment to carry out the editing of this book.

Our warmest thanks are due to all chapter authors, reviewers and publisher for their support and contribution to this book.

Last but not least we are using this opportunity to express our gratitude to everyone who supported throughout the course of this endeavour. we would like to thank those who directly or indirectly involved in bringing up this book successfully.

Butta Singh
Guru Nanak Dev University, India

Barjinder Singh Saini
Dr. B. R. Ambedkar National Institute of Technology, India

Dilbag Singh
Dr. B. R. Ambedkar National Institute of Technology, India

Anukul Pandey
Dumka Engineering College, India

Chapter 1
Reliable Medical Image Communication in Healthcare IoT:
Watermark for Authentication

Siva Janakiraman
Shanmugha Arts, Science, Technology, and Research Academy (Deemed), India

Sundararaman Rajagopalan
Shanmugha Arts, Science, Technology, and Research Academy (Deemed), India

Rengarajan Amirtharajan
Shanmugha Arts, Science, Technology, and Research Academy (Deemed), India

ABSTRACT

Images have been widely used in the medical field for various diagnostic purposes. In the field of healthcare IoT, secure communication of a medical image concerned with an individual is a crucial task. Embedding patients' personal information as an invisible watermark in their medical images helps to authenticate the ownership identification process. Reliable communication of medical image can be thereby ensured concerning authentication and integrity. Images in DICOM format with a pixel resolution of 8-bit depth are used for medical diagnostics. This chapter deals about the development of a lightweight algorithm to insert patients' identities as an invisible watermark in random edge pixels of DICOM images. This chapter describes the implementation of the proposed lightweight watermarking algorithm on a RISC microcontroller suitable for healthcare IoT applications. Imperceptibility level of the watermarked medical image was analyzed besides its lightweight performance validation on the constrained IoT platform.

DOI: 10.4018/978-1-5225-7952-6.ch001

INTRODUCTION

Internet of Things (IoT) finds its applications in diverse fields such as home automation, pollution monitoring, agriculture, and health care. Images have been predominantly used in medical diagnostic applications. The major aspects of security include confidentiality, integrity, and authentication. Due to the inevitable bondage of IoT devices with internet for data sharing via storage in the cloud, any data communication via IoT device is vulnerable to attacks. In the field of health care IoT, secure communication of a medical image concerned with an individual is a crucial task. Images such as human face can be easily distinguished and identified to authenticate the entry of a person in a restricted area.

In contrast, medical images cannot be distinguished unless it contains unique information about a patient. Information hiding on an image is a process that insets secret information into an image in an undetectable manner with a negligible loss in the original image quality. This work can be accomplished using techniques such as steganography or watermarking. A medical image with a patient's private information embedded as invisible watermark helps to identify the ownership and to authenticate. Thereby, authentication via watermark ensures the reliable communication of medical image.

Digital Imaging and Communications in Medicine (DICOM) is the widely used image format for medical diagnostics. These DICOM images can have a pixel resolution of 8-bit or 16-bit depth. Most of the existing watermarking schemes are designed for implementation on software platform like Matlab. To incorporate reliability on medical images used in healthcare IoT applications, it is necessary to device lightweight watermarking schemes that can be fit into the constrained devices such as microcontrollers used in IoT modules. Using less complex operations that take fewer clock cycles, minimal memory footprint and less power are the major requirements to be addressed while developing lightweight algorithms (Janakiraman, Thenmozhi, Rayappan, & Amirtharajan, 2018). Higher imperceptibility and a good level of randomness in the selection of image pixels for watermark insertion process are the significant parameters to make sure the reliability feature of the watermarking algorithms.

Edges are the pixels in the image that shows a visible disparity in their intensity levels. Identifying the edges of an image helps to locate an object and to know the borderline of a specific entity in an image. There are steganography algorithms that suggest embedding more information on edges to improve the embedding capacity while maintaining a good level of imperceptibility. Sobel mask, Quick mask, and Canny are some of the algorithms that can be used to accomplish edge detection on images. These algorithms decide the edges in an image by processing each pixel value with its surrounding pixels in all direction and by comparing the result with the set threshold values. Setting a threshold too high or too low may have a drastic impact on the ability of an algorithm to detect accurate edges.

This chapter describes the development of a lightweight algorithm in spatial domain that inserts the patient's identity as an invisible watermark in the edge pixels of the DICOM image. Further, this chapter also discusses the implementation aspects of the developed lightweight watermarking algorithm on a constrained microcontroller device suitable for health care IoT applications. Considering the memory constrains on IoT devices, DICOM images with 8-bit depth will be used for the implementation. Watermark information will be embedded in randomly chosen edge pixels of the medical image. Random edge detection will be carried out by applying the quick mask on the medical image with varying threshold values obtained from a Pseudo Random Number Generator (PRNG). Standard metrics such as Mean Average Error (MAE), Mean Square Error (MSE), Laplacian Mean Square Error (LMSE), Peak Signal to Noise Ratio (PSNR), Structural Similarity Index Measure (SSIM) and Normalised Cross Correlation (NCC) are to be analyzed to observe the imperceptibility level of the watermarked medical image.

Memory footprint and execution cycles of the watermarking algorithm while implemented on a constrained device will be analyzed to validate its lightweight properties. This chapter will explore a means for reliable medical data communication in IoT based healthcare applications through authentication and data integrity offered by the lightweight watermarking algorithm. The integrity part of reliability serves as proof to ensure the transfer of data in the unaltered form via an open channel even in the existence of any unauthorized persons. Additionally, the authentication side of reliability confirms the origin of information and its connectivity with a patient.

The major idea behind this chapter is to propose a novel method to identify random positions of edge pixels that can be effectively utilized for the insertion of patient's personal information as an invisible watermark in images used for medical diagnostic applications. Also, this chapter aims at analyzing the feasibility and limitations of embedded microcontrollers in handling medical image watermarking algorithms.

BACKGROUND

With the development in the arena of information technology and medicine, there is an increasing need for transmission of medical images over the public medium. In such a scenario, the medical images can be intentionally or unintentionally tampered during transmission. Therefore, it is highly essential to verify the trust within the medical images before taking any diagnostic decisions. Digital watermarking is the promising technique to ensure authentication and integrity of the medical images (Mousavi, Naghsh, & Abu-Bakar, 2014). In medical applications, authentication refers the ability to assure origin of information and the data is intended for the correct patient. Integrity refers to the ability to detect and manage the information from manipulations. In a wider sense, the medical image watermarking can be classified into three classes; classical schemes, Region of Interest (ROI) and Region of Non-Interest (RONI) schemes and reversible watermarking schemes.

In classical methods, the conventional way of data embedding based on the Least Significant Bit (LSB) is done (Coatrieux, Lecornu, Sankur, & Roux, 2006). When the last few planes of the medical image are replaced with watermarks, the image may perceptually change. These distorted medical images became unusable for the next diagnostic actions. Hence, the concept of ROI and RONI based embedding has come into the scene. Initially, the ROI and RONI concept is proposed by (Coatrieux, Maitre, & Sankur, 2001). The ROI is the portion which contains the most significant information for diagnosis, and the RONI contains insignificant/ less significant portion for diagnosis. Eventually, a single pixel change in ROI will lead to the wrong diagnosis; this region is usually exempted from watermark embedding. Though this class avoids the drawbacks of classic methods, the watermarked image with the watermark embedded in RONI suffers from the limitation of lesser bit embedding which ultimately depends on RONI size. This can be overcome by using the third class, i.e., reversible watermarking. Since, the embedding happens reversibly the quality of the medical image is protected for the next diagnostic actions (Honsinger, Jones, Rabbani, & Stoffel, 2001). Several works based on histogram shifting, difference expansion, and data compression are proposed under this class (Feng, Lin, Tsai, & Chu, 2006).

Cellular Automata (CA) is an important technique which is most widely used for random number generation. It can be designed with different length and dimensions. The one – dimensional (1D) cellular automata are an array of cells which are all interconnected and each cell depends on previous, present and past cell values. Generally, the CA is formed with the concept of rules which are framed by considering the neighboring cells. The rules define and decide the characteristics and operations of CA. For a k – bit CA, 2^k rules are possible. For example, an 8-bit CA consists of $2^8 = 256$ CA rules (Nayak, Patra, & Mahapatra, 2014). Among these Rule 90, Rule 150 and Rule 42 are more frequently used in image encryption applications due to it high randomness, large keyspace and to model complex systems (Sarkar, 2000; Rajagopalan, Rethinam, Arumugham, Upadhyay, Rayappan, & Amirtharajan, 2018; Rajagopalan, Sivaraman, Upadhyay, Rayappan, & Amirtharajan, 2018) Eq. (1-3) denotes the CA-90, CA-150 and CA-42 rules respectively.

$$x_i\left(t+1\right) = x_{i-1}\left(t\right) \oplus x_{i+1}\left(t\right) \tag{1}$$

$$x_i\left(t+1\right) = x_{i-1}\left(t\right) \oplus x_i\left(t\right) \oplus x_{i+1}\left(t\right) \tag{2}$$

$$S_i^{t+1} = \left(\overline{S_i^t} \wedge S_{i+1}^t\right) \oplus \left(\overline{S_{i-1}^t} \wedge S_i^t \wedge S_{i+1}^t\right) \tag{3}$$

where, $\left(i-1\right)$ represents the previous state, i, the present state and $\left(i+1\right)$ represents the next state.

Major techniques for image security can be broadly classified as steganography, image encryption and watermarking. These techniques are being implemented on pure software platforms, embedded software, and reconfigurable hardware platforms. Among the resource-constrained devices, reconfigurable systems like Field Programmable Gate Arrays (FPGAs) have been preferred over microcontrollers for image-based applications. Microcontrollers are the primary choice to perform computations in any embedded device. The processing devices for IoT applications demand additional features such as higher processing speed, low power consumption, wired / wireless connectivity to internet and support for a real-time kernel. The choice for IoT boards has Arduino boards in their lower end and powerful single board computers like raspberry-pi on the higher end. In the mid-level, Cortex-M4 based microcontrollers like STM32F4 family supports access to Universal Serial Bus (USB) hosts, Ethernet and multitasking real-time kernel with Wireless Fidelity (WiFi) link to wireless stack for internet connectivity. Edge detection algorithms such as Quick edge and Sobel edge are widely used for faster edge extraction. Sobel edge detection was implemented on reconfigurable devices (Nausheen, Seal, Khanna, & Halder, 2018) with an aim to further reduce the architecture from 10-bit to 8-bit. The suitability of STM32 Advanced RISC Machines (ARM) microcontroller to implement the Sobel filer was analyzed by Francisco Ordonez, & Onate (2016). Implementing image security algorithms on microcontrollers will serve for medical diagnostic in the field of healthcare IoT.

PROPOSED METHODOLOGY

This chapter aims to develop a lightweight algorithm that incorporates the personal details of the patient as a watermark on their medical images. The developed algorithm has been realized as using embedded

C language and implemented on a microcontroller with Cortex-M4 core. The proposed algorithm will serve for securing the communication of medical images.

Medical Image Watermarking Using Microcontroller

The proposed algorithm for image watermarking deploys lightweight operations, and it was implemented on MCBSTM32F400 evaluation board containing Cortex-M4 based STM32F407IG microcontroller with the intention to make the algorithm suitable for IoT applications. A patient's medical image of size 256×256 in DICOM format with 8-bit pixel values shall be chosen. An alphanumeric string of 25 bytes in length with the following details about a patient shall be chosen as watermark information as given in Table 1.

An 8-bit PRNG circuit constructed using the rule 90 and 150 of cellular automata as shown in the pseudo code given below. The circuit takes an 8-bit value as initial input (seed) to generate the next number in a pseudo-random manner. The first 25 numbers generated by the PRNG are used to encrypt the 25 bytes of watermark information through Ex-Or operation. Embedding the watermark bits only on the edges improves the imperceptibility. Sobel mask operator is applied in the input DICOM image to find the edge pixels. Here, the edge detection process did not consider the two LSBs that are manipulated during the watermark insertion process thereby facilitating the detection of identical pixels of the watermarked image as edges. Threshold selection plays a vital role in the edge detection process as the mask results that are greater than the threshold alone are accepted as edges. Instead of fixing a constant threshold, fixing a dynamic threshold value provides randomness in the edge detection process. Choosing the dynamic threshold from the output of the CA-based PRNG facilitates to enhance the randomness in the edge selection for watermark insertion. This algorithm excludes any pixel in the border from entering into the edge detection process. Also, the proposed algorithm avoids any two subsequent watermark insertion process to occur on the edge pixels detected from the same row or same column line thereby providing yet another style of randomness. Further, the edge detection process is terminated once all the watermark bits are completely embedded in the input image. The block diagram of the proposed edge based watermark embedding scheme is shown in Figure 1.

Pseudo Code for 8-Bit PRNG Using Rule 90 and 150 of 1D Cellular Automata

```
Select an 8-bit seed value S between 00 to FF;
Declare q_p and q_n to store the present and next state values of PRNG;
Initialize q_p with the seed value S;
for i in 0 to 255 loop
```

Table 1. Description of watermark information

Byte No.	Patient Information	No. of Bytes
0-6	Seven digit ID Number	7
7-8	Age	2
9	Gender: M / F	1
10-24	Name	15

Figure 1. Block diagram of proposed image watermarking

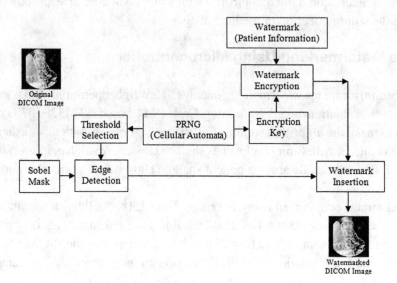

```
        q_n(0) = q_p(1);
        q_n(1) = q_p(2) ⊕ q_p(1) ⊕ q_p(0);
        q_n(2) = q_p(3) ⊕ q_p(1);
        q_n(3) = q_p(4) ⊕ q_p(3) ⊕ q_p(2);
        q_n(4) = q_p(5) ⊕ q_p(3);
q_n(5) = q_p(6) ⊕ q_p(5) ⊕ q_p(4);
        q_n(6) = q_p(7) ⊕ q_p(5);
        q_n(7) = q_p(6);
        Assign q_n as q_p for next iteration;
end for;
```

The flowchart in Figure 2 depicts the pictorial representation of the proposed watermark embedding procedure.

Steps for Watermark Embedding

Step 1: Input 1: DICOM Image I of size 256×256 with 8-bit pixel resolution.

Step 2: Input 2: Patient's information P of length L bytes as invisible watermark to be inserted in the DICOM image I.

Step 3: Implement an 8-bit pseudo-random number generator using the Rules 90 and 150 of Cellular Automata as said in the pseudo code.

Step 4: Generate an 8-bit key K using the CA-based PRNG.

Step 5: Encrypt a watermark data byte by performing Ex-Or operation with key K obtained from Step4.

Step 6: Repeat the Steps 4 and 5 until L bytes of Patient's information is encrypted to produce L bytes of watermark data W.

Figure 2. Flowchart for the proposed watermark embedding process

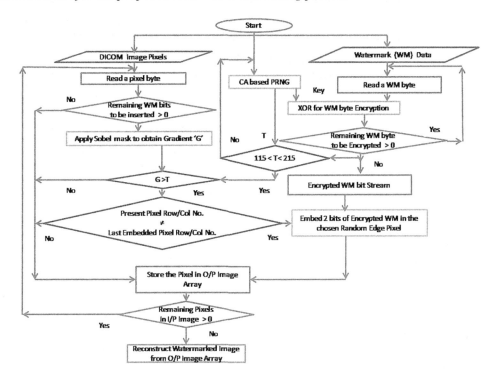

Step 7: Select a threshold T by running the CA-based PRNG until its 8-bit output comes in the range of 115 to 215.

Step 8: For pixels in the border (first and last row/column) of the input image, store the pixel value of the input image as an output image.

Step 9: Select a 3×3 sub-window S for the pixel N from the surrounding pixels of the input DICOM image I by masking two LSBs.

Step 10: Obtain the Gradient value G by applying the 3×3 Sobel mask operator on the sub-window S.

Step 11: Identify the edge pixel by comparing the value of G obtained from step 8 with the chosen threshold value, T.

Step 12: Regard the pixel N as an edge if G > T else regard the pixel N is a non-edge.

Step 13: Edge: If the detected edge pixel is in the same row or column number of the previously embedded edge pixel then store the pixel value of the input image as output image and Go to Step7 else Go to Step15.

Step 14: Non-edge: Store the pixel value of input image as output image then Go to Step7.

Step 15: Edge: Embed two bits of encrypted watermark data from W in the LSBs of the pixel N.

Step 16: Remaining watermark data to be embedded is not zero: Go to Step7.

Step 17: Remaining watermark data to be embedded is zero: Store the pixel value of input image as output image.

Step 18: Size of watermarked output DICOM image is less than the size of input image: Go to Step16.

Step 19: Size of watermarked output DICOM image is equal to the size of input image: stop the

Steps for Watermark Extraction

Step 1: Input: Watermarked DICOM Image WI of size 256 × 256 with 8-bit pixel resolution.

Step 2: Implement an 8-bit pseudo-random number generator using the Rules 90 and 150 of Cellular Automata as said in the pseudo code.

Step 3: Run the CA-based PRNG to generate an 8-bit key K and store the first 25 keys for later usage during the decryption phase.

Step 4: Continue running the CA-based PRNG until its 8-bit output comes in the range of 115 to 215 to select a threshold T.

Step 5: Exclude the pixels in the border of the watermarked image and select a 3×3 sub-window S for the pixel N from the surrounding pixels of the image WI by masking two LSBs.

Step 6: Obtain the value G by applying the 3×3 Sobel mask operator on the sub-window S.

Step 7: Identify the edge pixel by comparing the value of G obtained from Step6 with the chosen threshold value T.

Step 8: Regard the pixel N as an edge if G > T else regard the pixel N is a non-edge.

Step 9: Edge: If the detected edge pixel is in the same row or column number of the previously embedded edge pixel then store the pixel value of the input image as output image and Go to Step4 else Go to Step11.

Step 10: Non-edge: Go to Step4.

Step 11: Edge: Extract the two bits data from the pixel N and accumulate them to get the watermark data bytes in encrypted form.

Step 12: Size of extracted watermark data bytes in encrypted form is less than L: Go to Step4.

Step 13: Patient's information P of length L bytes is obtained by the decryption process that performs Ex-Or operation between the encrypted watermark data bytes and keys K obtained from Step3.

SOLUTIONS AND RECOMMENDATIONS

The edge-based random watermark embedding algorithm proposed in this chapter facilitates reliable communication of medical images. The work has been implemented on a microcontroller having Cortex-M4 core. The embedded software for the proposed work has been developed with embedded C language and compiled under Keil MDK µvision4 integrated development environment. Various analyses on security and performance aspects of the implementation have been carried out and presented in this section.

Visual Similarity Analyses

The proposed edge based random watermark insertion algorithm was tested on three different 8-bit DICOM images of size 256×256. As a process of ensuring the selection of right values as a threshold to detect true edges, edge detection was carried out on the entire image within the selected threshold range of 115 to 215. Considering the insertion of 200 watermark bits (25 bytes) as 2-bit information in the chosen edge pixels, the algorithm requires only 100 edge pixels to complete the watermark insertion process. The number of edge pixels in the chosen input images ranges from few hundred to several hundred. Therefore; the position of watermark embedded random edges on each image was identified to observe the random distribution of watermark information in the entire image area. The resemblance of the watermarked images with their respective original images can ensure visual imperceptibility. The input image, the edge detected image, watermark embedded edge pixel positions on the image and watermarked image are shown respectively in Figures 3-22.

On observing the input images in Figures 3-7 and their corresponding edge detected images in Figures 8-12, the input image in Figure 3 and Figure 5 has number of edges compared to other input images. It can be noticed in Figures 13-17, the watermark embedded edge pixels were chosen from different regions of the edge image arbitrarily. The watermarked images in Figures 18-22 did not show any discernible distortion against their original input images.

Error Estimation

The role of the proposed algorithm is to provide reliable communication of medical images by the insertion of patient's personal information in their medical images as an invisible watermark. Hence, imperceptibility is a vital parameter that validates the security aspect of the proposed algorithm. Imperceptibility can be quantified by measuring the distortion created in the watermarked image. The standard parameters to measure the distortion on images include Mean Absolute Error (MAE), Mean Square Error (MSE) and Root Mean Square Error (RMSE) given by the Eqs. (4) to (6). The average of absolute difference estimated between the pixels of original and watermarked image defines the value of MAE. The loss original information in the watermarked image will be zero when the value of MAE is zero. While MAE

Figure 3. Input image DICOM-1 without watermark

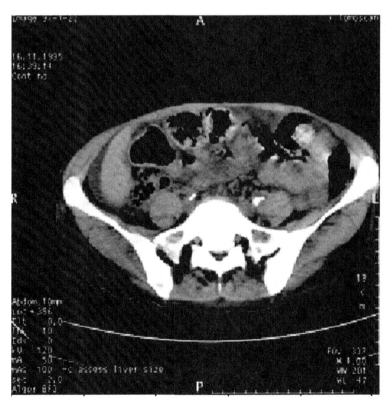

Figure 4. Input image DICOM-2 without watermark

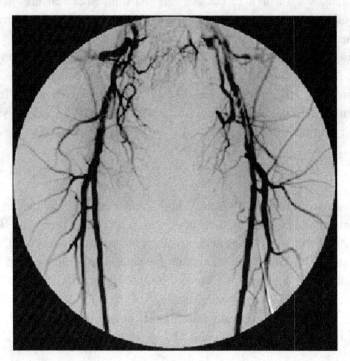

Figure 5. Input image DICOM-3 without watermark

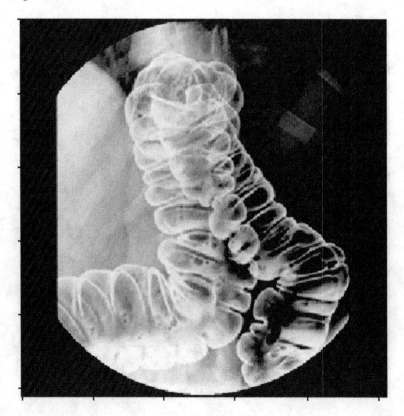

Figure 6. Input image DICOM-4 without watermark

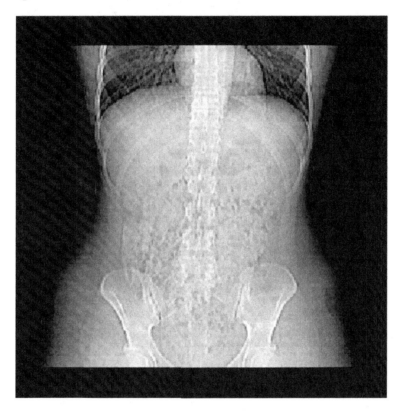

Figure 7. Input image DICOM-5 without watermark

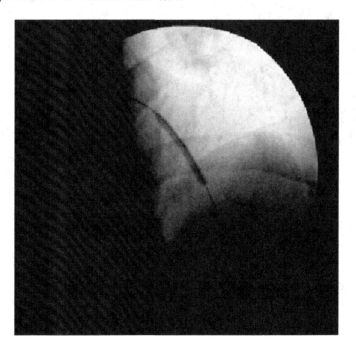

Figure 8. Edge detected image DICOM-1

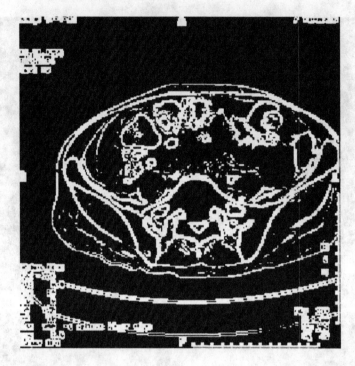

Figure 9. Edge detected image DICOM-2

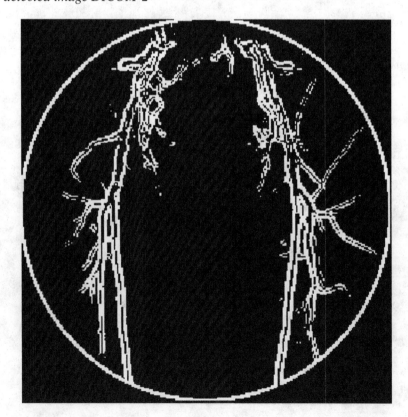

Figure 10. Edge detected image DICOM-3

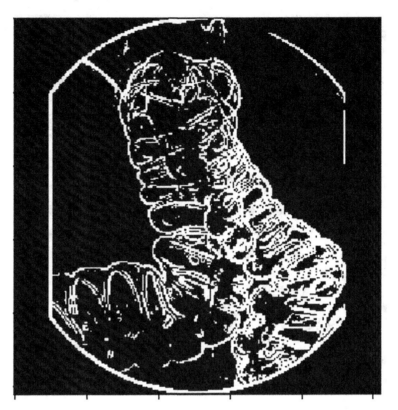

provides the error as an absolute value, the mean squared error value if given by MSE. RMSE provides the square root value of MSE. As the proposed algorithm selects the edge pixels on the images to insert watermark information, Laplacian Mean Square Error (LMSE) as given in Eq. (7) is a measure that exactly quantifies the distortion on edges. The minimal distortion on watermarked images should result in a value of MAE, MSE, RMSE, and LMSE being closer to zero (Bucerzan, & Raţiu, 2016).

Mean Average Error,

$$\text{MAE} = \frac{1}{MN} \sum_{x=1}^{M} \sum_{y=1}^{N} \left| WI_{x,y} - I_{x,y} \right| \tag{4}$$

Mean Square Error,

$$\text{MSE} = \frac{1}{MN} \sum_{x=1}^{M} \sum_{y=1}^{N} (WI_{x,y} - I_{x,y})^2 \tag{5}$$

Root Mean Square Error,

Figure 11. Edge detected image DICOM-4

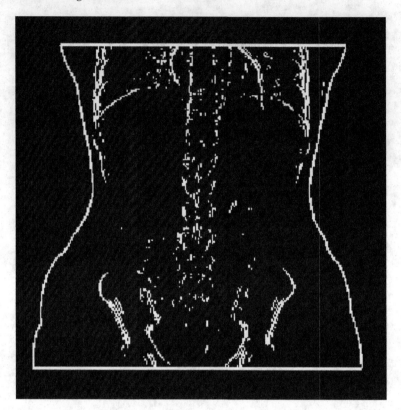

Figure 12. Edge detected image DICOM-5

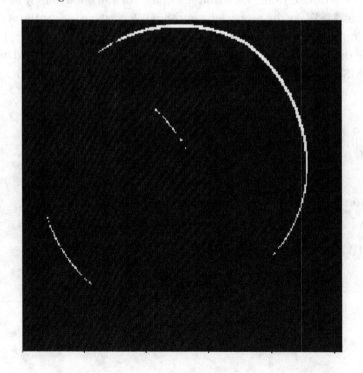

Figure 13. Watermark embedded edge pixels in DICOM-1

Figure 14. Watermark embedded edge pixels in DICOM-2

Figure 15. Watermark embedded edge pixels in DICOM-3

Figure 16. Watermark embedded edge pixels in DICOM-4

Figure 17. Watermark embedded edge pixels in DICOM-5

$$\text{RMSE} = \sqrt{MSE} \tag{6}$$

Laplacian Mean Square Error,

$$\text{LMSE} = \frac{\sum_{X=1}^{M}\sum_{y=1}^{N}\left[L\left(WI_{x,y} - I_{x,y}\right)\right]^2}{\sum_{X=1}^{M}\sum_{y=1}^{N}\left[L\left(I_{x,yj}\right)\right]^2} \tag{7}$$

The Laplacian operators $L\left(I_{x,y}\right)$ and $L\left(WI_{x,y}\right)$ are given by Eqs. (8) and (9)

$$L\left(I_{x,y}\right) = I_{x+1,y} + I_{x-1,y} + I_{x,y+1} + I_{x,y-1} - 4I_{x,y} \tag{8}$$

$$L\left(WI_{x,y}\right) = WI_{x+1,y} + WI_{x-1,y} + WI_{x,y+1} + WI_{x,y-1} - 4WI_{x,y} \tag{9}$$

Figure 18. Output - watermarked image DICOM-1

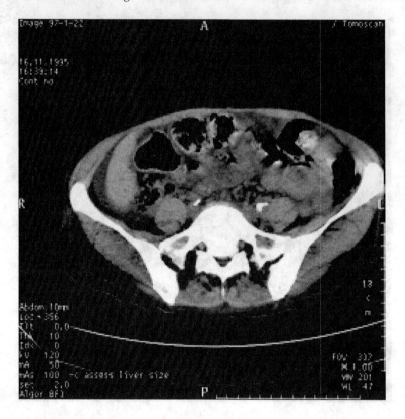

where, $I_{x,y}$ and $WI_{x,y}$ denotes the pixels of input and watermarked DICOM images respectively with x, y indicating one of the M rows and N columns in the images correspondingly.

The inference from Table 2 indicates the amount of error measured in various watermarked images and the number of edges detected based on the threshold range chosen by the algorithm. While the MAE and MSE values are trivial and nearly equal for the DICOM images 1, 2 and 3, it is comparatively a bit more for images 4 and 5. A significant difference can be noticed in the value of LMSE for DICOM images 4 and 5. As the watermark embedding was done only on the edges, a slightly higher distortion on edges (LMSE value) can be observed on the image DICOM-5 which contains the least number of edges among the DICOM images used for the analysis.

Statistical and Structural Similarity Analysis

Peak Signal to Noise Ratio (PSNR) measured in decibels as given by Eq. (10) quantifies the closeness of the watermarked image concerning the original image. Normalized Cross Correlation (NCC) as given by Eq. (11) is a metric that demonstrates the dimension of likeness between the images before and after the insertion of a watermark. Structural Similarity Index Measure (SSIM) is yet another parameter that confirms the resemblance of watermarked images against the input (original) images. The structural similarity given by Eq. (12) is a product of Luminance, Contrast, and Structure values.

Peak Signal to Noise Ratio (PSNR),

Figure 19. Output - watermarked image DICOM-2

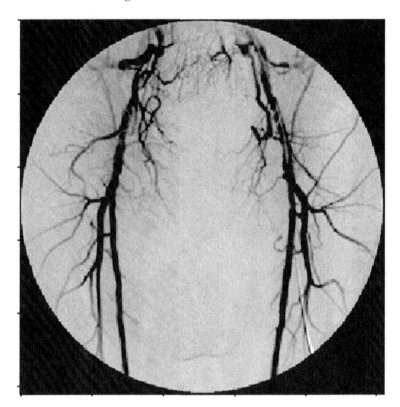

$$\text{PSNR} = 10 \log_{10} \{ B_{\max}^2 / MSE \} \text{ dB} \tag{10}$$

As the chosen DICOM images have 8-bit pixel depth, their maximum pixel intensity level $B_{\max}$ is 255.

Normalized Cross Correlation (NCC),

$$NCC = \frac{\sum_{X=1}^{M} \sum_{Y=1}^{N} WI_{XY} \cdot I_{XY}}{\sum_{X=1}^{M} \sum_{Y=1}^{N} WI_{XY}^2} \tag{11}$$

Structural Similarity Index Measure (SSIM),

$$SSIM = Luminance \times Conrast \times Structure \tag{12}$$

Similarity index of -1 indicates the null-matching whereas similarity value close to 1 substantiates the highest level of similarity between the original and watermarked image. NCC estimation of zero

Figure 20. Output - watermarked image DICOM-3

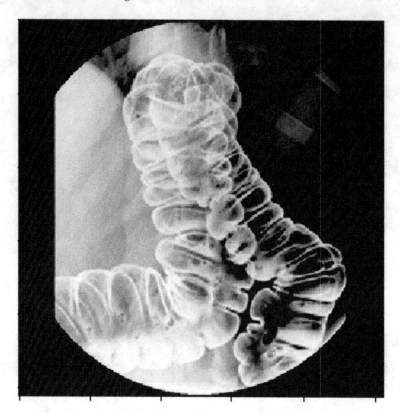

demonstrates an invalid similitude between the pictures while -1 shows comparable pictures with inverse signs. Estimation of NCC being one show signs of identical pictures.

According to Bucerzan, & Raţiu (2016), PSNR of more than 40 dB is good enough to maintain the quality of a stego image. From Table 3, the achieved PSNR for all watermarked images being more than 67 dB statistically quantifies the similarity with original images. Equally, attaining the SSIM and NCC values closer to 1 (more than 99.99% similarity) substantiates the structural similarity level between the watermarked and original images.

To showcase the efficiency of the proposed work, the major results of this chapter have been compared against an earlier work carried out by Selvam, P., Balachandran, S., Iyer, S.P., & Jayabal, R. (2017) on revisable watermarking technique for medical images. The SSIM and PSNR values calculated between the original and watermarked DICOM images 2, 3 and 4 are chosen for comparison. From the graph shown in Figure 23, the SSIM values presented by Selvam et al. (2017) for various DICOM images struggle to get closer to 1 (100% similarity on structure). In contrast, in Figure 23, SSIM values obtained for the same DICOM images in the proposed work are almost nearer to the theoretical maximum. This comparison proves the efficiency of the proposed work to insert a watermark on DICOM images without affecting the properties of the original image such as luminance, structure, and contrast.

As yet another aspect of proving the efficiency of the proposed work, the obtained PSNR values are compared against the PSNR values obtained by Selvam et al. (2017) for the same set of DICOM images. As shown in Figure 24 while the maximum PSNR value reported by Selvam et al. (2017) is <65dB,

Figure 21. Output - watermarked image DICOM-4

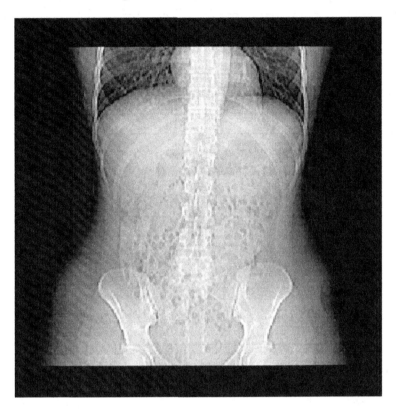

Figure 22. Output - watermarked image DICOM-5

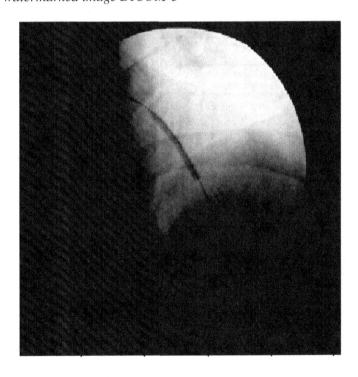

Table 2. Error estimation for watermarked images

Error Metrics	DICOM-1	DICOM-2	DICOM-3	DICOM-4	DICOM-5
MAE	1.79515	1.43013	1.02323	5.14610	3.59030
MSE	0.00013	0.00257	0.00135	0.01034	0.00045
RMSE	0.01140	0.05069	0.03674	0.10168	0.02121
LMSE	4.03296×10^{-9}	0.12886×10^{-9}	0.81852×10^{-9}	26.52778×10^{-9}	81.59623×10^{-9}
Edge count	13310	7605	11014	3479	711

Table 3. Error estimation for watermarked images

Error Metrics	DICOM-1	DICOM-2	DICOM-3	DICOM-4	DICOM-5
PSNR (dB)	86.7531	74.0167	76.8017	67.9833	81.5243
SSIM	0.9999	0.9997	0.9997	0.9998	0.9999
NCC	0.9999	0.9998	0.9998	0.9997	0.9999

Figure 23. Comparison on the efficiency of watermark embedding algorithm based on SSIM

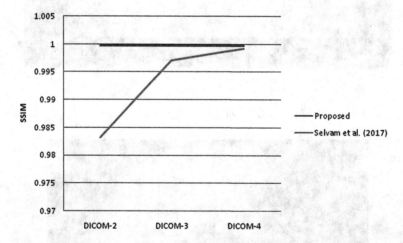

the minimum value of PSNR obtained in the proposed work is ≈68dB with a maximum value of PSNR is >76dB. This comparison ensures the efficiency of the proposed to work to embed a watermark on DICOM images with a highly imperceptible level of distortion.

Performance Analyses on Embedded Platform

Performance of embedded software for micro-programmed devices like microprocessors and microcontrollers are measured regarding its demand on memory space and the time taken to produce the results. A 32-bit microcontroller STM32F407IG with Cortex-M4 core having 512 KB of on-chip Flash memory and 192 KB of on-chip Static Random Access Memory (SRAM) has been chosen as target device. The 20-pin J-Link real-time debugger from Segger has been used to analyze the memory and timing related

Figure 24. Comparison of the efficiency of watermark embedding algorithm based on PSNR

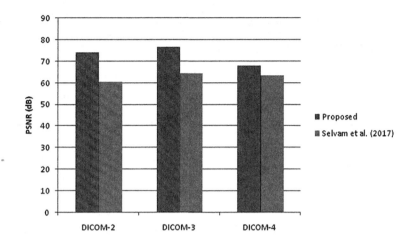

parameters. The Flash code area indicates the memory space required to store the application code. As the extraction algorithm does the same set of operations carried out during the watermark embedding process, the required size of code storage for the embedding and extraction process remains nearly equal. On considering the available on-chip Flash memory of the chosen microcontroller, the memory footprint of both the watermark embedding and extraction algorithms are much less than 1% of the available Flash area. For evaluation, the original DICOM image as input for watermark embedding algorithm and the watermarked image as input for the watermark extraction algorithm are stored as two-dimensional look-up tables in the code memory. This process contributes to the size of Flash data denoted in Table 4. The embedding algorithm requires more SRAM data space as it stores the entire watermarked image in it. The extraction algorithm needs fewer SRAM bytes as it has stores only the extracted watermark in SRAM along with the keys used by the algorithm to decrypt the extracted information.

For the calculation of computational time, the device's maximum operating frequency of 168 MHz has been used. From Table 4, time for extraction is about 1.5 ms less than the time to complete the watermark embedding process when using the DICOM-1 as input image. Embedding algorithm needs to process the entire pixels of the image to produce the watermarked image. In contrast, the extraction algorithm no longer needs to process the remaining pixels after it receives all the embedded watermark bits. As a result of this, the CPU cycles and computational time is taken by the extraction algorithm will always be less than the watermark embedding algorithm. Further, the difference in computational time between the watermark embedding and extraction algorithms is highly dependent on the parameters the seed value used to generate the PRNG sequence and the distribution of edge pixels in the original image.

The Novelty of the Present Work

The strength of any watermarking algorithm relies on the level of imperceptibility it offers. The proposed work inserts watermark bits only on the selective edges of the input image. The edge pixels of the image used to have an intensity level that is distinct from its surrounding pixels. Therefore, any change that happens in the intensity level of edge pixel due to watermark insertion will not be visually discernible. The edge detection algorithm used in this work applies a Sobel mask to find the gradient value

Table 4. Analyses on embedded software for DICOM image watermarking

Target Device	STM32F407IG Microcontroller with Cortex-M4 Core	Watermark Embedding Algorithm	Watermark Extraction Algorithm
Operating frequency	168 MHz		
On-chip Memory utilization (Bytes)	Flash Code	1244	1240
	Flash Data	65960	65960
	SRAM Data	67312	180
Performance Metrics	CPU cycles	32594292	32334528
	Computational Time (ms)	194.013	192.467

and compares it with a preset threshold value to identify the edge pixels. Although the distribution of edge pixels in an image tends to be random, in medical images the possibility of similarity will be high. The proposed work dynamically chooses a random value as a threshold for the edge selection process thereby making the selection of pixel positions for a watermark embedded almost a unique one for every input image. This special feature makes the proposed work to be distinct from others by offering higher imperceptibility to the watermarked medical images.

Limitations of the Present Work

- The proposed embedded platform implementation imposes a restriction on the input image size based on the available on-chip SRAM space of the chosen target device
- To use DICOM images with 16-bit pixel resolution as input to the same algorithm on the proposed embedded device, further compromise has to be made on the input image size
- The random edge pixel selection feature of the proposed algorithm may not allow completing the watermark insertion process when higher payload (more watermark bytes) need to be embedded on input images having a fewer number of edges

FUTURE RESEARCH DIRECTIONS

Image security applications such as steganography or image encryption developed using spatial domain techniques lag concerning robustness against the methods in the transform domain. Designing image security applications involving transform domain techniques like Discrete Cosine Transform (DCT), Discrete Wavelet Transform (DWT), etc. and their implementation analysis on embedded microcontroller and reconfigurable platforms such as Field Programmable Gate Arrays (FPGAs) can be a worthy topic for future research.

CONCLUSION

The proposed watermark insertion algorithm on medical images was implemented on STM32F407IG microcontroller having Cortex-m4 core. The algorithm embeds the watermark information on randomly chosen edges of the image and provides the minimal error regarding MAE and MSE. Although the LMSE value for the input image DICOM- is slightly higher due to the unavailability of more edges in it, the imperceptibility of the same image is substantiated by its higher values of PSNR and SSIM. This work has managed to use larger input image size with its on-chip memory by utilizing the part of Flash memory as data storage. The code size for the embedding and extraction algorithm remains constant while their execution time slightly differs due to the difference in the availability of edges in the input DICOM images. As this chapter elaborates yet another kind of image security application using a microcontroller, this will open-up more usage of constrained devices like microcontrollers for image-based security implementations on IoT platforms.

ACKNOWLEDGMENT

This research received no specific grant from any funding agency in the public, commercial, or not-for-profit sectors.

REFERENCES

Bucerzan, D., & Raţiu, C. (2016). Reliable Metrics for Image LSB Steganography on Mobile Platforms. *International Workshop Soft Computing Applications*, 517-528.

Coatrieux, G., Lecornu, L., Sankur, B., & Roux, C. (2006). A review of image watermarking applications in healthcare. *IEEE 28th Annual International Conference on Engineering in Medicine and Biology Society*, 4691-4694.

Coatrieux, G., Maitre, H., & Sankur, B. (2001). Strict integrity control of biomedical images. International Society for Optics and Photonics: Security and watermarking of multimedia contents, 4314, 229-240.

Feng, J. B., Lin, I. C., Tsai, C. S., & Chu, Y. P. (2006). Reversible watermarking: Current status and key issues. *International Journal of Network Security*, 2, 161–170.

Francisco Ordonez, J., & Onate, L. (2016). Edge detection image using arm microcontroller. *Ingenius-. Revista de Ciencia y Tecnología*, 16, 30–35. doi:10.17163/ingenius.n16.2016.04

Honsinger, C.W., Jones, P.W., Rabbani, M., & Stoffel, J.C. (2001). *Lossless recovery of an original image containing embedded data.* US Patent 6,278,791.

Janakiraman, S., Thenmozhi, K., Rayappan, J. B. B., & Amirtharajan, R. (2018). Lightweight chaotic image encryption algorithm for real-time embedded system: Implementation and analysis on 32-bit microcontroller. *Microprocessors and Microsystems*, 56, 1–12. doi:10.1016/j.micpro.2017.10.013

Mousavi, S. M., Naghsh, A., & Abu-Bakar, S. (2014). Watermarking techniques used in medical images: A survey. *Journal of Digital Imaging*, 27(6), 714–729. doi:10.100710278-014-9700-5 PMID:24871349

Nausheen, N., Seal, A., Khanna, P., & Halder, S. (2018). A FPGA based implementation of Sobel edge detection. *Microprocessors and Microsystems*, 56, 84–91. doi:10.1016/j.micpro.2017.10.011

Nayak, D. R., Patra, P. K., & Mahapatra, A. (2014). *A Survey on Two Dimensional Cellular Automata and Its Application in Image Processing.* arXiv Preprint ar Xiv:1407.7626

Rajagopalan, S., Rethinam, S., Arumugham, S., Upadhyay, H. N., Rayappan, J. B. B., & Amirtharajan, R. (2018). Networked hardware assisted key image and chaotic attractors for secure RGB image communication. *Multimedia Tools and Applications*, 1–34.

Rajagopalan, S., Sivaraman, R., Upadhyay, H. N., Rayappan, J. B. B., & Amirtharajan, R. (2018). ON-Chip Peripherals are ON for Chaos--an Image fused Encryption. *Microprocessors and Microsystems*, *61*, 257–278. doi:10.1016/j.micpro.2018.06.011

Sarkar, P. (2000). A brief history of cellular automata. *ACM Computing Surveys*, *32*(1), 80–107. doi:10.1145/349194.349202

Selvam, P., Balachandran, S., Iyer, S. P., & Jayabal, R. (2017). Hybrid transform based reversible watermarking technique for medical images in telemedicine applications. *Optik-International Journal for Light and Electron Optics*, *145*, 655–671. doi:10.1016/j.ijleo.2017.07.060

Chapter 2
Robust Steganography in Non-QRS Regions of 2D ECG for Securing Patients' Confidential Information in E-Healthcare Paradigm

Neetika Soni
Guru Nanak Dev University, India

Indu Saini
Dr. B. R. Ambedkar National Institute of Technology, India

Butta Singh
Guru Nanak Dev University, India

ABSTRACT

The upsurge in the communication infrastructure and development in internet of things (IoT) has promoted e-healthcare services to provide remote assistance to homebound patients. It, however, increases the demand to protect the confidential information from intentional and unintentional access by unauthorized persons. This chapter is focused on steganography-based data hiding technique for ECG signal in which the selected ECG samples of non-QRS region are explored to embed the secret information. An embedding site selection (ESS) algorithm is designed to find the optimum embedding locations. The performance of the method is evaluated on the basis of statistical parameters and clinically supportive measures. The efficiency is measured in terms of embedding capacity and BER while key space measures its robustness. The implementation has been tested on standard MIT-BIH arrhythmia database of 2 mins and 5 mins duration and found that the proposed technique embarks the proficiency to securely hide the secret information at minimal distortion.

DOI: 10.4018/978-1-5225-7952-6.ch002

INTRODUCTION

The advancement in communication technology has brought revolution in almost every sphere of life. It is so permeated into human lives that every job is a click away and the whole world is confined to a small city. In addition to numerous applications, modern telecommunication infrastructure significantly helped the medical industry to generate e-healthcare paradigm that delivers quality health care to the patients without the physical presence of medical experts. Some of the advantages of e-healthcare services include

- Improved medical assistance: patients' can seek advice from the world's specialised doctors at any geographical area via remote healthcare assistance.
- Fast medical access: In case of emergency services, patient's medical reports (physiological signals, medical images and other metadata) can be immediately sent to the doctor and appropriate actions can be taken without any delay.
- Convenient and cost effective: monitoring patients through tele-services reduce the traffic in hospitals to great extent and also cuts the transportation cost.

Along with the medical information, it is required to transmit patients' personal information and other details such as his medical history and pathological reports for the purpose of identification and early diagnosis. But transmitting this confidential information over the unsecured public network is a matter of concern as any illegitimate personnel can access and tamper it that may cause erroneous diagnosis. Therefore safety and security of patients' vital information are the prime concerns in tele-health services. Various methods are reported in the literature to conceal the confidential information such as cryptography, steganography, watermarking *etc.* (Subhedar & Mankar, 2014) but steganography being the economical way of hiding information is preferred in which the sensitive information is interleaved into less sensitive features of the host media without disturbing its features (Johnson & Jajodia, 1998). In case of medical media (medical images or physiological signals) also, it is highly preferred because of following advantages:

1. Any doctor can diagnose the stego-signal but only the authorised administrative personnel can extract the hidden secret information.
2. It provides data security.
3. It provides efficient memory utilization.
4. Storing different information of the patient in same file avoids mismatching of information.
5. Steganography restrains false claim of health insurance, as the patients' personal details are already embedded into his physiological signal or medical image.

The selection of host media depends upon the nature of ailment for which the patient seeks the doctor's opinion. For *e.g.* in case of orthopaedic ailments, medical images such as X-ray, Positron Emission Tomography (PET), Computed Tomography (CT) scans, *etc.* are essential for diagnosis while in case of neurological disorders, Electroencephalograph (EEG) signals are required. It is preferred that the host media should have sufficient redundancy to accommodate adequate amount of secret information without destroying its diagnosability features. The commonly used host media in e-healthcare services include Magnetic Resonance Imaging (MRI) (Dmour HA & Ani AA, 2016) CT scans (Nambaksh, Ahmadian & Zaidi, 2011), PET (Nambaksh, Ahmadian & Zaidi, 2011) images, EEG (Rubio, Alesanco & García,

2013), Electromyogram (EMG) (Shiu, Lin, Chien, Chiang & Lei, 2017), Electrocardiogram (ECG) (Ibaida & Khalil, 2013; Jero, Ramu & Ramakrishnan, 2014) *etc.* However, ECG is the prime signal for diagnosis and analysis, of various diseases *e.g.* cardiovascular diseases (Berkaya, Uysal, Gunal, Ergin, Gunal & Gulmezoglu, 2018), blood pressure (Seera, Lim, Liew, Lim & Loo 2015), sleep apnea (Trinder, Kleiman, Carrington, Smith, Breen, Tan & Kim, 2001), stress detection (Berkaya, Uysal, Gunal, Ergin, Gunal & Gulmezoglu, 2018), pre-surgeries (Algeria-Barrero & Algeria-Ezquerra, 2008) *etc.,* hence used as the host media to conceal the confidential information.

The major focus of this chapter is to camouflage the confidential information in ECG signal using steganography while achieving the optimum trade-off amongst its major attributes viz. imperceptibility, robustness and payload.

BACKGROUND

The steganography techniques can be broadly classified into two categories; spatial domain and transform domain (Subhedar & Mankar, 2014). Each domain has its own advantages and disadvantages in regard to its embedding capacity, robustness and execution time. In spatial domain, the secret information is directly embedded into the host media whereas in transform domain, the host media is initially converted from spatial domain to frequency domain by using some transform technique and then the information bits are embedded into the transformed coefficients. Various steganography techniques in spatial domain that are used for reversible data hiding are: Least Significant Bit (LSB) Substitution (Chan & Cheng, 2004; Yang, Sun & Sun, 2009; Wang, Yang & Niu, 2010; Kanan & Nazeri, 2014), Vector Quantization method (Chang, Tai & Lin, 2006; Chen & Chang 2010), Quantization Index Modulation (Phadikar, 2013), Pixel Pair Matching (Hong & Chen, 2012) *etc.* while the examples in transform domain include Discrete Cosine Transform (DCT) and similar to DCT with modified stages (Lin, 2012; Lima, Madeiro & Sales, 2015), Discrete Wavelet Transform (DWT) (Wang, Lu & Hu, 2013; Ibaida & Khalil, 2013; Chen, Guo, Huang, Kung,Tseng & Tu, 2014; Jero, Ramu & Ramakrishnan, 2014), Integer to Integer wavelet Transform(Lee, Yoo & Kalker, 2007), Curvelet Transform (Jero, Ramu & Ramakrishnan, 2015) *etc.* Based on these techniques, tremendous research has been reported in field of data, image and multimedia steganography. Since steganography causes irreparable loss to the cover media hence its application in medical field is still in its infancy. A brief literature review of ECG steganography techniques is discussed in Table 1.

Chaotic Map Based ECG Steganography

In an effort to provide intense security to patients' confidential information, chaotic maps are employed in the process of ECG steganography. The chaotic maps are the non-linear functions that produce random like signals which are unpredictable yet deterministic and can be easily reproduced using the same initial conditions and control parameters (Kanso & Smaoui, 2009; Zhou, Bao & Chang, 2014). The exclusive features of chaotic maps makes them suitable in the design of steganographic algorithms.

In this work, Combined Logistic-Sine (CLS) map is used which exhibits uniform chaotic distribution over the entire range of b_o (Zhou, Bao & Chang, 2014; Hua, Zhou, Pun & Chang, 2015; Martinez-

Table 1. Literature review of ECG steganography techniques

Sr. No	Author Name/Year	Journal/ Conference	Work Done	Results
1	Koszat SS, Vlachos M, Lucchese C, Herle HV(2009)	Journal of Medical Systems	Watermark bits are initially processed using hash function and hamming code and then embedded in the ECG signal using spread spectrum technique. The method proposed two types of watermarking; robust and fragile to provide additional security to meta data.	The efficacy of metadata retrieval and watermark detection was tested under various data transformations such as vertical shifts, re-sampling (upsampling or downsampling) and cropping and found an effective method for watermarking.
2	Ibaida, Khalil & Al-Shammary, 2010.	32nd Annual International Conference on the IEEE Engineering in Medicine and Biology Society	Data hiding in ECG signal using spatial domain where secret bits were embedded in ECG samples according to some special range of numbers The results show that for embedding 32 secret bits, the number of possible locations were 2.1475×10^9 thus making it extremely difficult for intruders to identify locations of secret bits.	Embedded 2500 bits in 2500 ECG samples with Percentage Residual Difference (PRD) of 0.0247% and 0.0678% for normal and abnormal ECG segments respectively.
3	Nambaksh, Ahmadian & Zaidi, 2011.	Computer Methods and Programs in Biomedicine	The ECG signal and the text image are used as watermark and are embedded in selected texture regions of PET image using wavelet decomposition.	For 25 different PET images of size 256 x 256, average Peak Signal to Noise Ratio (PSNR) between the original image and the watermarked image is 47.43dB with ECG signal of size 1kB.
4	Rubio, Alesanco & García, 2013.	Journal of Biomedical Informatics	This approach performed steganography on compressed 1D biomedical signal. The signal is initially compressed using 1D SPIHT algorithm and information is then embedded into it. The work includes digital signature to implement security and attribute-level encryption to support role-based access control.	The results show high Embedding Capacity (EC) of 3 KB in resting ECGs, 200 KB in stress tests and 30 MB in ambulatory ECGs. The compression ratio achieved is 3 in real-time transmission and 5 in offline operation.
5	Ibaida & Khalil, 2013.	IEEE Transactions on Biomedical Engineering	The Haar Wavelet Transform was used to decompose the signal and the encrypted secret bits were embedded in the subbands of wavelet coefficients of ECG signals.	The average PRD for Normal, Ventricular Tachycardia and Ventricular Fibrillation ECG segments of 10 seconds comes out to be 0.47129, 0.27599 and 0.56718 respectively with data size of 2.4Kb
6	Jero, Ramu & Ramakrishnan, 2014.	Journal of Medical Systems	Performed data hiding in 2D ECG signal where 2D ECG was decomposed with DWT and then Singular Value Decomposition (SVD) approach is applied to embed secret information in a selected subband.	The method was applied on 76800 ECG samples from MIT-BIH Arrhythmia database with payload of 350 bytes and achieved PSNR, PRD and Kullback Leibler Divergence (KL-Divergence) of 50.44, 0.0059 and 0.15 respectively at zero Bit Error Rate (BER)
7	Jero, Ramu & Ramakrishnan, 2015	Biomedical Signal Processing and Control	Proposed Curvelet Transform based 2D ECG steganography to identify and then modify less significant ECG coefficients according to 0 and 1 of secret bits.	This method achieved PSNR 75.56 dB, PRD 3.27×10^{-4} and zero BER but at very low EC of 83 bytes.
8	Liji, Indiradev & Anish Babu, 2015.	International Conference on Emerging Trends in Engineering, Science and Technology (ICETEST - 2015)	ECG steganography technique used lifting scheme based Integer-to-Integer wavelet transform to conceal the patient information in LSB locations. The secret data is scrambled inside the ECG signal through scrambling matrix and shared key.	The PRD of 0.4% is obtained between original and watermarked ECG signal with zero BER.
9	Jero, Ramu & Ramakrishnan, 2016	Expert Systems with Applications	Utilized DWT to decompose the cover ECG signal. SVD and quantization approach was used for watermarking and Continuous Ant Colony Optimization algorithm was used to generate multiple scaling factors to improve the trade-off between PSNR and robustness.	Embedded watermark bits of 0.89Kb at PSNR of 62.87 dB and PRD of .0018 with zero bit error rate.
10	Yang & Wang, 2016	Journal of Medical Systems	Proposed ECG steganography in time-domain and discussed two methods of data hiding based on co-efficient alignment.	The Lossy method has average Signal to Noise Ratio (SNR) of 56.34dB and payload of 7.5Kb with bundle size of 4 whereas the reversible data hiding method has average SNR and Mean Absolute Error (MAE) of 42.27dB and 1.84 with payload of 14.7Kb for lead I and SNR and MAE of 46.31dB and 1.49 respectively with payload of 14.5 Kb for lead II.
11	Pandey, Saini, Singh & Sood, 2017.	Journal of Medical Systems	Presented integrated approach using chaotic maps and sample value differencing where difference between the sample values was used to hide the secret bits and chaotic maps were used to determine the embedding locations.	The method achieved PSNR, PRD and Wavelet based Weighted PRD (WWPRD) of 55.49, 0.26 and 0.10 respectively

Gonzalez, Mendez, Luengas, 2016; Ravichandran, Praveenkumar, Rayappan & Amirtharajan, 2016). The mathematical expression for CLS map is given as

$$C(a_o, b_o, l) : a_{n+1} = \left[b_o a_n \left(1 - a_n \right) + \left(4 - b_o \right) \sin \left(\frac{\pi a_n}{4} \right) \right] \mathrm{mod}\, 1 \tag{1}$$

where a_{n+1} and a_n are $n+1^{th}$ and n^{th} values of chaotic sequence C and a_0 the initial value and b_o is the control parameter and l is the length of the sequence. With the help of bifurcation diagram in Figure 1, it is analysed that CLS map shows pure chaotic behaviour over the entire range of b_0 within $\left(0, 4\right]$.

METHODOLOGY USED

This method of ECG steganography works in spatial domain where confidential information is secretly stored in the ECG samples by modifying their amplitudes according to the values of chaotic maps. The complete framework for embedding and extracting the secret bits in ECG signal is illustrated in Figure 2 and 3 respectively. The process includes the detection of R-peaks in ECG signal and conversion of 1D ECG signal into 2D image (*Im*), ciphering the patient's personal information, concealing secret data and side information in *Im*, convert 2D stego-image (*Im*_{stego}) back to 1D stego-ECG signal (*ECG*_{s}) and finally transmitting it over the channel. At receiver, the reverse steps are followed to extract the secret information. The description of each step is given as:

R-Peak Detection

The raw input signal acquired from the MIT-BIH database is initially processed to detect R-peaks. There are several methods reported in the literature to detect the QRS complex (Pan& Tompkins,1985; Li,

Figure 1. Bifurcation diagram of combined Logistic–Sine (CLS) map

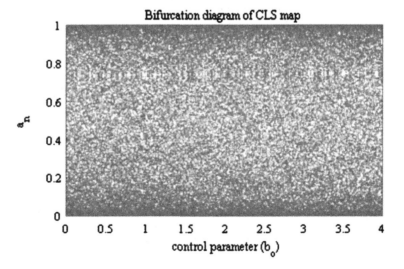

31

Zheng & Tai, 1995; Benitez, Gaydecki, Zaidi & Fitzpatrick, 2001; Slimane and Ali, 2010; Saini, Singh & Khosla, 2013) however in the present work Pan Tompkins algorithm has been employed to remove noise (artifacts and baseline issues) and to identify R-peaks (Pan & Tompkins,1985). The digital signal processes involved in the algorithm includes:

1. Bandpass filtering in order to attenuate noise
2. Differentiation to get slope of QRS complex
3. Squaring augments the slope of frequency response curve of the derivative and helps to detect false positive caused by T-wave higher than usual spectral energies.
4. Integration produces a signal that includes information about both the slope and width of the QRS complex.

Figure 4 shows the R-peaks detected from the ECG signal. Once the R-peaks are detected, each ECG beat from R-peak to R-peak are stacked one over the other using cut and align approach (Lee & Buckley, 1999). The length of each beat is normalised with zero-padding as shown in Figure 5 (Chou, Chen, Shiau & Kuo, 2006).

Figure 2. Structure of ECG steganography at transmitter side

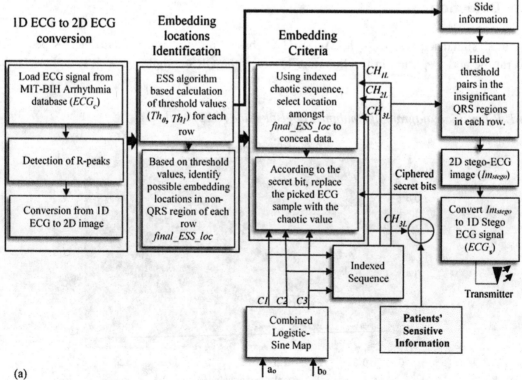

(a)

Figure 3. Structure of ECG steganography at receiver side

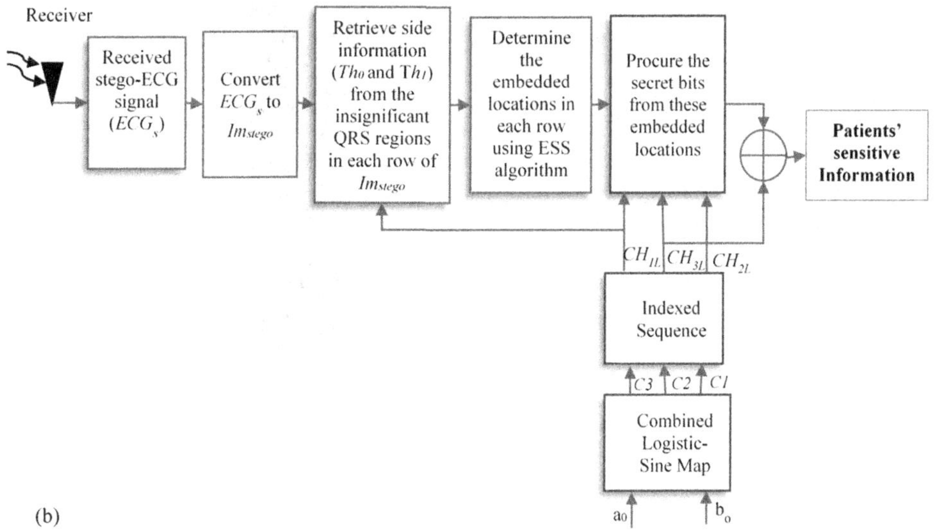

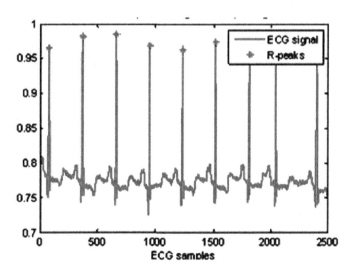

(b)

Figure 4. Detection of R-peaks in record 100 of MIT-BIH arrhythmia database using Pan-Tompkins algorithm

Conversion of Confidential Information to Cipher Text

In order to provide two fold protection to the confidential information, the chaos based ciphering is performed on the secret information prior to embedding in ECG signal. The XOR operation is performed between the indexed chaotic sequence (*CH*) and *secret_bits* to produce the *ciphered_bits* as explained in Figure 6.

Figure 5. Illustration of 2D ECG array of record 100 formed using cut and align beats with zero-padding.

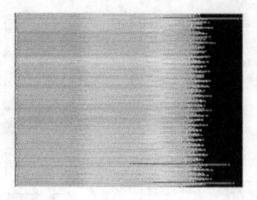

Figure 6. Flowchart to cipher the sensitive information

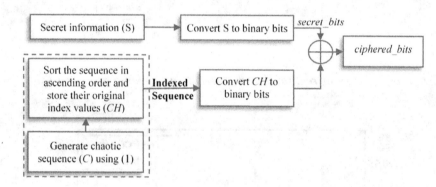

Identification of Optimum Embedding Locations in Non-QRS Region

Selection of optimal embedding locations to hide the secret bits is an important factor that affects the performance of steganography. The novel method of ECG steganography is discussed in this chapter which exploits the non-QRS region of the ECG signal to embed the secret information and avoid any perturbations in the sensitive QRS region. The number of ECG samples that are occupied by QRS complex depends upon the sampling frequency and duration of the QRS complex which are determined by (2) as

$$Number\ of\ QRS\ samples\left(n_R\right) = \left(fs * \max imum\ duration\ of\ QRS\ complex\right)/2 \qquad (2)$$

where fs is the sampling frequency of an ECG signal. For normal ECG the duration of QRS complex is 0.08-0.10 sec (Carr & Brown, 2004). In case of MIT-BIH Arrhythmia database, fs = 360 Hz the number of samples that represents QRS complex are 18 samples on each side of R-peak. However in order to avoid any error due to prolonged QRS (up to 0.165sec), 30 ECG samples on each side of R-peak are left out from embedding the secret bits.

To effectively conceal the information in non-QRS region, an Embedding Site Selection (ESS) algorithm has been designed which selects maximum possible locations that can act as optimum hosts. The procedure of threshold selection and recognising the embedding locations using ESS algorithm is well explained in the flowchart shown in Figure 7. The detailed view of the embedding and non- embedding regions in the second ECG train (*i.e.* row 2 of ECG image (*Im*)) of record 100 of MIT-BIH Arrhythmia database is illustrated in Figure 8. The algorithm identify the groups in non-QRS region of an ECG beat that have consecutive five ECG samples whose magnitude lying between thresholded R-peak amplitude ($th_0*RR\_amp_{i+1}$ and $th_1*RR\_amp_{i+1}$). Amongst the five samples of a group, embedding is done in the last three ECG samples based on the average of the amplitude of first two samples of that group. The algorithm starts identifying the embedding locations from the right end of the row towards the left side. As per the proposed algorithm if locations $L_{i,j}$ (j^{th} sample of ith ECG beat) $L_{i,j-1}$, $L_{i,j-2}$, $L_{i,j-3}$ and $L_{i,j-4}$ satisfy the ESS condition, then the positions $L_{i,j-2}$, $L_{i,j-3}$ and $L_{i,j-4}$ are suitable for embedding secret bits. As shown in Figure 8, R peaks in row 2 are lying at positions 1 and 293, therefore the regions 1 to 30 and 264 to 293 are prohibited to hide the secret bits. The ESS algorithm will identify embedding sites in the region from positions 31 to 263. The outcome of ESS algorithm is $final\_ESS\_loc_{m \times d}$ that holds the index values of the possible embedding locations and the side information (lower and upper threshold values) in Th_{0r} and Th_{1r} respectively.

Figure 7. Flowchart for selection of embedding locations in each row of 2D ECG image based on ESS algorithm

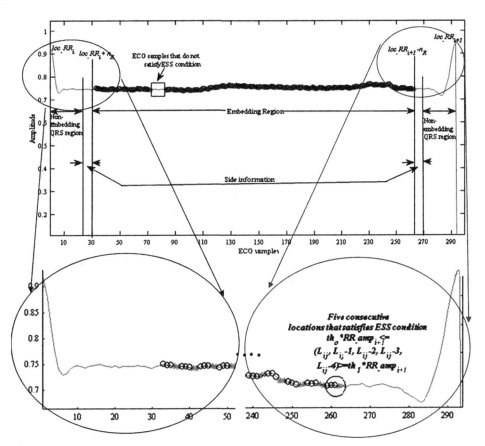

Figure 8. The detailed view of the embedding and non-embedding regions in second row of 2D ECG obtained from record 100 of MIT-BIH Arrhythmia database

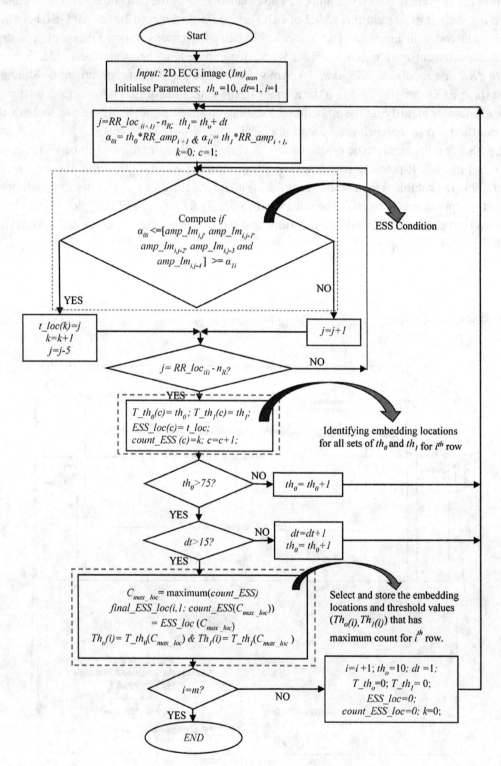

Thus each threshold pair is stored in seven consecutive ECG samples in the insignificant QRS region at each end of the chaotically picked row. For example, the binary bits of each $Th_0(i)$ and $Th_1(i)$ are stored in LSBs of ECG samples from locations 24 to 30 and 264 to 270 respectively in case of row 2 of record 100 of MIT-BIH Arrhythmia. Though it is obvious that embedding the side information in addition to the pivotal sensitive information adds onus on the stego-signal and affects the quality of the stego-ECG but hiding information using the mentioned approach has unnoticeable impact on the ECG signal. It can be viewed in Figure 8 that interleaving threshold values in the stego-ECG signal is negligible and it do not disturbs the attributes of an ECG signal.

Embedding Process

After identifying the embedding locations, the next step is to embed secret bits in these locations. The embedding process is crucial in steganography as it ensures security of the vital information while retaining its imperceptibility and robustness. The steganography method discussed in this chapter promises to keep diagnostic features intact inspite of high embedding capacity at minimal distortion. For the protection of the secret_bits, chaotic maps are used in two distinct ways (i) Indexed chaotic sequences are used to arbitrarily select locations amongst the ESS locations stored in *final_ESS_loc* (ii) to replace the amplitude at embedding site with the chaotic value according to 0's and 1's of secret bits. Since, three bits are stored in three consecutive ECG samples of the group, the security is

enhanced by using different chaotic sequences to store bits in each sample of the group. The flowchart in Figure 9 illuminates the complete process of concealing the patients' confidential information as well as the side information.

EXTRACTION PROCESS

At receiver, the received stego-signal is sent to the concerned doctor as well as to the authorised administrative personnel. The doctor diagnose the signal while the administrative personnel fetches sensitive information from it. The correct information is recovered only if the personnel has the same key as was used at the transmitter side. The extraction of secret bits at the receiver follows the reverse procedure of what was performed on the transmitter side. The flowchart in Figure 10 demonstrates the procedure to extract the secret bits. The proposed method guarantees lossless extraction of information with zero BER.

To hide the side information (Th_0 and Th_1), LSB based steganography is used. This is one of the simplest technique to hide secret data in the LSBs of the signal samples (Chan & Cheng, 2004; Yang, Sun & Sun, 2009; Wang, Yang & Niu, 2010; Kanan & Nazeri, 2014). Since, the human eye is imperceptible to the minor changes at LSB level, hence effective method for steganography. In the chapter, the side information is the pair of threshold values (Th_0 and Th_1) computed from ESS algorithm (Figure 11) for all the rows. These values lies between 10 and 90 which can be easily represented by seven binary bits.

RESULTS AND DISCUSSION

Although steganography causes irreversible degradation in the cover ECG signal but the steganography method discussed in this chapter conceals the patients' confidential information without making any

Figure 9. Flowchart to embed secret bits and side information in 2D ECG image

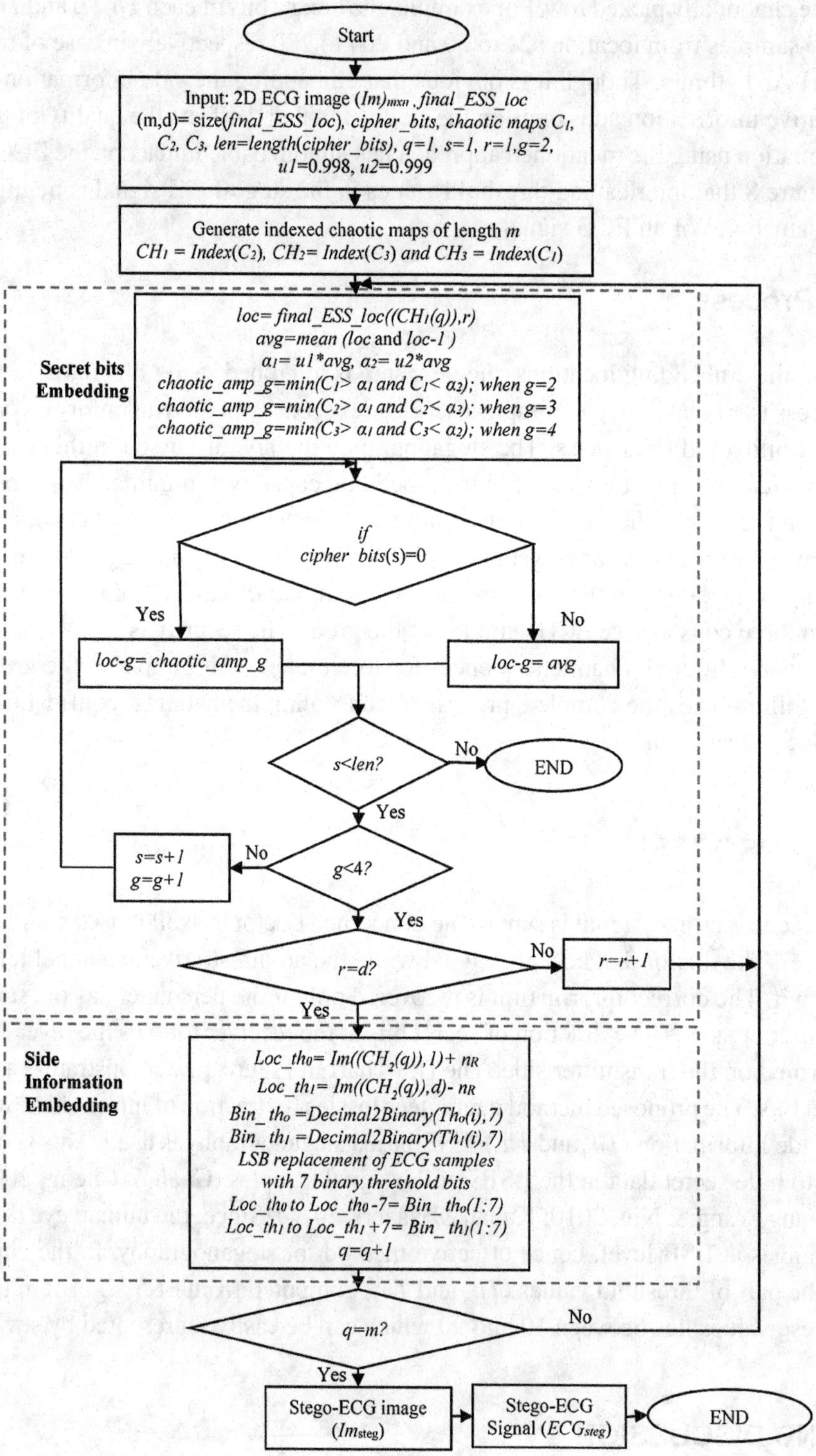

Figure 10. The flowchart to demonstrate the extraction process

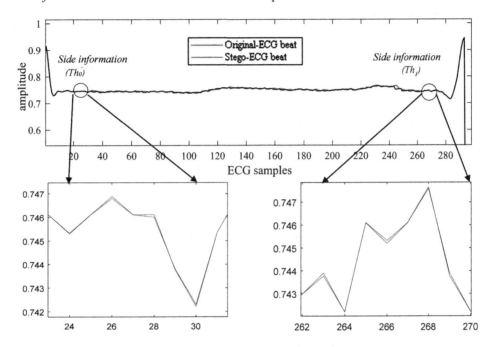

distinguishable change in its diagnostic features. Figure 12 shows the variation in amplitude of the second beat of original and stego-ECG of record 100 of MIT-BIH Arrhythmia database. Figure 13 shows that the error between the two signals is negligible to influence the diagnosis.

The proposed method is thoroughly tested on the basis of statistical measures such as PRD (Ibaida & Khalil, 2013), PRD1024(Pandey, Saini, Singh & Sood, 2016), PRDN (Pandey, Saini, Singh & Sood, 2016), RMS(Pandey, Saini, Singh & Sood, 2016), SNR(Pandey, Saini, Singh & Sood, 2016), PSNR (Jero, Ramu & Ramakrishnan, 2014) and KL-distance(Jero, Ramu & Ramakrishnan, 2014). However, the statistical parameters distributes the error equally over whole ECG signal and misleads the diagnostic elucidation (Fahoum & Ishijima, 1993; Chen & Itoh, 1998; Fahoum, 2006; Manikandan & Dhanpat, 2007). Therefore clinically authentic methods such as WWPRD (Ibaida & Khalil, 2013; Fahoum, 2006) and Wavelet Energy based Diagnostic Distortion (WEDD) (Manikandan & Dhanpat, 2007) are used additionally to assess the stego-ECG. These clinical parameters monitors the local distortion and estimates the weighted significant features. Moreover, the embedding efficiency is measured in terms of number of bits embedded, BER and Embedding Capacity. These performance evaluation metrics are applied on all the 48 records of MIT-BIH Arrhythmia database of 2 min and 5 min long durations. Each ECG signal is digitised at sampling frequency of 360 Hz with 11-bit resolution over a 10mV range.

The complete results given in Table 2 and Table 3 displays that the average PRD, PRD1024, PRDN, RMS, SNR, PSNR, KL-Divergence, WWPRD and WEDD comes out to be 0.0049, 0.0553, 0.078, 4.74, 47.9052, 50.98, 2.56×10^{-5}, 0.189 and 0.046 at EC of 0.4013 and zero BER for 2 minutes ECG signal and 0.0050, 0.05558, 0.075, 4.85, 47.05, 50.29, 2.22×10^{-5}, 0.1812 and 0.046 at embedding capacity of 0.3988 for 5 min respectively. It can be exhibited from the results that the proposed approach of steganography can accommodate plethora of confidential information at a very nominal error.

Figure 11. Effect of concealing the side information in insignificant QRS region of row 2 of record 100 of MIT-BIH Arrhythmia database

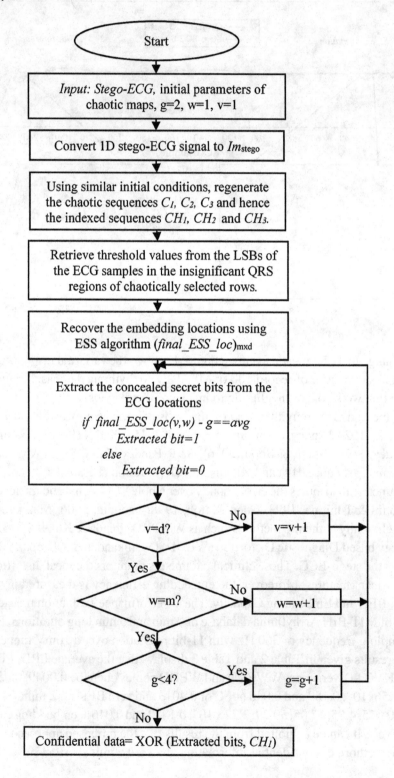

Figure 12. Comparison between the original ECG beat and stego-ECG beat

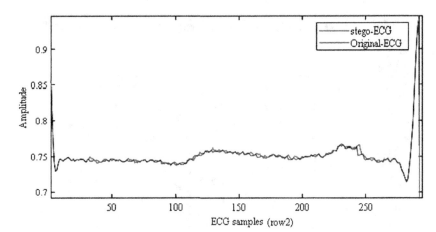

Figure 13. Error signal calculated between the original and stego-ECG beat for row 2 of record 100

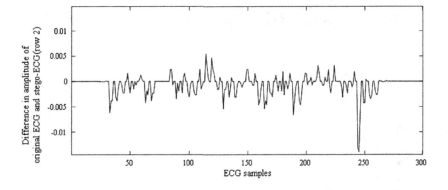

Effect of Signal Duration

The steganography methodology discussed in this paper is further analysed for varying lengths of ECG signals. Figure 14 and Figure 15 depicts an average PRD and average embedding capacity respectively for signal durations of nine different lengths when recorded on all 48 signals of Arrhythmia database. It has been found that although the number of bits embedded increases with increase in duration but the average PRD and average embedding ratio remains almost constant. From this, we can pre-determine the length of the ECG signal required to transmit the desired amount of secret information.

Effect of Scaling Factors (u1 and u2)

The amount of variation between amplitudes of the original ECG sample and the stego-ECG sample is controlled by the scaling factors *u1* and *u2*. Since the deciding parameters (α_1 and α_2) used in ESS condition for optimal location selection are determined by these scaling factors, the right choice of scaling factors ensues minimum variation in amplitude at the embedding site after embedding. To achieve good results it is required that the values of u1 and u2 should be near but less than equal to 1. Figure 16

Figure 14. Effect of varying durations of ECG signal on average embedding capacity

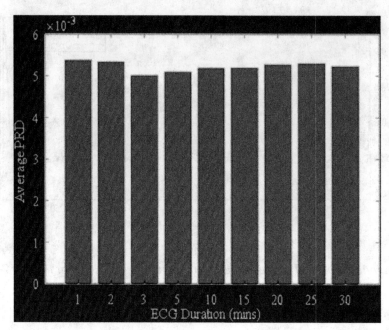

Figure 15. Effect of varying durations of ECG signal on average PRD all the 48 records of MIT-BIH Arrhythmia database

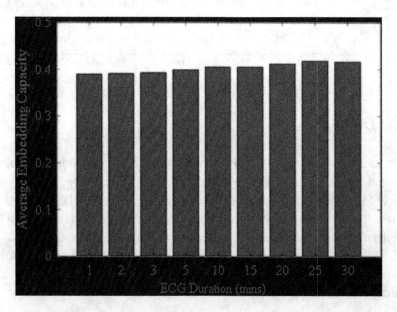

depicts the amount of variation occur in the original and stego-ECG signal for different values of u1 and u2. It has been found that the error is high when the difference between u1 and u2 is large (Figure 16(a)) and they are far from 1 whereas the error is minimal when their difference is less and both the factors (u1and u2) are closer but less than 1 (Figure 16(d)). In this chapter, the results are calculated with u1 and u2 taken as 0.998 and 0.999 respectively.

Key Space Analysis

The length of the key is an important parameter that makes the system invulnerable to any stego attacks. Therefore in the proposed steganography approach, the key space is kept sufficiently large that curtails the risk of illicit access of the sensitive information by intruders. The key consists of the initial parameters (a_0, b_0 and L) used to generate CLS maps and the scaling factors u1 and u2 as shown in Table 4. If the initial parameters of three CLS maps are set to precision of 14 decimals and the scaling factors *u1* and *u2* are set to 3 decimals then as per IEEE 754 standard of converting decimal numbers into binary (Rajaram, 2016), the length of the key is calculated as $2^{64*6+64+32*2}$ that is almost equal to 2^{484} bits. This length of key is sufficiently large to avoid any malicious attack.

PERFORMANCE COMPARISON WITH EXISTING TECHNIQUES

To review the performance of the proposed method, comparison has been made with the existing techniques is shown in Table 5.

Computational Complexity

The experimentation of the proposed technique is performed on the Intel Core i5–4210U CPU @ 1.70GHz 2.40 GHz processor. The average time elapsed to embed secret bits in ECG records of all 48 records of MIT-BIH Arrhythmia database of 5min duration at average EC of 0.4 comes out to be 40.215113 seconds whereas average time taken to extract the secret bits from the stego-signal comes out to be time 10.74978 seconds.

Table 4. Structure of the key used in ECG steganography

a_{01} (64 bits)	b_{01} (64 bits)	a_{02} (64 bits)	b_{02} (64 bits)	a_{03} (64 bits)	b_{03} (64 bits)	L (64 bits)	u_1 (32 bits)	u_2 (32 bits)

Table 2. Performance evaluation metrics of the proposed method for 48 records from MIT-BIH Arrhythmia database of 2min duration

Samples	PRD	PRD1024	PRDN	RMS	SNR	PSNR	KL-Divergence	WWPRD	WEDD	Bits embedded	EC	BER
100	0.002676	0.034586	0.072816	2.566759	51.45175	53.74355	3.43×10^{-6}	0.147845	0.052825	20292	0.469722	0
101	0.00504	0.05999	0.083842	4.883267	45.95123	49.36283	1.26×10^{-5}	0.18571	0.050736	20256	0.468889	0
102	0.003118	0.046233	0.079066	3.029842	50.12129	52.64378	4.88×10^{-6}	0.145266	0.053331	19710	0.45625	0
103	0.003705	0.046846	0.057084	3.637128	48.62443	51.90975	6.67×10^{-6}	0.121319	0.04056	20508	0.474722	0
104	0.006956	0.09856	0.126169	6.832486	43.15256	46.12487	2.47×10^{-5}	0.205428	0.077945	13973	0.323449	0
105	0.004114	0.054049	0.065264	4.048459	47.71387	50.8816	8.46×10^{-6}	0.172059	0.042456	19668	0.455278	0
106	0.005535	0.070429	0.078638	5.489493	45.13772	48.52018	1.53×10^{-5}	0.163065	0.057925	20028	0.463611	0
107	0.006936	0.039431	0.040883	6.882436	43.17783	47.24026	2.44×10^{-5}	0.094175	0.027872	15164	0.351019	0
108	0.026137	0.440638	0.765897	25.54002	31.6549	33.72401	0.000689	2.148554	0.293878	2528	0.058519	0
109	0.00404	0.039512	0.045746	3.948865	47.87247	50.85554	8.36×10^{-6}	0.128855	0.030407	19191	0.444236	0
111	0.003465	0.056592	0.067149	3.439501	49.20566	51.56898	5.94×10^{-6}	0.183787	0.041727	18975	0.439236	0
112	0.003851	0.01851	0.073202	3.286384	48.28873	50.47768	7.35×10^{-6}	0.170022	0.048991	19458	0.450417	0
113	0.005527	0.059151	0.061845	5.531026	45.15	48.83204	1.46×10^{-5}	0.12062	0.046125	20133	0.466042	0
114	0.00158	0.003842	0.000603	0.015686	96.0274	96.98818	1.27×10^{-10}	0.00143	0.000314	498	0.011528	0
115	0.003018	0.021669	0.038743	2.778019	50.406	54.40045	4.36×10^{-5}	0.078665	0.025963	21183	0.490347	0
116	0.007354	0.027629	0.050928	6.207699	42.66935	47.95362	2.7×10^{-5}	0.086606	0.037245	19890	0.460417	0
117	0.003671	0.018673	0.068904	3.164713	48.7043	50.30051	6.63×10^{-6}	0.175087	0.04042	18957	0.438819	0
118	0.006052	0.024877	0.060263	5.094152	44.36215	47.61419	1.82×10^{-5}	0.134287	0.037003	20232	0.468333	0
119	0.005726	0.023894	0.04709	4.889776	44.8433	49.75918	1.66×10^{-5}	0.119445	0.032546	20013	0.463264	0
121	0.002941	0.014996	0.051297	2.539834	50.62866	53.41483	4.15×10^{-6}	0.166338	0.021949	21159	0.489792	0
122	0.004585	0.019949	0.051748	3.886041	46.77353	50.02207	1.06×10^{-6}	0.137454	0.03184	19338	0.447639	0
123	0.004692	0.023349	0.061548	4.061032	46.57351	50.97036	1.09×10^{-6}	0.143321	0.040732	21879	0.506458	0
124	0.003319	0.016221	0.039162	2.873436	49.58113	53.41932	5.5×10^{-6}	0.107784	0.02274	22209	0.514097	0
200	0.005288	0.063327	0.067095	5.285779	45.53375	48.71713	1.4×10^{-6}	0.172259	0.041029	10035	0.232292	0
201	0.002435	0.046606	0.061355	2.413682	52.26874	54.17974	2.87×10^{-6}	0.149792	0.039678	19188	0.444167	0
202	0.003464	0.059314	0.071875	3.437709	49.20852	51.73204	5.84×10^{-6}	0.197663	0.046449	21681	0.501875	0
203	0.007635	0.07188	0.076844	7.571183	42.34399	45.75716	3.01×10^{-5}	0.177389	0.041177	11472	0.265556	0
205	0.002638	0.03278	0.069706	2.523817	51.5747	53.72865	3.32×10^{-6}	0.137026	0.046324	19197	0.444375	0
207	0.006008	0.078505	0.084744	5.994076	44.42605	47.03935	3×10^{-5}	0.300984	0.03192	6780	0.156944	0
208	0.005096	0.052468	0.053986	5.123722	45.85585	49.27784	1.36×10^{-5}	0.136084	0.035249	11919	0.275903	0
209	0.003755	0.065865	0.07937	3.730941	48.50704	50.86252	6.89×10^{-5}	0.157781	0.058522	18858	0.436528	0
210	0.002674	0.04612	0.051517	2.672342	51.45805	53.78767	3.57×10^{-6}	0.138096	0.029618	16770	0.388194	0
212	0.005293	0.074291	0.081266	5.27915	45.52536	48.52694	1.38×10^{-5}	0.164408	0.060853	19035	0.440625	0
213	0.008243	0.0605	0.069574	7.96157	41.67795	45.74171	3.41×10^{-5}	0.150341	0.051782	14706	0.340417	0
214	0.006565	0.065532	0.071125	6.497247	43.65538	47.07401	2.24×10^{-5}	0.175037	0.038995	19719	0.456458	0
215	0.004808	0.077875	0.086547	4.801768	46.36015	49.94576	1.15×10^{-5}	0.183192	0.060037	15645	0.362153	0
217	0.005444	0.042757	0.044205	5.440612	45.28108	48.68641	1.46×10^{-5}	0.104809	0.03031	15750	0.364583	0
220	0.003365	0.022747	0.046557	3.058798	49.46071	53.1117	5.6×10^{-6}	0.079442	0.035255	20475	0.473958	0
221	0.003314	0.047851	0.056096	3.28102	49.59204	52.32502	5.51×10^{-6}	0.145015	0.036726	19950	0.461806	0
222	0.003457	0.093761	0.118268	3.463129	49.22725	51.10005	5.8×10^{-6}	0.233742	0.077352	16019	0.37081	0

continued on following page

Table 2. Continued

Samples	PRD	PRD1024	PRDN	RMS	SNR	PSNR	KL-Divergence	WWPRD	WEDD	Bits embedded	EC	BER
223	0.003224	0.02188	0.037045	2.960298	49.83308	53.34566	5.26×10^{-6}	0.08753	0.024658	19824	0.458889	0
228	0.004438	0.057208	0.064985	4.392693	47.0571	50.97999	1×10^{-5}	0.19634	0.034003	14159	0.327755	0
230	0.00424	0.052581	0.056886	4.223891	47.45193	50.80843	9.29×10^{-5}	0.123432	0.03865	20040	0.463889	0
231	0.003635	0.051868	0.062557	3.588153	48.78887	51.7816	6.31×10^{-6}	0.126344	0.045754	21375	0.494792	0
232	0.003576	0.076024	0.128811	3.529172	48.93205	50.3656	6.44×10^{-6}	0.255122	0.078067	16479	0.381458	0
233	0.006955	0.059411	0.061501	6.955783	43.15439	46.6168	2.47×10^{-5}	0.149086	0.035934	17409	0.402986	0
234	0.003099	0.044447	0.049472	3.084755	50.17623	53.11329	4.75×10^{-6}	0.112156	0.032276	18942	0.438472	0
Average	**0.004972**	**0.055374**	**0.078679**	**4.741673**	**47.90504**	**50.98999**	**2.56×10^{-5}**	**0.189293**	**0.046328**	**17336.27**	**0.401303**	**0**
SD	**0.003436**	**0.0598**	**0.101595**	**3.412869**	**7.798474**	**7.45892**	**9.61×10^{-5}**	**0.286813**	**0.038562**	**4649.335**	**0.107623**	**0**

Table 3. Performance evaluation metrics of the proposed method for 48 records from MIT-BIH Arrhythmia database of 5min duration

Sample	PRD	PRD1024	PRDN	RMS	SNR	PSNR	KL-Div	WWPRD	WEDD	Bits Embedded	EC	BER
100	0.002625	0.034444	0.071767	2.520774	51.6187	54.06589	3.31×10^{-6}	0.145566	0.051903	48742	0.451315	0
101	0.004904	0.054778	0.072345	4.754352	46.18946	50.0262	1.2×10^{-6}	0.170097	0.042467	50791	0.470287	0
102	0.00283	0.043158	0.072877	2.754807	50.96311	53.47036	4.03×10^{-6}	0.13541	0.049061	39616	0.366815	0
103	0.003674	0.046032	0.056058	3.605379	48.69799	52.07635	6.59×10^{-6}	0.118564	0.039621	50071	0.46362	0
104	0.010628	0.138881	0.175704	10.41381	39.47111	42.68745	5.76×10^{-6}	0.301461	0.100862	41401	0.383339	0
105	0.003635	0.046747	0.056723	3.572114	48.79027	51.97502	6.67×10^{-6}	0.149816	0.036098	45304	0.419478	0
106	0.005317	0.069178	0.077028	5.279031	45.4862	48.85974	1.39×10^{-6}	0.164961	0.057494	48565	0.449672	0
107	0.011851	0.068871	0.071821	11.72436	38.52459	42.61332	0.000101	0.166332	0.04497	27676	0.256257	0
108	0.019536	0.324469	0.509399	19.13139	34.18309	36.2335	0.00038	1.399486	0.207432	26768	0.247852	0
109	0.003788	0.037978	0.04296	3.719722	48.43239	51.37478	7.35×10^{-6}	0.122305	0.028192	41428	0.383589	0
111	0.003649	0.060713	0.074591	3.61426	48.7576	51.1385	6.49×10^{-6}	0.194675	0.046941	41701	0.386117	0
112	0.003752	0.018234	0.066061	3.211803	48.51528	51.28793	7.02×10^{-6}	0.164025	0.042905	45352	0.419922	0
113	0.006064	0.063242	0.066537	6.054649	44.34429	48.07473	1.7×10^{-5}	0.128976	0.048668	47368	0.438589	0
114	0.00057	0.013648	0.019429	0.566711	64.88815	66.16182	1.59×10^{-7}	0.044818	0.012587	6648	0.065259	0
115	0.003033	0.022549	0.039626	2.803635	50.36343	54.35046	4.41×10^{-6}	0.076907	0.027618	50359	0.466283	0
116	0.007239	0.026708	0.049015	6.094527	42.8063	48.31821	2.64×10^{-5}	0.083999	0.035975	45337	0.419783	0
117	0.004419	0.022221	0.079507	3.804505	47.09351	49.01412	9.28×10^{-5}	0.202445	0.05459	44035	0.407728	0
118	0.005606	0.025201	0.057516	4.803113	45.02666	48.30774	1.55×10^{-5}	0.129338	0.033294	43982	0.407241	0
119	0.006552	0.027694	0.051598	5.630999	43.67222	48.53325	2.37×10^{-5}	0.132885	0.036612	51499	0.476843	0
121	0.003122	0.015357	0.047018	2.686673	50.11116	53.43689	4.71×10^{-5}	0.157379	0.019148	47629	0.441005	0
122	0.004417	0.020293	0.051461	3.780986	47.0967	50.36523	9.86×10^{-6}	0.136566	0.032106	45028	0.416926	0
123	0.004506	0.022528	0.06323	3.895935	46.92412	51.33085	9.96×10^{-6}	0.142824	0.042562	52879	0.489616	0
124	0.003308	0.015632	0.033406	2.865847	49.60766	54.04027	5.55×10^{-6}	0.094354	0.018515	53269	0.493227	0
200	0.006804	0.085011	0.089706	6.813139	43.3443	46.85488	2.33×10^{-6}	0.226019	0.053223	38863	0.359839	0
201	0.002366	0.045587	0.06075	2.343806	52.521	54.51193	2.7×10^{-6}	0.149388	0.039198	45331	0.419728	0

continued on following page

Table 3. Continued

Sample	PRD	PRD1024	PRDN	RMS	SNR	PSNR	KL-Div	WWPRD	WEDD	Bits Embedded	EC	BER
202	0.003454	0.057048	0.071857	3.41537	49.23289	51.89923	5.79×10^{-6}	0.19701	0.046874	51955	0.48106	0
203	0.007146	0.071217	0.075883	7.102779	42.91904	46.51061	2.98×10^{-6}	0.194179	0.044429	35935	0.332728	0
205	0.002768	0.03368	0.070402	2.645955	51.15524	53.38169	3.69×10^{-6}	0.141515	0.047482	44758	0.414422	0
207	0.006571	0.076995	0.083634	6.531717	43.64674	46.95074	3.56×10^{-6}	0.335525	0.032295	28657	0.269785	0
208	0.00474	0.049476	0.051927	4.735317	46.48529	49.96257	1.16×10^{-6}	0.131929	0.034849	42811	0.396394	0
209	0.004523	0.072876	0.085162	4.493582	46.89149	49.75202	1.01×10^{-5}	0.167035	0.06332	43588	0.403589	0
210	0.005305	0.086367	0.100659	5.273586	45.50578	47.9033	1.44×10^{-5}	0.223393	0.0529	43372	0.401589	0
212	0.005122	0.0724	0.079402	5.107523	45.81066	48.82018	1.29×10^{-5}	0.159444	0.059879	44338	0.410533	0
213	0.008375	0.057631	0.063434	8.152195	41.54048	45.93796	3.58×10^{-6}	0.144184	0.046976	41464	0.383922	0
214	0.005765	0.059689	0.062845	5.754005	44.78355	48.36286	1.75×10^{-5}	0.164955	0.038737	45001	0.416672	0
215	0.006543	0.106118	0.117833	6.534493	43.6851	47.26955	2.15×10^{-5}	0.23205	0.081942	38767	0.35895	0
217	0.005779	0.046374	0.048098	5.768442	44.76339	48.28907	1.74×10^{-6}	0.116442	0.03319	36493	0.337895	0
219	0.003881	0.023134	0.039112	3.515574	48.222	52.0336	7.82×10^{-6}	0.083536	0.025976	46546	0.430977	0
220	0.002852	0.020205	0.041817	2.604608	50.89707	54.50787	4.08×10^{-6}	0.074161	0.03077	48370	0.447866	0
221	0.003031	0.043299	0.049954	3.004783	50.36715	53.43428	4.66×10^{-6}	0.132855	0.031448	41206	0.381534	0
222	0.003119	0.07621	0.10707	3.105487	50.12085	52.04683	4.73×10^{-6}	0.220128	0.07222	38512	0.358812	0
223	0.003572	0.024816	0.042409	3.285703	48.94228	52.7132	6.31×10^{-6}	0.101819	0.027618	49534	0.458644	0
228	0.005178	0.064162	0.069661	5.154844	45.71624	49.5903	1.34×10^{-5}	0.214252	0.033332	41956	0.388478	0
230	0.003878	0.047501	0.052214	3.850805	48.2287	51.66481	7.46×10^{-6}	0.113644	0.036549	44608	0.413033	0
231	0.00346	0.049287	0.059626	3.414281	49.21751	52.465	5.74×10^{-6}	0.121201	0.043603	50242	0.465199	0
232	0.003238	0.078427	0.108754	3.224859	49.79458	51.28948	5.19×10^{-6}	0.225996	0.068235	39881	0.369228	0
233	0.006928	0.060269	0.062839	6.911244	43.18816	46.6726	2.46×10^{-6}	0.154155	0.041747	44779	0.414617	0
234	0.003051	0.04165	0.047142	3.026262	50.31248	53.65702	4.63×10^{-6}	0.10965	0.030856	44080	0.408144	0
Average	**0.005052**	**0.055583**	**0.075997**	**4.855411**	**47.0595**	**50.29634**	**2.22×10^{-5}**	**0.181201**	**0.046401**	**43051.98**	**0.398842**	**0**
SD	**0.002951**	**0.046845**	**0.068073**	**2.91757**	**4.483976**	**4.193421**	**5.48×10^{-5}**	**0.186**	**0.028365**	**9071.601**	**0.083996**	**0**

CONCLUSION

The chapter proposed a novel method of ECG steganography in spatial domain in which the non-QRS region of ECG signal is exploited to embed the confidential information. An ESS algorithm has been designed to select the optimum embedding locations and then replace the amplitudes of these ECG samples with the chaotic values according to 0 and 1 of secret bits. The performance of the proposed method is measured in terms of statistical and clinical measures and found that the average PRD, PRD1024, PRDN, RMS, SNR, PSNR, KL-Divergence, WWPRD and WEDD comes out to be 0.0049, 0.0553, 0.078, 4.74, 47.9052, 50.98, 2.56×10^{-5}, 0.189 and 0.04 at average embedding capacity of 0.4 when measured for all the 48 records of standard MIT-BIH Arrhythmia database of 2 mins. This error is nominal to affect the diagnosability of the ECG signal. Moreover, the method supports the lossless extraction of the embedded information with zero BER. Chaotic maps employed in the method strengthens the key space and keep the embedded information safe and secure. Hence, the proposed method is competent to conceal the personal information without loss of diagnosability.

Figure 16. The amount of error occurred for different combinations of scaling factors (u1 and u2)

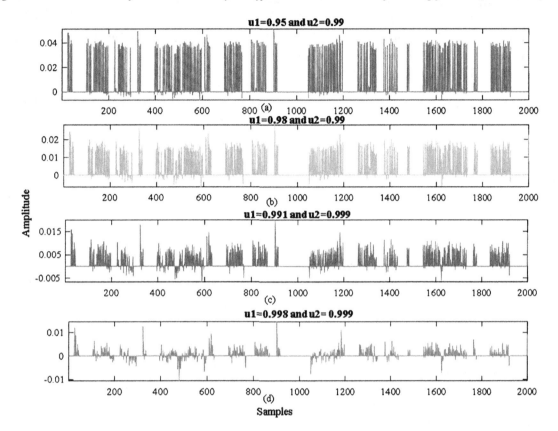

Table 5. Comparison of the proposed method with the existing techniques

ECG Steganography Method	Database Used	Parameters Studied	Existing Method/ Proposed Method
DWT and SVD (2014) [Jero SE, Ramu P, Ramakrishnan S (2014)]	MIT-BIH Arrhythmia 76800 samples	PSNR	69.13/**50.65**
		PRD	0.06/**4.8x10^{-2}**
		Payload (bytes)	350/**4012**
		KL-Div	6.84x10^{-5}/**2.52 x10^{-5}**
Curvelet Transform [Jero SE, Ramu P, Ramakrishnan S (2015)]	MIT-BIH Normal Sinus Rhythm (128 trains)	PSNR	43.44/**47.17**
		PRD	0.013/0.009
		Payload (bytes)	502/**725**
		KL-Div	0.144/**1.13x10^{-4}**
DWT with SVD and CACO [Jero SE, Ramu P, Ramakrishnan S (2016)]	MIT-BIH Normal Sinus Rhythm	PSNR	34.46/**47.12**
		PRD	0.06/**0.0032**
		Payload (Kb)	3.07/**4.398**
		KL-Div	2.04/**0.00061**
CMSaVD [Pandey A, Saini BS, Singh B, Sood N (2017)]	MIT-BIH Arrhythmia 20 mins samples	PRD	0.26/**0.00503**
		Payload (bits)	0.4/**0.423**
		KL-Div	3.34 x10^{-6}/ **2.53x10^{-5}**
		PSNR	55.49/**50.2**

REFERENCES

Al-Fahoum, A. S. (2006). Quality assessment of ECG compression techniques using a wavelet-based diagnostic measure. *IEEE Transactions on Information Technology in Biomedicine*, *10*(1), 182–191. doi:10.1109/TITB.2005.855554 PMID:16445263

Al-Fahoum, A. S., & Ishijima, M. (1993). Fundamentals of the decision of optimum factors in the ECG data compression. *IEICE Transactions on Information and Systems*, *E76-D*(12), 1398–1403.

Algeria-Barrero, E., & Algeria-Ezquerra, E. (2008). When to perform pre-operative ECG. European Society of Cardiology, 7(3).

Benitez, D., Gaydecki, P. A., Zaidi, A., & Fitzpatrick, A. P. (2001). The use of the Hilbert transform in ECG signal analysis. *Computers in Biology and Medicine*, *31*(5), 399–406. doi:10.1016/S0010-4825(01)00009-9 PMID:11535204

Berkaya, S. K., Uysal, A. K., Gunal, E. S., Ergin, S., Gunal, S., & Gulmezoglu, M. B. (2018). A survey on ECG Analysis. *Biomedical Signal Processing and Control*, *43*, 216–235. doi:10.1016/j.bspc.2018.03.003

Carr, J. J., & Brown, J. M. (2004). *Introduction to biomedical equipment technology* (4th ed.). Pearson Education.

Chan, C. K., & Cheng, L. M. (2004). Hiding data in images by simple LSB substitution. *Pattern Recognition*, *37*(3), 469–474. doi:10.1016/j.patcog.2003.08.007

Chang, C. C., Tai, W. L., & Lin, C. C. (2006). A reversible data hiding scheme based on side match vector quantization. *IEEE Transactions on Circuits and Systems for Video Technology*, *6*(10), 1301–1308. doi:10.1109/TCSVT.2006.882380

Chen, C. C., & Chang, C. C. (2010). High capacity SMVQ-based hiding scheme using adaptive index. *Signal Processing*, *90*(7), 2141–2149. doi:10.1016/j.sigpro.2010.01.018

Chen, J., & Itoh, S. (1998). A wavelet transform-based ECG compression method guaranteeing desired signal quality. *IEEE Transactions on Biomedical Engineering*, *45*(12), 1414–1419. doi:10.1109/10.730435 PMID:9835190

Chen, S. T., Guo, Y. J., Huang, H. N., Kung, W. M., Tseng, K. K., & Tu, S. Y. (2014). Hiding patients confidential data in the ECG signal viaa transform-domain quantization scheme. *Journal of Medical Systems*, *38*(6), 1–8. doi:10.100710916-014-0054-9 PMID:24395031

Chou, H. H., Chen, Y. J., Shiau, Y. C., & Kuo, T. S. (2006). An effective and efficient compression algorithm for ECG signals with irregular periods. *IEEE Transactions on Biomedical Engineering*, *53*(6), 1198–1205. doi:10.1109/TBME.2005.863961 PMID:16761849

Dmour, H. A., & Ani, A. A. (2016). Quality optimized medical image information hiding algorithm that employs edge detection and data coding. *Computer Methods and Programs in Biomedicine*, *127*, 24–43. doi:10.1016/j.cmpb.2016.01.011 PMID:27000287

Hong, W., & Chen, T. S. (2012). A novel data embedding method using adaptive pixel pair matching. *IEEE Transactions on Information Forensics and Security*, *7*(1), 176–184. doi:10.1109/TIFS.2011.2155062

Hua, Z., Zhou, Y., Pun, C. M., & Chang, C. L. P. (2015). 2D Sine Logistic modulation map for image encryption. *Information Sciences*, *297*, 80–94. doi:10.1016/j.ins.2014.11.018

Ibaida, A., & Khalil, I. (2013). Wavelet-based ECG steganography for protecting patient confidential information in point-of-care systems. *IEEE Transactions on Biomedical Engineering*, *60*(12), 3322–3330. doi:10.1109/TBME.2013.2264539 PMID:23708767

Ibaida, A., Khalil, I., & Al-Shammary, D. (2010) Embedding patients confidential data in ECG signal for healthcare information systems. *32nd Int. conf. of IEEE Buenos Aires, Argentina*, 3891-3894. 10.1109/IEMBS.2010.5627671

Jero, S. E., Ramu, P., & Ramakrishnan, S. (2014). Discrete wavelet transform and singular value decomposition based ECG steganography for secured patient information transmission. *Journal of Medical Systems*, *38*(10), 132. doi:10.100710916-014-0132-z PMID:25187409

Jero, S. E., Ramu, P., & Ramakrishnan, S. (2015). ECG steganography using curvelet transform. *Biomedical Signal Processing and Control*, *22*, 161–169. doi:10.1016/j.bspc.2015.07.004

Jero, S. E., Ramu, P., & Ramakrishnan, S. (2016). Imperceptibility—Robustness trade-off studies for ECG steganography using continuous ant colony optimization. *Expert Systems with Applications*, *49*, 123–135. doi:10.1016/j.eswa.2015.12.010

Johnson, N. F., & Jajodia, S. (1998). Exploring steganography: Seeing the unseen. *Computers*, *31*(2), 26–34. doi:10.1109/MC.1998.4655281

Kanan, H. R., & Nazeri, B. (2014). A novel image steganography scheme with high embedding capacity and tunable visual image quality based on a genetic algorithm. *Expert Systems with Applications*, *41*(14), 6123–6130. doi:10.1016/j.eswa.2014.04.022

Kanso, A., & Smaoui, N. (2009). Logistic chaotic maps for binary numbers generations. *Chaos, Solitons, and Fractals*, *40*(5), 2557–2568. doi:10.1016/j.chaos.2007.10.049

Koszat, S. S., Vlachos, M., Lucchese, C., & Herle, H. V. (2009). Embedding and Retrieving Private Metadata in Electrocardiograms. *Journal of Medical Systems*, *33*(4), 241–259. doi:10.100710916-008-9185-1 PMID:19697691

Lee, H., & Buckley, K. M. (1999). ECG data compression using cut and align beats approach and 2-D transforms. *IEEE Transactions on Biomedical Engineering*, *46*(5), 556–564. doi:10.1109/10.759056 PMID:10230134

Lee, S., Yoo, C. D., & Kalker, T. (2007). Reversible image watermarking based on integer-to-integer wavelet transform. *IEEE Transactions on Information Forensics and Security*, *2*(3), 321–330. doi:10.1109/TIFS.2007.905146

Li, C., Zheng, C., & Tai, C. (1995). Detection of ECG characteristic points using wavelet transforms. *IEEE Transactions on Biomedical Engineering*, *42*(1), 21–28. doi:10.1109/10.362922 PMID:7851927

Liji, C. A., Indiradevi, K. P., & Anish, B. K. K. (2015) Integer wavelet transform for embedded lossy to lossless image compression. *International Conference on Emerging Trends in Engineering, Science and Technology, Procedia Technology*, *24*, 1039–47.

Lima, J. B., Madeiro, F., & Sales, F. J. R. (2015). Encryption of medical images based on the cosine number transform. *Signal Processing Image Communication, 35*, 1–8. doi:10.1016/j.image.2015.03.005

Lin, Y. K. (2012). High capacity reversible data hiding scheme based upon discrete cosine transformation. *Journal of Systems and Software, 85*(10), 2395–2404. doi:10.1016/j.jss.2012.05.032

Manikandan, M. S., & Dandapat, S. (2007). Wavelet energy based diagnostic distortion measure for ECG. *Biomedical Signal Processing and Control, 2*(2), 80–96. doi:10.1016/j.bspc.2007.05.001

Martínez-González, R. F., Díaz Méndez, J. A., Palacios-Luengas, L., López-Hernández, J., & Vázquez-Medina, R. (2016). A steganographic method using bernoulli's chaotic maps. *Computers & Electrical Engineering, 54*, 435–449. doi:10.1016/j.compeleceng.2015.12.005

Nambakhsh, M. S., Ahmadian, A., & Zaidi, H. (2011). A contextual based double watermarking of PET images by patient ID and ECG signal. *Computer Methods and Programs in Biomedicine, 104*(3), 418–425. doi:10.1016/j.cmpb.2010.08.016 PMID:20934773

Pan, J., & Tompkins, W. J. (1985). A real-time QRS detection algorithm. *IEEE Transactions on Biomedical Engineering, BME-32*(3), 230–236. doi:10.1109/TBME.1985.325532 PMID:3997178

Pandey, A., Saini, B. S., Singh, B., & Sood, N. (2016). A 2D electrocardiogram data compression method using a sample entropy-based complexity sorting approach. *Computers & Electrical Engineering, 56*, 36–45. doi:10.1016/j.compeleceng.2016.10.012

Pandey, A., Saini, B. S., Singh, B., & Sood, N. (2017). An integrated approach using chaotic map & sample value difference method for electrocardiogram steganography and OFDM based secured patient information transmission. *Journal of Medical Systems, 41*(12), 187. doi:10.100710916-017-0830-4 PMID:29043502

Phadikar, A. (2013). Multibit quantization index modulation: A high-rate robust data-hiding method. *Journal of King Saud University-Computer and Information Sciences, 25*(2), 163–171. doi:10.1016/j.jksuci.2012.11.005

Rajaraman, V. (2016). IEEE standard for floating point numbers. *Resonance, 21*(1), 11–30. doi:10.100712045-016-0292-x

Ravichandran, D., Praveenkumar, P., Rayappan, J. B. B., & Amirtharajan, R. (2016). Chaos based crossover and mutation for securing DICOM image. *Computers in Biology and Medicine, 72*, 170–18. doi:10.1016/j.compbiomed.2016.03.020 PMID:27046666

Rubio, O., Alesanco, A., & García, J. (2013). Secure information embedding into 1D biomedical signals based on SPIHT. *Journal of Biomedical Informatics, 46*(4), 653–664. doi:10.1016/j.jbi.2013.05.002 PMID:23707304

Saini, I., Singh, D., & Khosla, A. (2013). QRS detection using K-Nearest Neighbor algorithm (KNN) and evaluation on standard ECG databases. *Journal of Advanced Research, 4*(4), 331–344. doi:10.1016/j.jare.2012.05.007 PMID:25685438

Seera, M., Lim, C. P., Liew, W. S., Lim, E., & Loo, C. K. (2015). Classification of Electrocardiogram and Auscultatory blood pressure signals using machine learning models. *Expert Systems with Applications*, *42*(7), 3643–3652. doi:10.1016/j.eswa.2014.12.023

Shiu, H. J., Lin, B. S., Chien, H. H., Chiang, P. Y., & Lei, C. L. (2017). Preserving privacy of online digital physiological signals using blind and reversible steganography. *Computer Methods and Programs in Biomedicine*, *151*, 159–170. doi:10.1016/j.cmpb.2017.08.015 PMID:28946998

Slimane, Z. E. H., & Naït-Ali, A. (2010). QRS complex detection using empirical mode decomposition. *Digital Signal Processing*, *20*(4), 1221–1228. doi:10.1016/j.dsp.2009.10.017

Subhedar, M. S., & Mankar, V. H. (2014). Current status and key issues in image steganography: A survey. *Computer Science Review*, *13-14*, 95–113. doi:10.1016/j.cosrev.2014.09.001

Trinder, J., Kleiman, J., Carrington, M., Smith, S., Breen, S., Tan, N., & Kim, Y. (2001). Autonomic activity during human sleep as a function of time and sleep stage. *Journal of Sleep Resolution*, *10*(4), 253–264. doi:10.1046/j.1365-2869.2001.00263.x PMID:11903855

Wang, K., Lu, Z. M., & Hu, Y. J. (2013). A high capacity lossless data hiding scheme for JPEG images. *Journal of Systems and Software*, *86*(7), 1965–1975. doi:10.1016/j.jss.2013.03.083

Wang, S., Yang, B., & Niu, X. (2010). A secure steganography method based on genetic algorithm. *Journal of Information Hiding and Multimedia Signal Processing*, *1*(1), 28–35. www.physionet.org/cgi-bin/atm/ATM

Yang, C. Y., & Wang, W. F. (2016). Effective electrocardiogram steganography based on coefficient alignment. *Journal of Medical Systems*, *40*(3), 66. doi:10.100710916-015-0426-9 PMID:26711443

Yang, H., Sun, X., & Sun, G. (2009). A high-capacity image data hiding scheme using adaptive LSB substitution. *Wuxiandian Gongcheng*, *18*(4), 509–516.

KEY TERMS AND DEFINITIONS

Chaotic Maps: The mathematical functions used to generate random sequences.
Ciphertext: The encrypted data.
Clinical Distortion: Distortion in the physiological signal that can affect the diagnosis.
Key Space: The length of the key used to extract the hidden information.
Steganography: An art of hiding some sensitive information into the insensitive features of host media.

Chapter 3
Implementation and Performance Assessment of Biomedical Image Compression and Reconstruction Algorithms for Telemedicine Applications:
Compressive Sensing for Biomedical Images

Charu Bhardwaj
Jaypee University of Information Technology, India

Shruti Jain
Jaypee University of Information Technology, India

Urvashi Sharma
Jaypee University of Information Technology, India

Meenakshi Sood
Jaypee University of Information Technology, India

ABSTRACT

Compression serves as a significant feature for efficient storage and transmission of medical, satellite, and natural images. Transmission speed is a key challenge in transmitting a large amount of data especially for magnetic resonance imaging and computed tomography scan images. Compressive sensing is an optimization-based option to acquire sparse signal using sub-Nyquist criteria exploiting only the signal of interest. This chapter explores compressive sensing for correct sensing, acquisition, and reconstruction of clinical images. In this chapter, distinctive overall performance metrics like peak signal to noise ratio, root mean square error, structural similarity index, compression ratio, etc. are assessed for medical image evaluation by utilizing best three reconstruction algorithms: basic pursuit, least square, and orthogonal matching pursuit. Basic pursuit establishes a well-renowned reconstruction method among the examined recovery techniques. At distinct measurement samples, on increasing the number of measurement samples, PSNR increases significantly and RMSE decreases.

DOI: 10.4018/978-1-5225-7952-6.ch003

INTRODUCTION

With the advancement in information and communication technology, data traffic generates noticeably massive amount of information data especially in biomedical area. Radiological medical imaging methods (MRI and CT-Scan experiments) are used to inspect and analyze the inner structure of human body. These methods generate a large amount of scientific information which is digitally stored in the form of medical image that can be easily accessible. Clinical imaging records are significantly high as a typical hospital generates terabytes of information per year (Ravishankar & Breler, 2011). Clinical imaging data is certainly excessive and needs more storage space thus medical image compression is essential. Compression is a proficient solution for illustrating compact and robust data representation to facilitate efficient transmission and storage. File size is reduced, less bandwidth is utilized and the transmission speed is accelerated using compression techniques. Predominant goal of compression is to lessen the redundant and irrelevant bits of data for efficient data storage and transmission. Compression may be extensively categorised into two classes, Lossy and Lossless Compression. Lossy compression is appropriate for the applications where a slight loss of information is permissible like for natural pictures, text images, etc. For lossy compression techniques, compression ratio is high but the image quality is low. In case of lossless compression, the reconstructed image is the exact replica of the actual image as there is no data loss in lossless compression technique. Compression ratio achieved for this approach is not always high but the recovered image is of better-quality as compared to that of the lossy compression approach.

Data loss is not tolerable in scientific field like biomedical image processing as it can lead to wrong diagnosis. Many hospitals have small clinics situated in the far flung regions where distance is a vital issue to deliver the health care facilities. Patient residing in remote, rural and semi-urban areas find tough time to travel to far away hospitals particularly for diagnostic functions. For the convenience of patients suffering from severe diseases, the hospitals make use of telemedicine practices to provide health care facilitates in such areas. These tele-radiology applications allow the technician at the remote centres to capture a series of medical image data (MRI or CT scan) and transmit it to the principal health centre situated at the city where the diagnostic radiologist can examine the image and send back the diagnostic information to the clinical prognosis and the patients (Vijaykuymar, & Anuja, 2012).

In conventional image capturing systems, sampling is primarily based on Nyquist criteria wherein the original signal is sampled at a rate more than or equal to two times the maximum frequency of the signal. This sampling rate is too high for certain applications thereby increasing the complications in terms of complexity during compression. The increased rate of sampling adds directly to the complexity of the sensing hardware and this leads to wastage of power resources (Zhao, *et al.*, 2017; Wiegand, *et al.*, 2003). So, to facilitate the need of image compression for contemporary applications it is required to have a system with decreased acquisition complexity and flexible process for decoding. Compressive Sensing (CS) technique emerges as a new idea for signal acquisition, compression and reconstruction which has become main focus of researcher's interest. It is a far unique technique employing sub-Nyquist sampling criteria overcoming the drawbacks of the conventional strategies (Donoho, 2006; Candes, *et al.*, 2008; Romberg, *et al.*, 2006). CS utilizes the sparse signal recovery using fewer linear measurements and convex optimization approach for approximate recovery relative to standard schemes utilizing the complete ensemble of signal space (Candes & Romberg, 2007).

The concept of CS was at first introduced by Emmanuel Candes, collectively with Justin Romberg and Terry Tao (Donoho, 2006; Candes, *et al.*, 2008; Romberg, *et al.*, 2006; Candes, *et al.*, 2007). Signals fulfilling the requirement of sparsity in any domain can be recovered using CS approach, may it be an audio, image or a video signal. In (Nahar & Kolte, 2014) it was seen that CS was a progressive approach for signal acquisition and restoration. The key advantages of CS are faster data acquisition from very few sparse samples, reduced computational complexity, low power transmission, small traffic extent, etc. X. Zhang, *et al.* have used Orthogonal Matching Pursuit (OMP) reconstruction algorithm in (Zhang, Wen, Han, & Villasenor, 2011) applying the set of rules to recover an image. It was found that OMP has negligible additional complexity however enabling overall performance improvement in the reconstruction. Combined sparsifying transforms were used in (Qu, Cuo, Guo, Hu, & Chen, 2010) to achieve CS for MRI imaging by enforcing the sparsity of image using Total Variation (TV), wavelet approach, etc. It was seen that smooth L_0 norm method have NP hard problem which was then replaced by Basic Pursuit (L_1) norm minimization. Predefined information was used in (Liang & Ying, 2010) for CS reconstruction that utilises partially known spatial and temporal frequency domains from motion patterns of MR images. Reconstruction was done using L_1 norm minimization technique which was the best approach for image sample recovery. A real time MRI recovery technique was proposed in (Majumdar, Ward, & Aboulnasr, 2012) and the residual (the difference image between the previous and the current image) was taken. M.M Sevak, *et al.* (Sevak, Thakkar, Kher, & Modi, 2012) have implemented wavelet transform for the generation of a set of sparse components and CS approach for compression and later they combined the two techniques. Various Non- Linear Mapping Techniques are compared with OMP technique in (Zhang & Wen, 2012). As compared to the other convex optimization approaches, OMP was less complex approach providing faster running speed, lower power consumption and optimal reconstruction. Guaranteed reconstruction was however provided by convex optimization based recovery algorithms. Scan time for MR image acquisition was improved by T.D.Tran *et al.* (Tran, Duc, & Bui, 2010). In this paper authors combines CS approach along with the wireless transmission mechanism which was based on 802.11 providing bit rate requirement at 11Mbps. An improvised L_1 norm reconstruction method for CS-MRI was proposed in (Chang & Ji, 2010) investigating the previously developed approaches like SMASH and SENSE recovery algorithms. A better recovery algorithm; L_1 norm minimization approach was used in this paper to provide precise details, sharp edges and accurate recovery for MRI image reconstruction. This approach yields lower Normalised Mean Square Error (NMSE) producing a better quality recovered image with less computation complexity. A new set of parameters consisting of different auxiliary measurements, low pass filter coefficients, ordering index, etc. are proposed in (Lakshminarayana & Sarvagya, 2016) for improving the performance of CS algorithm. Authors (Lakshminarayana & Sarvagya, 2016) show that L_1 reconstruction approach was used to recover the signal using the concept of sparsity. A better performance was achieved maintaining the trade-off between compression ratio and medical image quality as compared to the existing literature in this field. Some of the other state of the art literatures are summarized in Table 1.

The main motivation of this chapter is reduction in file size using CS approach for biomedical image compression so as to minimize the storage and bandwidth requirements. The main goal of this chapter is to find an efficient method for reconstruction of images and evaluate recovery algorithms to maintain the balance between image quality and compression ratio. A modified approach for better acquisition, compression and reconstruction using CS technique provides better reconstruction and least distorted compressed image.

Table 1. Literature review of CS techniques

S. No.	Authors	Utilized Techniques	Implication Drawn and Estimated Parameters	Demerits
1.	(Shiqian M., *et.al.*, 2008)	L_1- norm minimization, Total Variation approach and Wavelets	Error of image and Signal-to-Noise-Ratio	Requirement of better image quality and storage space.
2.	(Nagesh P., Baoxin L., 2009)	Compressed sensing Technique (CS)	Recognition rate and percentage of storage space	Multiple views of scenes are used.
3.	(Wright J., *et.al.*, 2009)	L_1- minimization technique for sparse representation	Sparsity Concentration Index (SCI)	Detection of object is also required.
4.	(Sen P., Darabi S., 2011)	Compressive rendering for finding pixel values	MSE is evaluated. Scheme gives better quality reconstruction.	Sampling densities employed are very less.
5.	(Jing C., Wang Y., & Hanxiao W., 2012)	Real time video surveillance CS tracking and motion detection algorithm	Better recovery at high resolution for fast tracking utilizing less storage space.	Outcomes are not evaluated on benchmark datasets.
6.	(Hemalatha R., *et.al.*, 2013)	BinDCT and Noiselet based CS approach is utilized for Energy consumption analysis	Compression ratio, PSNR and reduced bit rate	More energy consumption reduction is required.
7.	(Yipeng L., *et.al.*, 2013)	Biomedical signal recovery using L_1- Total Variation approach and Nuclear norm minimization	Technique employed provide accurate signal recovery and Mean L_1 error is evaluated	Outcomes are not evaluated on benchmark datasets.
8.	(Tremoulheac B., *et.al.*, 2014)	L1 norm minimization with Fourier transform in temporal direction and Alternating Direction Methods of Multipliers (ADMM)	Normalized MSE for intensity and motion	Method is not optimized and run-time elapsed is more.
9.	(Xie S., Guan C., & Lu Z., 2015)	ADMM with variable splitting strategy	MSE is calculated	Datasets are not standardized and approach is computationally complex
10.	(Zhang Q., *et.al.*, 2016)	CS theory is applied from down-sampled l-space data and a wavelet tree-based recovery algorithm is proposed	SNR is calculated for MR images	Can be extended for recovery of dynamic MR sequences
11.	(Bilala M., *et.al.*, 2017)	L1 norm approximations are employed	SSIM, Gaussian noise level in MR images, RMSE of recovered MR images	Complex architecture
12.	(Shrividya G. & Bharathi S.H., 2018)	CS-MRI technique is used along with Total Variation algorithm	MSE, PSNR, SSIM and Sampling percentage of MR images	SSIM value can be improved more to get quality

COMPRESSIVE SENSING

CS plays a significant role in numerous fields like biomedical, scientific imaging and satellite imaging to reconstruct the signal using fewer samples (Foucart, *et al.*, 2013; Madhukumar, *et al.*, 2015). CS techniques produces better results in terms of high imaging speed, high Compression Ratio (CR) and better quality image (Wang, Bresler, & Ntziachristos, 2011). This technique exploits the samples of sparse signal of interest rather than collecting the entire ensemble of signal samples (Baraniuk, 2007). CS approach intend to acquire sensing and compression in a single step by converting the sensing paradigm (Madhukumar & Baiju, 2015). Figure 1 shows the block diagram of CS technique which is the combination of sensing and compression.

Figure 1. Block diagram of Compressive sensing

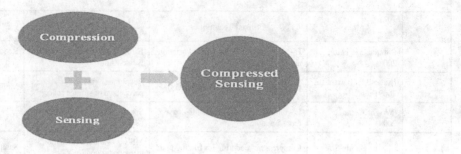

Sensing and Sampling

Sensors are used to sample and analyse the signal by taking a linear measurement of signal space. The whole ensemble of this signal space is not exploited for CS recovery but the CS technique works on alternating present vectors using already known vector space. This sampling consists of measurement samples having decreased dimensions than the original signal. Let the highest frequency component f (in hertz) is maximum for an analog signal then according to Nyquist, the sampling criteria should be at least $2 \times f_{max}$, or twice the highest frequency component. If the sampling criteria is not fulfilled or if the sampling rate is less than the twice of maximum frequency component then highest frequency components does not provide the correct representation of an analog input signal.

The sub-Nyquist sampling has involved a lot of concentration in both fields of mathematics and computer science. Sub-Nyquist sampling, also known as compressed sensing refers to the problem of recovering the signal by its samples. It can also recover the signal from the fewer samples than required by Nyquist sampling criteria. Recovery principles involved in Compressed Sensing approach to recover the signals are briefed in the next section.

Principles of Compressive Sensing Reconstruction

The two recovery principles involved in CS recovery are Sparsity and Incoherence. To implement CS theory, signal of interest is represented by sparsity and an isometric property of incoherence which limits the sensing modality.

Sparsity

Sparsity expresses an idea, that a continuous time signal has the rate of information much lower than expressed by the signal bandwidth. Similarly for a discrete signal to be sparse, the degree of freedom should be much lower than the finite length of the signal. Sparse signals have many zero coefficients and few non-zero coefficients. Fewer non-zero coefficients consist of majority of signal information and the other coefficients are not exactly zero however having very less value. Signal estimation for a sparse signal is done by considering only the larger coefficients consisting of majority information and other least significant coefficients are ignored during computation (Park & Wakin, 2009). A signal can be sparse or compressible having a concise representation in a proper sparsifying (Ψ) basis. Thresholding algorithms also depend on sparsity to estimate the signal. For systems of linear equations, sparse approximation theory deals with sparse solutions. Several variations for sparse approximation problem are structured sparsity and collaborative sparse coding.

1. **Structured Sparsity:** In the original version of sparsity, any of the coefficients of the problem domain can be selected but in case of structured sparsity model, group of coefficients are chosen instead of picking individual coefficients (Eldar, Kuppinger, & Bolcskei, 2010).
2. **Collaborative or Joint Sparse Coding:** Original version of the problem is defined only for single signal but in collaborative sparse coding a set of signal is available and each of them is converged from the same set of coefficients (Tropp, Gilbert, & Strauss, 2006).

Incoherence

The duality between time and frequency domain is expressed by incoherence which basically presents the idea that the signal having sparse representation in sparsifying domain (Ψ) and must be spread out in the sampling domain in which they are acquired. Incoherence for sparse signals is implemented through isometric property. Coherence basically evaluates the maximum correlation between any two elements of entirely two different matrices. Incoherence refers to the property which signifies that there must be minimum correlation between the elements of two different matrices. Considering two different domains, a signal is considered to be compressible if it has high sparsity in Ψ domain and is incoherent in sampling domain (Baig, Lai, & Punchihewa, 2012). Low correlation enables the signal reconstruction of sparse signal with few samples whereas it is impossible for high correlation samples regardless of signal sparsity.

Imaging Modality

A particular imaging technique or a system in the area of Computed Tomography Scan (CT-Scan), nuclear medicine, ultrasound, projection radiography and Magnetic Resonance Imaging (MRI) is termed as imaging modality. Modalities like CT-Scan, projection radiography and nuclear medicine make use of ionization to visualize the interior human body structure. High frequency sound signals are fired into the human body for ultrasound imaging and the echoes are received from the structures within the body. High strength magnetic field and radio waves are combined to acquire MRI images and it exploits the property of nuclear magnetic resonance. The main tool used in biomedical imaging field for acquiring the interior structure of human body is MRI. Notable visualization of human body and its contrast mechanism is employed to obtain the body structure using MRI scan (Ravishankar & Breler, 2011). MRI is different from CT-Scan as this process does not use radiations and CT-Scan uses ionizing radiations which can harm the human body. MRI provides the detailed view of human body which is not indicated in X-Ray, CT-Scan or ultrasound images. Magnetic resonance imaging approach provides better contrasted image and clear diagnostic quality than other imaging modalities like X-Ray and CT- Scans.

MRI Scan

MRI imaging utilizes magnetic resonance scanners exhibiting the properties of Nuclear Magnetic Resonance (NMR). The nucleus of the hydrogen atom tends to align itself in the presence of strong magnetic field. As the vast numbers of hydrogen atoms are present in the human body, it leads to net magnetization of the human body structure. Selective excitation of different regions within the body is also possible by inclining the group of these magnets away from the magnetic field direction. General categories of MR-Scanners are functional MRI (*f*MRI) and Magnetic Resonance Spectroscopic Imaging.

1. **Functional MRI (fMRI):** This scanner, images the blood oxygenation of the human brain by using oxygenation sensitive pulse sequence. fMRI employing an advance MRI in such a way that blood flow is increased to activate regions of brain. Standard MRI-Scanners do not actually detect blood flow as fMRI.

2. **Magnetic Resonance Spectroscopic Imaging:** It is termed as a non-invasive imaging technique as it gives spectroscopic information along with the image. Besides imaging the hydrogen atom, other nuclei are used for magnetic resonance spectroscopic imaging. This can be used to infer the cellular activity information from the human body. Different MRI scan images (leg, foot and brain) are shown in Figure 2.

CT-Scan

CT-Scans make use of X-Rays which are collimated (restricted in their geometrical spread) to travel in a 2D 'fan-beam' approximation. Tissues in the 2D cross-section of the human body create the X-Ray beam which is detected by a number of small detectors. The projections of X-Ray beam are collected from varying angular orientations of the detectors and the X-Ray tube as they rotate around a stationary subject (patient). Different CT-Scan modalities are helical CT and multi-slice CT which are currently being used for 3D imaging.

1. **Helical CT:** This CT-Scan modality is named as helical CT because the X-Ray tube slices out a helix. The detectors and the X-Ray tubes rotate around a circle and the patient is also continuously moving through the circle's center. It can acquire 3D Scan of the whole body very rapidly (in less than a minute).

Figure 2. Different MRI images (a) Leg MRI, (b) Foot MRI, (c) Brain MRI

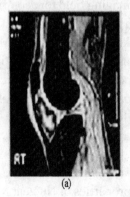 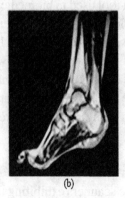 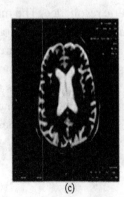

(a) (b) (c)

2.   **Multi-Slice CT:** It consists of several rows of detectors to speedily gather a cone of X-Ray data which comprises of 2D projection of patients. The quick rotation of X-Ray source and the detectors helps to produce 3D images using CT-Scanners. The different types (leg, foot and brain) of CT scan images are shown in Figure 3.

Compressive Sensing for Medical Images

Biomedical technology is progressing and clinics need to store huge volume of medical data in the form of images and signals to diagnose the current condition of the patients. A standard 12 bit X-ray of size 2048×2560 pixels interpreting 10,485,760 bytes of file size is very huge (ME, et al., 2012). Storage and transmission problem of higher quantity of data can get a breakthrough if the biomedical images are compressed in such a way that not only better quality image is obtained but also less transmission time is required without utilizing high bandwidth.

CS shows the considerable development in the field of biomedical engineering. As an improved framework for sampling and recovery, it is implemented on sparse signal of interest (Liu, Liang, Liu, & Zhang, 2012). In widespread mechanism, radiological images are captured from coupled devices which differentiate it from other information capturing mechanism. Because of presence of external artifacts, massive quantity of noisy data is also present within the informative data which is not required for diagnostic process. As the data is subjected to compression, medical information is compressed along with the undesirable noisy data, but in case of CS, only the desired information is decomposed (Wang, et al., 2011). Medical images like MRI and CT scan takes a long scanning time and these scans are indicative of patient's coronary heart rate, breathing pattern and position which may change time to time leading to degraded diagnosis quality. CS might also reduce poor effects of heart rate variation, pattern of respiration and also reduces the imaging time providing appreciated involvement in medical imaging field (Sevak, *et al.*, 2012).

After applying CS for compression the original medical image is also needed to be recovered and its quality is to be assessed so that these images can be utilized for diagnosis purpose. For this reason different recovery algorithms are implemented and their performance is assessed based on image quality parameters and compression ratio.

Figure 3. Different CT-scan images (a) Leg_CT Scan, (b) Foot_CT Scan and (c) Brain_CT Scan

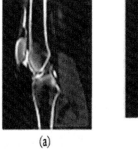 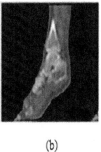 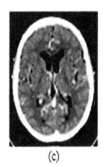

(a)   (b)   (c)

Recovery Algorithms

For optimal reconstruction of signal certain key requirement which should be satisfied are stability, speed, uniform guaranteed reconstruction and efficient performance. Convex optimization technique has gained the popularity due to its better efficiency, highly accurate reconstruction and guarantees the successful reconstruction (Liu, De Vos, Gligorijevic, Matic, Li, & Van Huffel, 2013). Numerous reconstruction strategies are available in the literature and they are detailed below.

Minimum L0 Norm Reconstruction

The exact solution of linear equations for minimum L_0 norm minimization is guaranteed by defining a set of rules. For a signal which is sparse in spasifying domain, the precise recovery is possible by using $2m$ random measurements. Every combination in m-sparse vector space is checked to find the exact solution in an N- dimensional space to satisfy the linear system of equations. This reconstruction technique is complex to implement and leads to NP-hard problem (Satyan, 2013).

$$\min \|x\|_0 \text{ subject to } y = \Phi \times x \tag{1}$$

here x is the original signal, y is the measurement vector which is obtained by multiplying measurement matrix Φ with the original signal x.

Basic Pursuit (L1 Minimization)

It is a convex optimization technique which is also termed L_1 minimization and it provides guaranteed recovery over sparse domain. L_1 minimization technique is not a speedy technique as massive numbers of iterations are involved in this method but it provides robustness for approximating the sparse signal. This technique is not optimally rapid but conversely it is a favourable approach as it gives better quality of reconstruction (Bhatt & Bamniya, 2015). As per the definition of the norm, L_1-norm of signal x is defined as,

$$\|x\|_1 = \sum_i |x_i| \tag{2}$$

L2 Norm Minimization

L_2 norm minimization reconstruction algorithm finds the minimum energy solution for minimizing the system of equations. This approach is easier to implement as compared to any other recovery algorithm but the solution provided by this approach is not accurate. Pseudo inverse is calculated to find the solution of L_2 norm but the calculated solution is far away than the optimally correct solution producing the undesired aliasing effect (Candes, *et al.*, 2006; Blumensath, *et al.*, 2009). L_2-norm is also well known as Euclidean norm, which is used to measure a vector difference and its equation is given by,

$$\|x\|_2 = \sqrt{\sum_i x_i^2} \qquad\qquad (3)$$

Minimum Total Variation Reconstruction

Total Variation (TV) minimization is a modification in L1 minimization technique that is especially successful in case of imaging applications. It is considered that the image is sparse in its gradient and therefore the image has very few variations in intensity.

$$\min \|s\|_{TV}, \text{ subject to } \|\Phi s - y\|_2 \leq \in \qquad\qquad (4)$$

Eq. (4) defines the TV-minimization reconstruction approach for recovering the gradient sparse signal and here s denotes the transform vector containing k non-zero coefficients, Φ is the measurement matrix, y is the measurement vector and ϵ denotes the upper bound of tolerance for reconstruction error energy (Candes, et al., 2006).

Greedy Method

Compressive sample matching pursuit, orthogonal matching pursuit and stage-wise orthogonal matching, etc. falls into the category of greedy algorithms. Greedy technique presents more rapid reconstruction than simple basic pursuit method but delivers least recoverable sparsity as compared to other reconstruction algorithms like L1 norm minimization. Greedy pursuit often provides uniform guarantee and stability but on the cost of quality. One of the most commonly used greedy algorithms for the recovery of nearly sparse signal is Orthogonal Matching Pursuit (OMP). For each of the new iteration, OMP works iteratively by initially choosing a column with the maximum projection onto the residual signal and then adding it to the already chosen columns. Once choosing a replacement column vector, representation coefficients with respect to the column vectors are chosen and observed through the least square optimization method. This method is not optimally stable but is a speedy reconstruction algorithm as compared to the other recovery approaches (Tropp, 2004).

For performance assessment of these recovery algorithms on medical images, various evaluation parameters are used and they are detailed in the next section.

Performance Evaluation Parameters

There are various performance assessment parameters. In this chapter we are using Mean Square Error (MSE), Peak Signal to Noise Ratio (PSNR), Compression Ratio (CR) and Structural Similarity Index (SSIM) for evaluation of CS recovery algorithms. PSNR is an image quality parameter calculated using MSE and these are inversely related to each other. Higher PSNR value indicates the higher quality of image. SSIM is based on arithmetical values of image and it is based on mean and variance and its value lies in between 0 to 1. The recovered image is structurally similar to the original image if its value leads toward 1. Ratio of compressed bits to the original image bits gives CR of an image (Bhardwaj, *et al.*, 2017; Ji, *et al.*, 2017).

Compressive Sensing: Scope and Its Applications

This section briefs about the various fields and applications where CS technique can be optimally used.

Biomedical Imaging

The technique of creating a visual perception or representation of internal body organs or tissues for medical evaluation and clinical intervention is referred as biomedical imaging. Clinical imaging seeks to reveal the inner body system detailing the pores, skin and bones which are used to diagnose and deal with the diseased body parts. Medical imaging additionally establishes a database of ordinary anatomy and body structure to make it viable to discover abnormalities. Thus better image compression is needed for screening and better diagnosis for biomedical imaging.

Telemedicine

Telemedicine practices allow the clinical services to be used from a distance by the means of modern telecommunication and information technology facilities. Electronic medical information is transferred over a distance to the main diagnostic centre where the information is processed and diagnosed.

Patients residing in the rural areas can take the benefit of medical care facilities without visiting the far away situated hospitals and this helps in removing the distance barriers. Therefore better image compression is required to serve this purpose of telemedicine facility without using much bandwidth and transmission time providing prompt clinical healthcare services.

Multimedia

Multimedia makes use of a combination of variety of contents like audio, video, images, text, animations, etc to make the multimedia applications more interactive. It is different from normal media applications, which makes use of basic conventional computer display like text-only, printed or hand-written material. Multimedia can be recorded, played, displayed, interacted with or accessed via facts content material processing gadgets, which includes automatic and digitally computerized gadgets, but also can be used as a part of live performances. Subsequently arising the need for better image compression to facilitate the multimedia applications to provide an ease to access various facilities.

Virtual Imaging or Digital Photography

An arrangement of electronic photo-detectors is used to capture images in virtual imaging or digital photography. This electronic photo detector is focused by a lens and is exposed on a photographic film to capture a digital photograph. The captured Images are digitized and stored as a computer file equipped with further digital processing, viewing, virtual publishing or printing equipments. Thus there is a need for higher image compression to aid virtual photography.

ALGORITHMS AND IMPLEMENTATION

In this chapter, CS technique is proposed for efficient compression, storage and transmission of MRI and CT-scan medical images. Dataset of MRI and CT-scan benchmark images is acquired from www.physionet.org to test the effectiveness of CS algorithm. For better image recovery different reconstruction algorithms are used and a comparative analysis is done. The following section gives a brief overview of CS algorithm and different recovery algorithms. Implementation and critical performance validation is also done in this section.

CS Algorithm

For the implementation of CS algorithm, consider an input image (x) of dimensions $n \times 1$ and a randomly generated measurement matrix (Φ) of dimensions $m \times n$. If Φ matrix is generated randomly, some useful information might become disoriented so Gaussian distribution is used for random variable generation having mean (μ) as 0 and variance (σ) as 1. Later x and Φ are multiplied to obtain the compressed sized measurement vector y having dimensions $m \times 1$. Steps followed for CS reconstruction are depicted in Figure 4.

Measurement vector y represents the CS sampling procedure and is computed by multiplying the measurement matrix Φ with the original image x.

$$y = \Phi \times x \tag{5}$$

The two main conditions which must be satisfied to recover an image using CS theory are illustrated below. Sampling process structure of CS matrices is depicted in Figure 5 and Figure 6 shows the complete arrangement of CS matrices.

Figure 4. Different steps for Compressive Sensing reconstruction

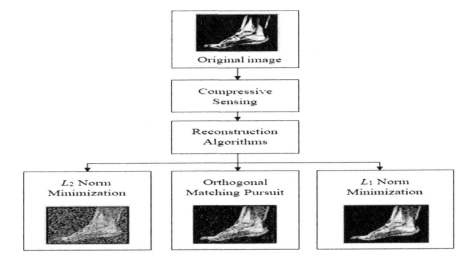

First Condition: Input image (x) should be sparse in some domain for the accurate image reconstruction utilizing few samples. For accurate recovery of an original image, x should fulfil the condition of sparsity i.e., it should be sparse in some domain. Let us consider a sparsifying matrix domain Ψ with dimensions (n× n) and a transform vector s having k significant non-zero coefficients (k<<n). The equation of sparisty is given by,

$$x = \Psi \times s \tag{6}$$

where, Ψ is the sparsifying matrix (n× n) and s is the transform vector containing k non-zero coefficients and k<<n.

Second Condition: The isometric property of incoherence should be satisfied by measurement matrix (Φ) and sparsifying matrix (Ψ) for CS recovery. Signal is more compressible if Ψ is incoherent to Φ and it is stated by the isometric property of incoherence [27]. Incoherence enables a sparse signal to be recovered using less number of samples. The condition of incoherence is denoted by θ in Eq. (7).

$$\theta = \Phi \times \Psi \tag{7}$$

The overall process of sampling is represented by θ' and it becomes,

$$\theta' = \Phi \times \Psi \times s \tag{8}$$

here, Φ is the measurement matrix, Ψ is sparsifying marix and s is transform vector.

Signal recovery for CS technique is achieved using minimization norm equation. By solving the Eq. (9), x can be recovered using sparse transform vector s,

$$x = \min \left\| \Psi^{-1} \times s \right\|_p \tag{9}$$

where, Ψ is sparsifying matrix, s is the sparse transform vector and p is the signal sparsity.

Figure 5. Sampling process structure of CS matrices

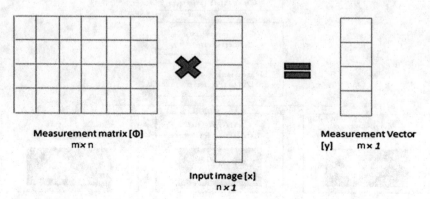

Figure 6. Complete arrangement of CS matrices

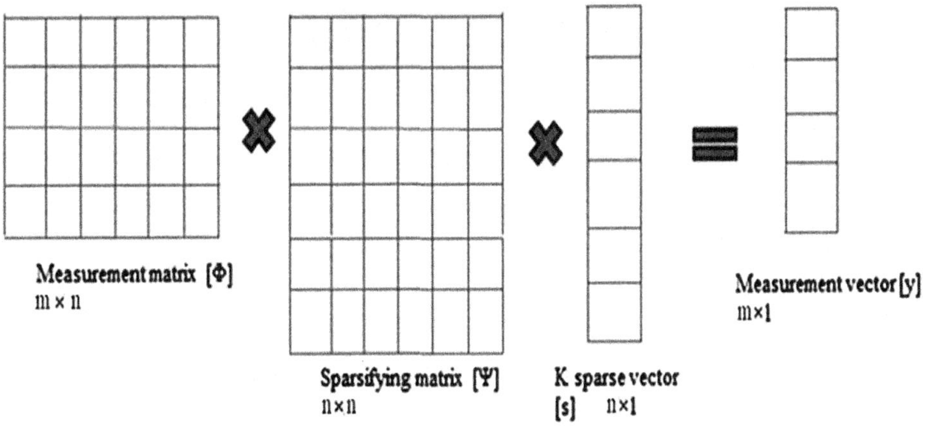

Measurement matrix [Φ]
$m \times n$

Sparsifying matrix [Ψ]
$n \times n$

K sparse vector
[s] $n \times 1$

Measurement vector [y]
$m \times 1$

The above equation is reduced to L_0 norm minimization if $p = 0$ but it leads to NP hard problem. To resolve this problem, L_1 norm minimization technique is used for reconstruction.

Before analyzing two dimensional (2D) signals, CS is applied on one dimensional (1D) signal to validate the CS algorithm. Consider a 1D signal generated on MATLAB 2013. CS technique is applied on 1D signal having total number of samples (n) = 256 and number of peaks (P) = 6 are considered in the original signal. Keeping n and P constant, measurement samples (m) are varied to recover the original signal using fewer samples than the total number of samples ($m \ll n$). Measurement Samples (m) are varied from 16 to 64 to analyze the accurate reconstruction and maintain a trade-off between the sampling rate and accuracy recovery.

Waveforms of 1D signal when CS recovery is applied are shown in Figure 7 to Figure 9 for measurement samples of 16, 32 and 64 respectively. In Figure 7 to Figure 9, x-axis denotes number of samples and y-axis denotes the amplitude of the signal. Three subplots in Figure 7 to Figure 9 represents the original signal, measurement samples considered and recovered signal respectively.

Signal reconstruction for varying number of measurement samples m is shown in Figure7 to Figure 9. It can be seen from Figure 7 that signal is reconstructed with visible distortions if m is considered as 16. On increasing the number of samples, accurate recovery is observed for m as 32 which can be seen in Figure 8. For the value of m ranging from 32 to 64, signal recovery is same as that of original signal. For better signal recover, m should be adjusted in such a way that there is balance between signal quality and sampling rate.

After analysis of CS technique on 1D signal it is applied on medical image samples (2D signal) and the images are recovered using three reconstruction algorithms (L_2 norm minimization, OMP technique and L_1 norm minimization). A detailed discussion of different reconstruction algorithms along with the results obtained are illustrated in the following sections.

CS Recovery Using Least Square Method (L2 Norm Minimization)

The commonly used method to solve the equation ($y = \Phi x$) and to find the minimum energy solution is L_2 norm minimization. The main advantage of this scheme is its simple implementation but it has a drawback that it does not provide the accurate solution producing the image with "aliasing-effect" [32,

Figure 7. Waveforms for m=16

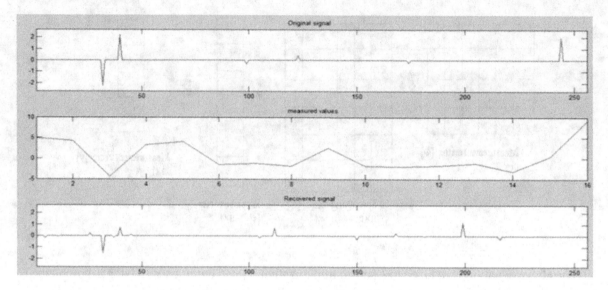

Figure 8. Waveforms for m=32

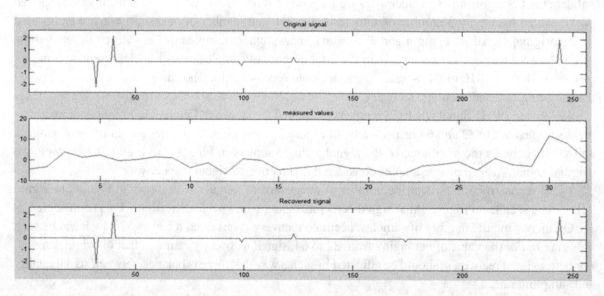

33]. This norm method works on the pseudo inverse based principle. L_2 norm minimization steps are detailed below;

1. Consider $y = \Phi x$ as the system of underdetermined linear equation where y is the measurement vector, x is the original signal, Φ is measurement matrix and $\Phi \in R^{m \times n}$ here ($m<n$).

2. One particular solution for L_2 norm is given by the following equation ;

Figure 9. Waveforms for m=64

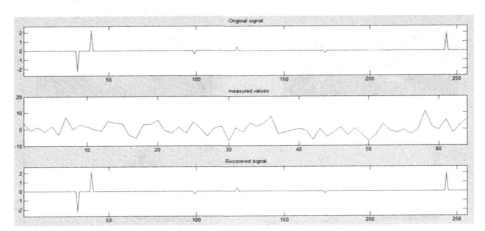

$$\tilde{x} = \Phi^T \left(\Phi \Phi^T \right)^{-1} \qquad (10)$$

here $\Phi \Phi^T$ is invertible since Φ is a full rank matrix.

$\breve{x}$ is the solution of $y = \Phi \times x$ that minimizes x and provides the solution of optimization problem.

Figure 10 (a) depicts the original foot MRI image and Figure 10 (b) depicts the reconstructed image obtained using Least Square method (L_2 norm minimization). Figure 10 (c) and Figure 10 (d) shows the respective histograms of original and reconstructed images respectively. In the Figure 10 (a), (b) and Figure 11 (a), (b) x axis and y axis shows horizontal and vertical dimensions of the image. Figure 10 (c), (d) and Figure 11 (c), (d) x axis shows dynamic range of grey scale ranging from 0 to 255 and y axis represents intensity value. Similarly, the original foot CT-Scan image and recovered image using L_2 norm minimization is depicted in Figure 11 (a) and Figure 11 (b) respectively. Figure 11 (c) and Figure 11 (d) shows histograms of original and reconstructed CT-Scan image respectively. It is clear from the

Figure 10. (a) Original image of foot MRI-scan, (b) reconstructed image obtained from Least Square (L_2) and (c) histogram of original image and (d) histogram of reconstructed image

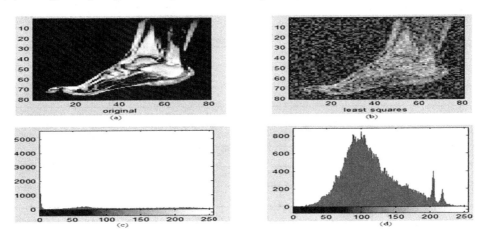

Figure 11. (a) Original image of foot CT-scan, (b) reconstructed image obtained from Least Square (L₂) and (c) histogram of original image and (d) histogram of reconstructed image

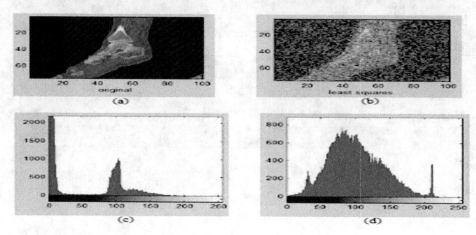

visual representation that the image recovered by L_2 norm minimization is not of better quality and this is further validated after calculating different performance assessment parameters obtained in Table 2. For evaluation purpose we have used 5 images of MRI and 5 images of CT-Scan.

RMSE calculated for L_2 reconstruction method gives a high RMSE value which in turn provides a lower value of PSNR in dB indicating poor image quality. SSIM index is human vision perception based structural similarity index and its value for L_2 norm method is more near 0 indicating less structural similarity to that of the original image.

CS Recovery Using Orthogonal Matching Pursuit (OMP)

Algorithms of matching pursuit like CS Matching Pursuit, Regularization Orthogonal Matching Pursuit and stage-wise Orthogonal Matching Pursuit all falls into the category of greedy algorithms. An estimated signal is obtained by finding the correlation between the columns of Φ measurement matrix and

Table 2. Different performance parameters obtained for L_2 recovery algorithm

Image Samples	RMSE	PSNR (dB)	SSIM
Img1_MR	55.82	12.62	0.43
Img2_MR	52.15	13.33	0.27
Img3_MR	89.79	10.89	0.20
Img4_MR	50.69	13.23	0.44
Img5_MR	46.33	14.65	0.31
Img1_CT	81.16	9.75	0.19
Img2_CT	43.60	14.40	0.21
Img3_CT	39.33	15.91	0.17
Img4_CT	90.12	8.87	0.20
Img5_CT	93.27	7.08	0.17

the measurement residual (r). The new estimated signal (x_k) is highly correlated with the residual [34, 35]. The steps of OMP algorithm are detailed as follows;

1. First of all the residual is initialize, $r_0 = y$ and Column C_0 is set as Φ for iteration count $k=1$.
2. Column vector Φ_{ck} of Φ is obtained using approximation a_c i.e., highly correlated with the residual and the equation is given by;

$$\Phi_{ck} = \max_c \left| \langle r_{k-1}, a_c \rangle \right|, c \in [n] \tag{11}$$

3. Least square problem is solved by:

$$x_k = \left\| y - \Phi_{ck} \times x \right\|_2 \tag{12}$$

4. To remove the contribution of a_c (approximation), the residual is updated by

$$r_k = y - \Phi_{ck} \tag{13}$$

5. Increase the iteration count k, and repeat steps 2-4 until stopping criterion is met.

Figure 12 (a) depicts the original foot MRI image and Figure 12 (b) depicts the reconstructed image obtained using Matching Pursuit method (OMP). Similarly, the original foot CT-Scan image and recovered image using OMP is depicted in Figure 13 (a) and Figure 13 (b) respectively. It is clear from the visual representation that the image recovered by OMP reconstruction method gives better recovered image as compared to the L_2 norm minimization and this is further validated after calculating different performance assessment parameters for OMP reconstruction algorithm obtained in Table 3.

Figure 12. (a) Original image of foot MRI-Scan, (b) reconstructed image obtained from Matching Pursuit (OMP) and (c) histogram of original image and (d) histogram of reconstructed image

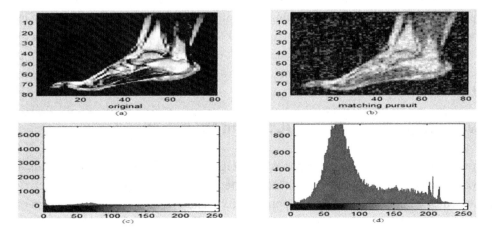

Figure 13. (a) Original image of foot CT-Scan, (b) reconstructed image obtained from Matching Pursuit (OMP) and (c) histogram of original image and (d) histogram of reconstructed image

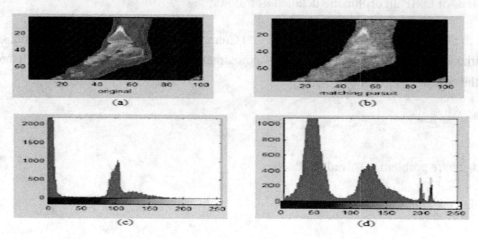

Table 3. Different performance parameters obtained for OMP recovery algorithm

Image Samples	RMSE	PSNR (dB)	SSIM
Img1_MR	39.19	15.84	0.51
Img2_MR	30.16	18.00	0.53
Img3_MR	41.32	15.42	0.49
Img4_MR	36.32	16.48	0.64
Img5_MR	31.26	17.53	0.46
Img1_CT	31.01	17.13	0.48
Img2_CT	14.39	22.32	0.51
Img3_CT	15.31	26.71	0.40
Img4_CT	37.74	16.17	0.44
Img5_CT	53.45	13.26	0.49

RMSE calculated for OMP was less than L_2 reconstruction method thus OMP recovery method provides greater value of PSNR in dB indicating better image quality. Structural similarity index is also near to 0.5 which shows that the recovered image is 50% similar to that of the original medical image. Image recovered using OMP reconstruction method gives better results as compared to L_2 norm minimization method in terms of image quality indicative by image pixel values and also in terms of visual perception based similarity parameter.

CS Recovery Using Basic Pursuit (L1 Norm Minimization)

The best established reconstruction technique is Re-weighted L_1 norm minimization that is used for CS image recovery in contrary to the other reconstruction technique. Uniform guaranteed recovery and stability is provided by L_1 norm minimization approach [32]. There is no linear bound on run time for this technique and it provides better recovery but it is optimally slow. On solving the following minimization problem, x is recovered by solving the equation,

$$x = \min \left\| \Psi^{-1} \times s \right\|_p \tag{14}$$

where, Ψ is sparsifying matrix, x is the original signal and p is the signal sparsity.

L_1 norm minimization recovery steps are as follows:

1. Weight (w) is initially given by $w_i^{(0)} = 1$, for $i = 1 \ldots N$. $w_i^{(0)}$ is the weights on pixels, the iterative count is set to 0.

2. By using equation (12), the weighted L_1 minimization problem is solved.

$$\min \left\| W \times s \right\|_1, \text{ s.t., } y = \Phi \times x \tag{15}$$

where W_s are the total number of weights in transform domain s.

3. Weights are then updated for $i = 1 \ldots N$,

$$w_i^{(j+1)} = \frac{1}{\left| \tilde{s}_i^{(j)} \right| + \epsilon} \tag{16}$$

Here, s is the sparse transform vector. ϵ is a positive number and use to prevent zero-valued denominator and j refers to number of iterations.

4. After that a specific maximum number of iteration j_{max} is attained by j and convergence terminates; otherwise increase j and repeat step 2-3.

Figure 14 (a) depicts the original foot MRI image and Figure 14 (b) depicts the reconstructed image obtained using Basic Square method that is L_1 norm minimization. Similarly, the original foot CT-Scan image and recovered image using L_1 norm minimization is depicted in Figure 15 (a) and Figure 15 (b) respectively. This is further validated after analysing the different performance assessment parameters for L_1 reconstruction algorithm obtained in Table 4.

Analysis of performance metrics like RMSE, PSNR and SSIM is done in Table 4 for different medical image samples recovered using L_1 recovery algorithm. L_1 recovery algorithm gives high value of PSNR and lower RMSE value as compared to the previously evaluated recovery methods; L_2 and OMP recovery techniques. Higher value of SSIM is obtained from the L_1 recovery technique out of three evaluated techniques. It is estimated that recovered image is much similar to the original image when L_1 recovery method is used and higher values of performance parameters are also obtained for L_1 reconstruction technique.

Figure 14. (a) Original image of foot MRI-Scan, (b) reconstructed image obtained from Basic Pursuit (L₁) and (c) histogram of original image and (d) histogram of reconstructed image

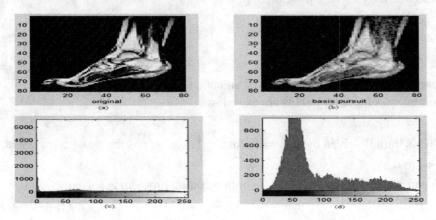

Figure 15. (a) Original image of foot CT-Scan, (b) reconstructed image obtained from Basic Pursuit (L₁) and (c) histogram of original image and (d) histogram of reconstructed image

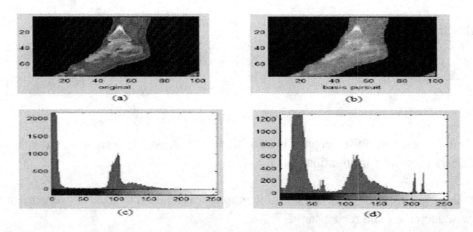

Table 4. Different performance parameters obtained for L₁ recovery algorithm

Image Samples	RMSE	PSNR (dB)	SSIM
Img1_MR	23.38	20.06	0.69
Img2_MR	19.61	21.87	0.65
Img3_MR	22.34	20.22	0.71
Img4_MR	20.15	21.17	0.72
Img5_MR	18.62	22.91	0.66
Img1_CT	21.34	20.05	0.61
Img2_CT	11.83	25.92	0.64
Img3_CT	9.03	28.87	0.60
Img4_CT	22.50	19.93	0.61
Img5_CT	36.31	17.49	0.64

Compression Ratio (CR) is calculated when CS is applied on image samples and it is obtained by taking the ratio of original image bits to the recovered image bits. There should be a trade-off between CR and image quality of an image. CR should be maintained in such a way that there is no degradation of reconstructed image quality. Space saving and CR for different compressed MRI images are graphically represented in Figure 16, graphical representation for different CT images is shown in Figure 17.

Effect of Measurement Samples on Different Image Samples

Foot MRI testing and recovery at varying measurement samples (m) employing L_1, L_2 and OMP reconstruction techniques is shown in Figure 18 to Figure 20 and it shows significant change in recovered images at different m samples. Previously, the effect of m measurement samples are verified for 1D signal and here in this section effect of varying m samples are verified for 2D signal (image). For an image, value of m measurement samples is considered less than the total number of pixels in an image.

Figure 16. Compression ratio and space saving from Compressive Sensing technique for different MRI images

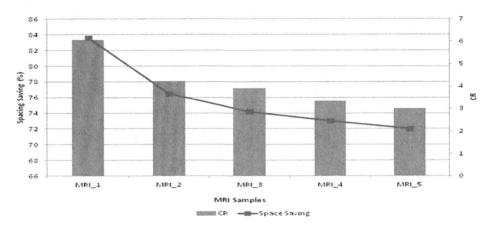

Figure 17. Compression ratio and space saving from Compressive Sensing technique for different CT images

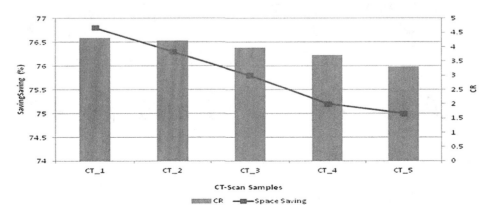

For e.g., for an image having dimension 80×80, *n* number of samples are 6400 and *m* can be any value less than 6400. To verify the effect of varying *m* measurement samples for better image recovery, *m* is considered 1000, 2000 and 4000 for an image of resolution 80×80. Only single brain MRI image analysis for varying measurement samples is shown in the following figures however the analysis is done for different image modalities.

It is clear from the above figures from Figure 20 to Figure 22 that quality of recovered image is improved when number of *m* samples is increased. In Figure 20, number of *m* samples is less i.e., *1000* so the recovered images from all three recovery techniques are of low quality. When number of samples (*m*) is increased from *1000* to *4000* as shown in Figure 21 and Figure 22, quality of recovered image

Figure 18. (a) Original MRI image of foot, reconstructed image using (b) Least Square (L_2), (c) Matching Pursuit (OMP) and (d) Basic Pursuit (L_1) reconstruction methods at measurement samples m=1000 samples over original image samples n=6400

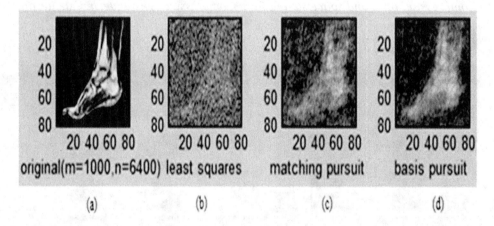

Figure 19. (a) Original MRI image of foot, reconstructed image using (b) Least Square (L_2), (c) Matching Pursuit (OMP) and (d) Basic Pursuit (L_1)reconstruction methods at measurement samples m=2000 samples over original image samples n=6400

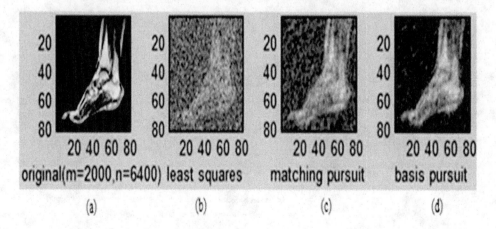

Figure 20. (a) Original MRI image of foot, reconstructed image using (b) Least Square (L_2), (c) Matching Pursuit (OMP) and (d) Basic Pursuit (L_1) reconstruction methods at measurement samples m=4000 samples over original image samples n=6400.

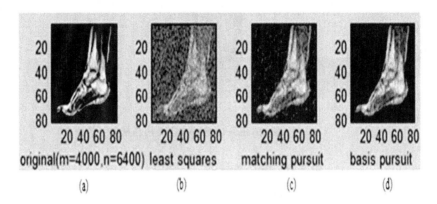

is improved. So number of samples (*m*) should be adjusted in such a way that there is balance between quality of recovered image *(PSNR)* and compression performance *(CR)*.

The effect of performance metrics PSNR and RMSE is seen with variation in measurement samples. At different measurement samples for MRI of brain, PSNR and RMSE are calculated. For all three recovery algorithms, PSNR is obtained at *m* = 1000, 2000 and then at 4000 when total number of samples (*n*) are 6400 (resolution of foot MRI) and *m* can be any number less than *n*. It is estimated that value of PSNR increase when number of measurement samples increases. Hence *m* should be selected such that the recovered image is of high quality with higher value of CR.

When *m* =*1000*, it is seen that PSNR value is around 9 to 15 dB and when it is varied from 1000 to 4000 then PSNR value increases with increase in *m*. Change in PSNR value for recovered images obtained using L_1, L_2 and OMP algorithms is shown in Figure 21 for varying number of samples from 1000 to 4000.

RMSE should be minimized to obtain better image quality. At *m*=1000, higher value of RMSE is obtained for all three recovery algorithms and when *m* is increased from 1000 to 4000, RMSE starts

Figure 21. Measurement samples v/s PSNR for brain MRI

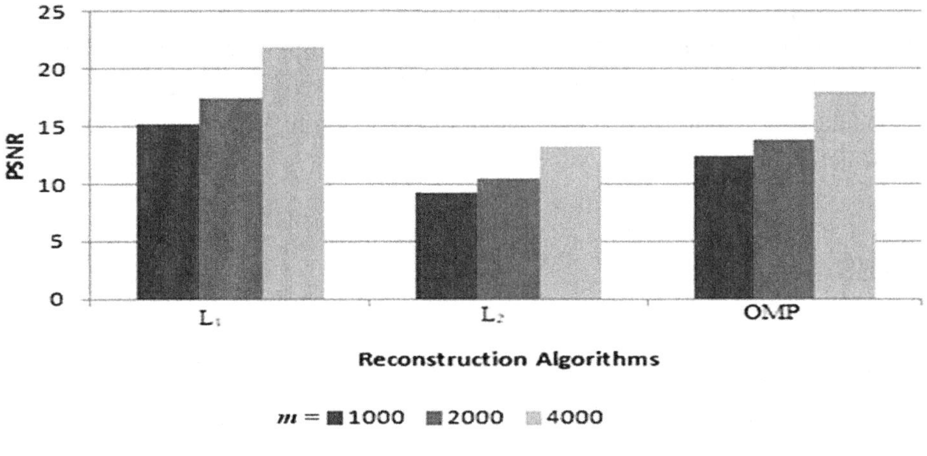

Figure 22. Measurement samples v/s RMSE for brain MRI

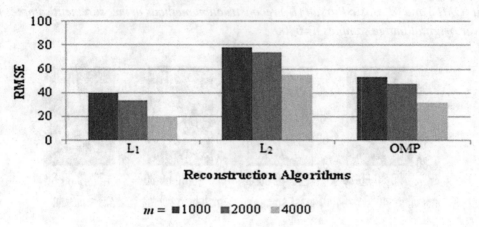

decreasing. RMSE values obtained for L_1, L_2 and OMP recovered images are graphically shown in Figure 22. Out of these three recovery algorithms, the image recovered using L_1 technique provides minimum RMSE value which indicates that the quality of image recovered by L_1 is better than other two algorithms.

CONCLUSION

CS performance is estimate for 1D signal and different medical image samples of MRI and CT- Scan. It is observed that the value of samples should be taken in such a way that there is appropriate balance between the recovered image quality and sampling rate. Quality metrics are obtained for L_1, L_2 and OMP algorithms for different image samples and it is estimated that L_1 technique is better than other reconstruction algorithms in terms of PSNR, RMSE, SSIM and CR. Perfect image recovery is possible by L_1 technique as it resembles more to the original image in comparison to L_2 and OMP reconstruction methods. It is concluded that all quality metrics are better obtained by L_1 and this is the best recovery technique among other implemented algorithms. Thus for a CS based system, L_1 recovery algorithm is considered as a good compression technique that enables a compromise between compression performance and recovered image quality. It is also concluded that the algorithm performance is also altered by the number of measurement samples taken for reconstruction. Value of PSNR increases with increase in number of measurement samples and RMSE value decreases. CS based recovery algorithms can also be implemented for various other medical samples of varying resolution and modality to obtain improved quality image by achieving higher value of PSNR. Compressed sensing concept can also be applied to video signals and the future scope in this field will focus on attaining maximum value of CR along with accurate reconstruction.

REFERENCES

Baig, M. Y., Lai, E. M., & Punchihewa, A. (2012). Compressive Video Coding: A Review of the State-Of-The-Art. In Video Compression. InTech.

Baraniuk, R. G. (2007). Compressive sensing. *IEEE Signal Processing Magazine, 24*(4), 118–121. doi:10.1109/MSP.2007.4286571

Bhardwaj, C., Ji, U., & Sood, M. (2017). Implementation and Performance Assessment of Compressed Sensing for Images and Video Signals. *Journal of Global Pharma Technology, 6*(9), 123–133.

Bhatt, M. U., & Bamniya, K. (2015). *Medical Image Compression and Reconstruction Using Compressive Sensing.* Academic Press.

Bilal, M., Ahmed, A. H., Shah, J. A., Kadir, K., & Ayob, M. Z. (2017, September). Comparison of L 1-norm surrogate functions used for the recovery of MR images. In *Engineering Technology and Technopreneurship (ICE2T), 2017 International Conference on* (pp. 1-4). IEEE.

Blumensath, T., & Davies, M. E. (2009). Iterative hard thresholding for compressed sensing. *Applied and Computational Harmonic Analysis, 27*(3), 265–274. doi:10.1016/j.acha.2009.04.002

Candes, E., & Romberg, J. (2007). Sparsity and incoherence in compressive sampling. *Inverse Problems, 23*(3), 969–985. doi:10.1088/0266-5611/23/3/008

Candès, E. J., Romberg, J., & Tao, T. (2006). Robust uncertainty principles: Exact signal reconstruction from highly incomplete frequency information. *IEEE Transactions on Information Theory, 52*(2), 489–509. doi:10.1109/TIT.2005.862083

Candes, E. J., & Tao, T. (2006). Near-optimal signal recovery from random projections: Universal encoding strategies? *IEEE Transactions on Information Theory, 52*(12), 5406–5425. doi:10.1109/TIT.2006.885507

Candès, E. J., & Wakin, M. B. (2008). An introduction to compressive sampling. *IEEE Signal Processing Magazine, 25*(2), 21–30. doi:10.1109/MSP.2007.914731

Chang, C. H., & Ji, J. (2010, August). Improved compressed sensing MRI with multi-channel data using reweighted l 1 minimization. In *Engineering in Medicine and Biology Society (EMBC), 2010 Annual International Conference of the IEEE* (pp. 875-878). IEEE.

Donoho, D. L. (2006). Compressed sensing. *IEEE Transactions on Information Theory, 52*(4), 1289–1306. doi:10.1109/TIT.2006.871582

Eldar, Y. C., Kuppinger, P., & Bolcskei, H. (2010). Block-sparse signals: Uncertainty relations and efficient recovery. *IEEE Transactions on Signal Processing, 58*(6), 3042–3054. doi:10.1109/TSP.2010.2044837

Foucart, S., & Rauhut, H. (2013). *A mathematical introduction to compressive sensing.* Basel: Birkhäuser.

Hemalatha, R., Radha, S., Raghuvarman, N., Soumya, B., & Vivekanandan, B. (2013). Energy Efficient Image Transmission over Bandwidth Scarce WSN using Compressed Sensing. *International Conference on IT and Intelligent Systems,* 57-61.

Ji, U., Bhardwaj, C., & Sood, M. (2017). Effectiveness of Reconstruction Methods in Compressive Sensing for Biomedical Images. *Journal of Global Pharma Technology, 6*(9), 134–143.

Jing, C., Wang, Y., & Hanxiao, W. (2012). A Coded Aperture Compressive Imaging Array and Its Visual Detection and Tracking Algorithms for Surveillance Systems. *Sensors (Basel), 12*(11), 14397–14415. doi:10.3390121114397 PMID:23202167

Lakshminarayana, M., & Sarvagya, M. (2016). Algorithm to balance compression and signal quality using novel compressive sensing in medical images. In *Software Engineering Perspectives and Application in Intelligent Systems* (pp. 317–327). Cham: Springer. doi:10.1007/978-3-319-33622-0_29

Liang, D., & Ying, L. (2010, August). Compressed-sensing dynamic MR imaging with partially known support. In *Engineering in Medicine and Biology Society (EMBC), 2010 Annual International Conference of the IEEE* (pp. 2829-2832). IEEE. 10.1109/IEMBS.2010.5626077

Liu, D. D., Liang, D., Liu, X., & Zhang, Y. T. (2012, August). Under-sampling trajectory design for compressed sensing MRI. In *Engineering in Medicine and Biology Society (EMBC), 2012 Annual International Conference of the IEEE* (pp. 73-76). IEEE.

Liu, Y., De Vos, M., Gligorijevic, I., Matic, V., Li, Y., & Van Huffel, S. (2013). Multi-structural signal recovery for biomedical compressive sensing. *IEEE Transactions on Biomedical Engineering, 60*(10), 2794–2805. doi:10.1109/TBME.2013.2264772 PMID:23715599

Madhukumar, N., & Baiju, P. S. (2015). Contourlet Transform Based MRI Image Compression using Compressed Sensing. *International Journal of Advanced Research in Electrical, Electronics and Instrumentation Engineering, 4*(7), 6434-6440.

Majumdar, A., Ward, R. K., & Aboulnasr, T. (2012). Compressed sensing based real-time dynamic MRI reconstruction. *IEEE Transactions on Medical Imaging, 31*(12), 2253–2266. doi:10.1109/TMI.2012.2215921 PMID:22949054

ME, M. S. S., Vijayakuymar, V. R., & Anuja, M. R. (2012). A survey on various compression methods for medical images. *International Journal of Intelligent Systems and Applications, 4*(3), 13.

Nagesh, P., & Baoxin, L. (2009). A Compressive Sensing Approach for Expression-Invariant Face Recognition. *IEEE Conference on Computer Vision and Pattern Recognition*, 1518-1525. 10.1109/CVPR.2009.5206657

Nahar, P. C., & Kolte, M. T. (2014). An introduction to compressive sensing and its applications. *Int J Sci Res Publ, 4*(6).

Park, J. Y., & Wakin, M. B. (2009, May). A multiscale framework for compressive sensing of video. In *Picture Coding Symposium, 2009. PCS 2009* (pp. 1-4). IEEE. 10.1109/PCS.2009.5167440

Qu, X., Cuo, X., Guo, D., Hu, C., & Chen, Z. (2010). Compress sensing MRI with combined sparisifying transforms and smoothed l0 norm minimization. *International Conference of IEEE*, 626-629.

Ravishankar, S., & Bresler, Y. (2011, August). Adaptive sampling design for compressed sensing MRI. In *Engineering in Medicine and Biology Society, EMBC, 2011 Annual International Conference of the IEEE* (pp. 3751-3755). IEEE. 10.1109/IEMBS.2011.6090639

Satyan, S. (2013). *The Use of Compressive Sensing in Video* (Doctoral dissertation).

Sen, P., & Darabi, S. (2011). Compressive Rendering: A Rendering Application of Compressed Sensing. *IEEE Transactions on Visualization and Computer Graphics, 17*(4), 487–499. doi:10.1109/TVCG.2010.46 PMID:21311092

Sevak, M. M., Thakkar, F. N., Kher, R. K., & Modi, C. K. (2012, May). CT image compression using compressive sensing and wavelet transform. In *Communication Systems and Network Technologies (CSNT), 2012 International Conference on* (pp. 138-142). IEEE. 10.1109/CSNT.2012.39

Shiqian, M., Wotao, Y., Yin, Z., & Chakraborty, A. (2008). An Efficient Algorithm for Compressed MR Imaging using Total Variation and Wavelets. *IEEE Conference on Computer Vision and Pattern Recognition*, 1-8. 10.1109/CVPR.2008.4587391

Shrividya, G., & Bharathi, S. H. (2018, February). A study of Optimum Sampling Pattern for Reconstruction of MR Images using Compressive Sensing. In *2018 Second International Conference on Advances in Electronics, Computers and Communications* (pp. 1-6). IEEE. 10.1109/ICAECC.2018.8479422

Tran, T. D., Duc, T. T., & Bui, T. T. (2010, November). Combination compress sensing and digital wireless transmission for the MRI signal. In *Micro-NanoMechatronics and Human Science (MHS), 2010 International Symposium* (pp. 273-276). IEEE.

Tremoulheac, B., Dikaios, N., Atkinson, D., & Arridge, S. R. (2014). Dynamic MR Image Reconstruction–Separation From Undersampled (k, t)-Space via Low-Rank Plus Sparse Prior. *IEEE Transactions on Medical Imaging, 33*(8), 1689–1701. doi:10.1109/TMI.2014.2321190 PMID:24802294

Tropp, J. A. (2004). Greed is good: Algorithmic results for sparse approximation. *IEEE Transactions on Information Theory, 50*(10), 2231–2242. doi:10.1109/TIT.2004.834793

Tropp, J. A., Gilbert, A. C., & Strauss, M. J. (2006). Algorithms for simultaneous sparse approximation. Part I: Greedy pursuit. *Signal Processing, 86*(3), 572–588. doi:10.1016/j.sigpro.2005.05.030

Wang, G., Bresler, Y., & Ntziachristos, V. (2011). Guest editorial compressive sensing for biomedical imaging. *IEEE Transactions on Medical Imaging, 30*(5), 1013–1016. doi:10.1109/TMI.2011.2145070 PMID:21692237

Wiegand, T., Sullivan, G. J., Bjontegaard, G., & Luthra, A. (2003). Overview of the H. 264/AVC video coding standard. *IEEE Transactions on Circuits and Systems for Video Technology, 13*(7), 560–576. doi:10.1109/TCSVT.2003.815165

Wright, J., Yang, A. Y., Ganesh, A., Sastry, S. S., & Ma, Y. (2009). Robust Face Recognition via Sparse Representation. *IEEE Transactions on Pattern Analysis and Machine Intelligence, 31*(2), 210–227. doi:10.1109/TPAMI.2008.79 PMID:19110489

Xie, S., Guan, C., Huang, W., & Lu, Z. (2015). Frame-based compressive sensing MR image reconstruction with balanced regularization. In *Engineering in Medicine and Biology Society (EMBC), 2015 37th Annual International Conference* (pp. 7031-7034). IEEE.

Yipeng, L., De, V. M., Gligorijevic, I., Matic, V., & Li, Y. (2013). Multi-Structural Signal Recovery for Biomedical Compressive Sensing. *IEEE Transactions on Biomedical Engineering, 60*(10), 2794–2805. doi:10.1109/TBME.2013.2264772 PMID:23715599

Zhang, Q., Zhang, J., & Sei-ichiro, K. (2016). Adaptive sampling and wavelet tree based compressive sensing for MRI reconstruction. In *Image Processing (ICIP), 2016 IEEE International Conference*, (pp. 2524-2528). IEEE.

Zhang, X., & Wen, J. (2012, September). Compressive video sensing using non-linear mapping. In *Image Processing (ICIP), 2012 19th IEEE International Conference on* (pp. 885-888). IEEE. 10.1109/ICIP.2012.6467002

Zhang, X., Wen, J., Han, Y., & Villasenor, J. (2011, February). An improved compressive sensing reconstruction algorithm using linear/non-linear mapping. In *Information Theory and Applications Workshop (ITA)*, 2011 (pp. 1-7). IEEE. 10.1109/ITA.2011.5743577

Zhao, C., Ma, S., Zhang, J., Xiong, R., & Gao, W. (2017). Video compressive sensing reconstruction via reweighted residual sparsity. *IEEE Transactions on Circuits and Systems for Video Technology*, *27*(6), 1182–1195. doi:10.1109/TCSVT.2016.2527181

Chapter 4
Shielding the Confidentiality, Privacy, and Data Security of Bio-Medical Information in India:
Legal Edifice

Varinder Singh
Guru Nanak Dev University, India

Shikha Dhiman
Panjab University, India

ABSTRACT

The framers of Indian Constitution were very much cognizant about the significance of human nobility and worthiness and hence they incorporated the "right to life and personal liberty" in the Constitution of India. Right to life is considered as one of the primordial fundamental rights. There is no doubt that Indian Judiciary has lived up to the expectations of the Constitution framers, both in interpreting and implementing Article 21 initially, but there are still a few complications left as to the viability of Article 21 in modern times. Looking at the wider arena of right to life, it can be articulated that broader connotation of "right to life" aims at achieving the norms of "privacy" as well.

PROLOGUE

Analysing the concept about biomedical information has become a complex and tedious issue. There is as such no prescribed definition or clear cut theoretical ground to extrapolate the term. Biomedical information and its privacy, security as well as confidentiality has been a topic of 'emerging field' since decades. Biomedical information can be understood as a field which is mainly concerned with the reasonable use of technology, so as to improvise public health, health care and biomedical research

DOI: 10.4018/978-1-5225-7952-6.ch004

("Medical Informatic and Telemedicine", n.d.). The medical information in India is being recorded in an old manual way of keeping records, instead of new methods coming up for securing one's data. The health care delivery systems in India has become a tool or a subject matter for concern, which now needs utmost priority. There have been many healthcare organisations who are working for protecting and securing the biomedical information since decades. Apart from these organisations, we have the Indian Medical Council Regulations states that every medical practitioner is required to maintain the patient-physician confidentiality as well as security. Data protection provides for various set of privacy rules, policies and procedures that ultimately focuses to reduce intrusion and interruption into person's privacy which might result by the collection, dissemination and storage of one's personal information.

The aspect which remains doubtful is that as to what all is to be covered under right to privacy for secreting biometric information and what not. The biometric informations so provided are important from the government's perspective and there lies a number of advantages like Aadhar based Direct Transfer Subsidy, Jan Dhan Yojna, Passport in 10 days, Digital locker, Voter Card Linking, Monthly Pension Provident Fund Opening new bank account, Digital Life Certificate and SEBI facilities (Ahmed et al, 2016). As it was rightly quoted by some renouned jurist that privacy has been considered a matter of interpretation and construction. It might take number of decades to decide as to what is the concrete form of privacy and security as the terms are itself very wide in their interpretation. Therefore, the term 'privacy' is quite a vague one to understand and comment upon.

GLOBAL PERSPECTIVE

The shielding and safeguarding of biomedical information has become a concern at global level. Every country focuses upon certain aspects of an individual to protect his or her information thereby securing his or her privacy, in whatever field so. Universally, many legislations have been made in order preserve such rights of the person. Few of the legislations of different nations are highlighted as under, as to how they deal with security and privacy provisions of their citizens or people residing in such countries.

United States of America

In United States of America, healthcare systems are viewed as one of the most appropriate factors in ensuring the security and privacy of one's life. In order to conduct any diagnose, patients are required to disclose their true medical information. But however, such information needs to be protected in any form. In order to protect and safeguard such information, there has been recently enacted Health Insurance Portability and Accountability Act (HIPAA) for providing healthcare applications to patients (Appari et al, 2010). Apart from HIPAA, United States healthcare systems have formed many other legislations such as Health Maintenance Organisation Act 1973. Moreover, there also have been Privacy and Security Rules for the protection of biomedical information formed under HIPAA in 1996. This is how the security and confidentiality of biomedical information is protected in a country like United States of America.

United Kingdom

In United Kingdom, the law with regard to the protection of bio-medical information as well as other information is thus provided under The Data Protection Act (DPA) of 1998. It has been in the latest updates that very soon the General Data Protection Regulation (GDPR) will replace the UK's Data Protection Act and will come up with some advanced as well as new provisions with regard to medical data protection. This change has to be brought into consideration because it is believed that everything now is changed with the assistance of new science and technology, so getting access to one's information is also becoming very easier. Hence, in order to keep everyone up to-date, there is a dire need for strengthening data protection laws in United Kingdom.

Australia

Maintaining health records and securing its privacy has been the most sensitive topic with respect to personal information of a person. It is for this reason that the Australian government have come up with drafting of the Privacy Act 1988. This Act of 1988 requires every organisation, whether big or small to deal with person's information very carefully and definitely needs the consent of a concerned person before such organisation is to take any health information from him or her ("Health Information and Medical Research", n.d.) However, with the passage of time this Act of 1988 has been amended and now the latest has come into force i.e. The Privacy Amendment (Enhancing Privacy Protection) Act 2012.

Turkey

The Personal Data Protection Law of 2016 and the Patients Rights Regulation (PRR) of 1998 are such laws which has been used and practised in Turkey for ascertaining the health of people. The Patients Rights Regulation of 1998 initially came into force in 1998 but has been recently updated in the year 2014, thereby collaborating the rights of both inpatients as well as outpatients in a legal aspect. Therefore, according to the legal mandate as stated in Turkey, the confidentiality clause of the patients does not only involve the assuring of patient's private information but in fact also encompasses the privacy of patient's body.

China

In order secure information in China, there has been two kinds of legislation, namely, the PRC Criminal Law and the PRC Trot Liability Law. Such laws enunciates that if any information is being shared by one person to another with respect to his/her privacy and if the latter disclose it to another, then the same can be held liable under either Criminal Law or Tort Liability Law. Recently, on 2nd January 2018, the SAC (Standardization Administration of China) has come up with framing of national standards for protecting the personal information i.e. Information Technology – Personal Information Security Specification, which came into force on 1st May 2018 (Luo et al, 2018). Such standards have been formed to safeguard the 'personal data and information' and 'sensitive personal information' which includes the information regarding banking details, identification card details, bio-medical information, credit details and many more of alike.

South Africa

The healthcare issues prevailing in South Africa does not provide much for their solutions or remedies. It has been just provided all the personal health information of the person concerned should be kept confidential for that matter. There was a legislation i.e. The National Health Act 2003 which allows the disclosure of information of the person only with the prior consent of the person/patient. In cases of minors, the consent can thus be given by the parents or guardian, in case it is required. In 2009, The Protection of Personal Information Bill (POPI) has been passed by the Parliament and is to come into force very soon. This Bill aims to give practicability and effect to the constitutional right to privacy which might usually get infringed, knowingly or unknowingly. This Bill is to safeguard the rights of the persons by shielding their personal and biomedical information (known as data subjects) which is maintained and processed by some public and private bodies (known as responsible parties). Few of the key features of The Protection of Personal Information Bill (POPI) are: duties of responsible parties are duly mentioned in the Bill itself, processing of personal health information is allowed to an extent; consent to be given for the purpose of processing one's information; responsibility of public as well as private bodies to secure the collected personal health information of the person; processing of information by third party as well as cross-border transfer of information; and also there will an Information Regulator as well as Information Officer for the purpose of receiving complaints with regard to any violations of the Bill. This is how the country is securing and keeping confidentiality maintained of their persons' health records and information.

It becomes crystal clear from analyzing the above provisions that many countries have framed and many are framing the legislations with respect to the privacy and confidentiality clauses of one's information and data security. The laws of the different countries are though not same in their provision but its core idea remains same as to secure the person's private data as well as his or her biomedical information. This has been made in order to make a cover for the one's whose information is being misused or there is violation of one's right to privacy.

CONSTITUTIONAL JURISPRUDENCE

Private life of a person, generally means, some of the secrets and hidden aspects of one's life, wherein the privacy and confidentiality is secured. Also the person usually wishes to stay alone in his internal world without being interfered by anyone else surrounding him. The term 'right to privacy' thereby inculcates security of any sort of personal information as well as data. It also involves the need for solitude without any internal disturbances and such requirements are mainly because of the highly accelerating growth and development of science and technology.

The Constitution of India does not *prima* facie talks about or grants right to privacy. This notion of protecting one's right to privacy under the domain of right to life has been enshrined under Part III of the Constitution (Fundamental Rights) which has duly taken from the American Constitution. The Constitution of India preserves and protects the rights of every person of the country as well as limits and restrains the States also as not to infringe the fundamental rights and fundamental freedoms guaranteed to the citizens. The right to privacy as to the data of a person has also been secured under the provisions of Universal Declaration of Human Rights, 1948. Even the Preamble to Universal Declaration of Human Rights, 1948 states:

Whereas recognition of the inherent dignity and of the equal and inalienable rights of all members of the human family is the foundation of freedom, justice and peace in the world.

This fundamental right to life under the Constitution of India even goes beyond the personal interest and is acquired under the societal domain. The meaning of the word 'life' as was defined in Munn v. Illinois (1876), wherein Field J. spoke very well by stating, 'by analyzing the word 'life', it amounts to something more than a mere animal existence. The inhibition against its deprivation extends to all those limbs and faculties by which life is enjoyed. The provision equally prohibits the mutilation of the body by the amputation of an arm or leg, or the putting out of an eye, or the destruction of any other organ of the body through which the soul communicates with outer world'.

The Constitutional perspective of right to life under Article 21 has been given a very wide interpretation. Therefore, in that context the term 'right to privacy' has been evolved from the term 'right to life'. Undoubtedly, Article 21 has been always understood in the light of living and dynamic Constitution thereby highlighting its various aspects and now, bringing 'privacy' under its ambit. Privacy, as understood, has to be given broader meaning so as to include the state of being apart from others, concealing one's presence from others, solitude and seclusion. Privacy in regard to biomedical information, therefore, means not to disclose one's information relating to its biomedicine. Relating the biomedical information to privacy and confidentiality to Article 21 of the Constitution brings into picture the protection of personal data in the field of health. Deprivation of right to privacy from the term 'right to life' will not only denude the actual meaning of the word 'life' but will also make it tedious and near to impossible for the people to live and survive, without their privacy being secured and protected. The right to privacy as such cannot be expressly added or inserted in the Constitution itself. The term has no exactitude in itself and hence it differentiates from person to person and if an attempt ever is made to make such right as an express fundamental right, it might result in war of litigations and conflicts.

CONSENT VIS-À-VIS PRIVACY AND CONFIDENTIALITY

Any treatment done to the person who infringes his confidentiality or privacy without the consent of the person concerned is technically an offence or a wrong which can be tried under criminal law or civil law, respectively. When it falls under the criminal law, it is dealt according to the provisions of Indian Penal Cade and when the issue comes under civil wrong, it is dealt under the Law of Torts.

The Indian Penal Code while dealing with such issues does specifically mentions about the age of a person who can validly give the consent. So the minimum age criteria for getting any health information, is little ambiguous in Indian Penal Code. There are different provisions as to understand the notion of 'consent'. Section 87 of the Indian Penal Code prescribes that a person of 18 years or above the age of 18 years can give a valid consent; whilst Section 89 of the same Code mentions that the child below the age of 12 years cannot be deemed to be giving of the valid consent. Moreover, there is one more legislation i.e. Indian Contract Act 1872 which states under Section 11 that every person who has attained the age of majority is competent to contract and is competent to give a valid consent. Now to understand as to which all persons are said to have attained the age of majority, there is Indian Majority Act which clearly provides under the provision of Section 3(1) of the Act that every person attains majority on completing the age of 18 years. This, clearly enunciates that no Indian legislation mentions about the notion of 'consent' of the person from 12 to 18 years of age. The question that arises are: whether the person falling under such category of age can give valid consent?, whether the person of that age can give his biomedical information without any objections?, whether the person of such an age, on obtaining his biometric information, may state that his prior consent was not taken? and many more. These are some the questions which remain unanswered because of the complexities and technicalities mentioned in the laws prevailing in India.

In order to treat a person, wherein it becomes emergency for his health then the law even prescribes to diagnose that person even without the consent of the person. In such cases even if any biomedical information needs to be disclosed and the person is in such a critical situation so as to cure him, then Section 92 of Indian Penal Code comes into picture. This is how Section 92 of the Indian Penal Code provides for lawful immunity to a registered medical practitioner to conduct the medical treatment of a person even without the consent of the person concerned in such extreme cases of emergency.

Similarly on the other side, the term 'right to confidentiality' ignites out. But what shall be the age at which the person can claim his or her right to confidentiality is yet not defined in any of the stature of legislations as of now. Let us take an instance, a girl of 15 years becomes pregnant and on her plea she wants to know from the medical practitioners about the contraceptive procedures. She claims her right to confidentiality as far as her biomedical information is concerned. But the question now sparks on here is that whether it would be feasible for the medical practitioner to inform the girl child of just 15 years about contraceptive procedures on the ground of her right to confidentiality or the medical practitioner should inform the parents of the child on some ethical and reasonable grounds. Such problem arises because of lack of presence of any legislation on this issue. Considering such problems and aspects in society, there are few of the legislations that criminalises sex below the age of 18 years even if it is done with the consent of the girl. Such laws does not expressly talks about the age for right to confidentiality but however provides punishment for such acts under prescribed age. Those legislations are:

1. Section 2(1)(d), 19(1) and 21(1) of the Protection of Children from Sexual Offences Act, 2012
2. Section 375 of the Indian Penal Code, 1860.

Such laws are being made keeping in view the actual present scenario of the country and in order to cope with such issues of confidentiality and privacy of biomedical information of a person.

However in the case of *Samira Kohli v. Dr. Prabha Manchanda (2018),* the Apex court of the country tried to state as to what the term 'consent' means when it comes to doctor patient relationship and maintaining of privacy in that relationship pertaining to the biomedical information of the patient. The Supreme Court of India stated that 'consent' means giving permission or allowing the doctor to conduct any diagnosis or any other treatment either through surgical or therapeutic procedure. At times, it becomes tedious for the doctors to take the consent of the patient because of some unavoidable circumstances or in cases of emergency, then consent can be taken impliedly even from the existing circumstances. The order was given by the Supreme Court regarding the principles of consent with respect to medical treatment of the person or pertaining to any biomedical information of the person concerned. Those principles were stated as follows:

1. The doctor is to mandatorily take the consent of the person concerned before starting up with the treatment. This is done so because the person whose consent is taken should actually know as what treatment is going to happen on him. This will ensure his confidentiality and the consent so taken shall be entirely valid as well as voluntary.
2. In cases, where the consent is taken for some diagnosis or some diagnostic procedure, the same cannot be deemed to be the consent taken for treatment to be done with his body. Similarly if consent is taken for some particular treatment, that consent shall be only for that particular treatment and

cannot be impliedly taken to be the consent for some other treatment as well. This would otherwise amount to violation of one's free consent.

3. The doctor is under the core duty to maintain a balance between the limit of disclosing the necessary and required information as well as the information which is to be kept entirely confidential. If this balance will shake, it will be an infringement of right to confidentiality because the patient discloses the information to the doctor on very trustful grounds and the same should be maintained and respected.

4. There can be, at times, common consent may taken for different procedures to be performed on the patient. That common consent can be given even for diagnosis as well as surgical treatment.

Therefore, consent needs to be taken before anything is to be done to the patient or even any information about the person is to be disclosed to the other person. If such consent, express or informed, not taken it will result in abridging their right to confidentiality with respect to their biomedical information.

LEGISLATIVE MEASURES

India, as such does not have concrete and precise legislation to deal with issues of biometric information. Whatsoever information is given needs some confidentiality, privacy and security for that matter. But the biometric information culls out to be protected by securing one's fundamental right to privacy. Therefore, though not any specific legislation with regard to protection of biomedical information, we have many laws in India that secures the same from being spoiled, damaged or misused. The term 'right to privacy' has been dealt variedly under different legislations in India. As discussed above, its genesis is from Article 21 of the Constitution of India. Apart from the Constitutional provision, there are many other such laws, that guarantees for the protection of data privacy, its confidentiality as well as its security; whether official data or any personal data.

The term 'privacy' has been given a very complex meaning and is subject to wider interpretations by many. In brief, it enunciates that about one's own capability to hide one's information. The term 'confidentiality' on the other side means the ability of one person to disclose his information to the third person without such information being disclosed or shared in public. Similarly, there is another term 'securing' i.e. the duty of another person to secure or hide the information of one person from letting it being disclosed to another. Therefore, it can be stated that all these terms are interlinked in one way or the other. The person claiming for his privacy needs his information to be kept confidential and secured from the public at large. The information relating to biomedical often relates to the information of the patients suffering from some diseases, which they themselves never want to disclose. With the advancement of science and technology, it has become quite easy for the people to upload the information on some electronic storage devices, which further makes it easier to circulate that information. Therefore, storing such information relating to biomedicine or person's individual health on electronic storage devices has lead to accelerate in the risk of one's identification being leaked out at multiple stages of data collection and data storage (Srinivas et al, 2012). Hence, there has been the enactment of Information Technology Act 2000. It was Latestly seen that the government had framed out the Information Technology (Reasonable Security Practices and Procedures and Sensitive Personal Data or Information) Rules 2011 i.e. IT Rules. Rule 6,7 and 8 specifies some of the security requirements with respect to sensitive personal data (SPD). Another Rule no.5 also mentions that prior consent is to be required of the person whose information is to be disclosed or used for any other purposes. Section 43, 43A, 66E and 72A of the Information Technology Act 2000 talks about privacy aspects. These are discussed as follows:

1. Section 43 of the Information Technology Act 2000 enunciates upon penalising the person who tries damage the computer system, even without the permission of the owner or any other person who is an in charge of the computer or computer system. This may result in accessing of any information, downloading or copying any information or even damaging or denying to access the information provided therein. It also encompasses to punish the wrongdoers who without the prior consent of owner or person in charge of the computer steals or conceals or alters or changes any information stored on the computer. This provision would result in providing compensation to the affected person by way of damages to be paid by the wrongdoer. This section 43 of the Act 2000 provides for civil liability.

2. Section 43A of the same Act 2000 provides that in case where a company or any other body corporate fails to handle and sensitive personal data (SPD) or any such related information with respect person's privacy and confidentiality or the body corporate fails to maintain reasonable standards to protection and maintenance of such information, then such body corporate or the company shall be liable to pay damages to the affected party by way of some compensation. Indian legislations are putting remarkable responsibility and duty upon the persons as well as companies who are handling sensitive personal data or information to come out with some justifiable and protective measures in order to safeguard such information.

3. Section 66E of the Information Technology Act 2000 states about the punishment for violation of privacy. As discussed earlier, the term 'privacy' may include any sort of privacy so even if someone's biomedical information is disclosed without his or her consent, that person will be held liable and punished for disclosing the same under this Section for the reason of infringing one's right to privacy. The Section provides that if any person (citizen or non citizen), intentionally or unintentionally, knowingly or unknowingly, captures, publishes or transmits any image of a private area of any person, without his or her consent, under such circumstances that tends to violate the privacy of a person, will be deemed guilty of privacy violation. Hence, the person shall be punished to an imprisonment which may be extended to a period of three years or with fine that may extend to two lakh rupees or even both. This section was basically brought after 2008 Amendment because there has increased number of electronic voyeurism. Voyeurism is basically an act of a person, who for some sexual desire and gratifying need, observes and captures the image of another person, without taking his or her consent. So in order to set aside this issue, which has been increasing with the information and technology, there arose a need to add such a provision in the Information Technology Act 2000 in order to protect one's privacy.

4. Section 72A of the Information Technology Act 2000 mentions that any sort of disclosure of the information, if done, irrespective of the fact that it is being done intentionally or unintentionally, knowingly or unknowingly, but done without the consent of the person involved or concerned with that information, shall be made punishable under this Act. The punishment may extend to the term of three years along with the fine extending to five lakh rupees.

But however, it is to be noted under the provisions of the Information Technology Act 2000 that it is never such that no personal information can ever be disclosed without the person's consent on the ground of its being infringing its right to privacy. There are always certain exceptions to the main provisions. Section 69 of the Act is an exception to the general rule of maintaining privacy and confidentiality of one's personal or biometric information. This implies that there are certain situations wherein the Government has the full power to know about the person's information. Such grounds are when the Government is satisfied that it is indispensable in the interest of:

1. Sovereignty or integrity of India;
2. Defence of India;
3. Security of the State;
4. Friendly relations with foreign state;
5. Public order;
6. Preventing incitement to the commission of any cognizable offence;
7. For investigation of any offence.

Therefore, this particular Section empowers the appropriate Government to monitor as well as decrypt the information (including personal or biometric) which is stored, maintained, received or transmitted in any of the computer resource. Thence it can be enunciated that more these technological advancements have been made to secure and record our personal information, the more these advancements are creating intrusion in one's right to privacy.

Another effort has been made by the legislature to bring in a new law especially for the protection of one's personal data. The draft Personal Data Protection Bill will introduce data protection and security regime that will maintain a balance between the data to be protected on one side and the data that can be used by the State and other private entities on the other side. The Personal Data Protection Bill has been passed in 2006 and still is continuing for discussions and debates in the Indian Parliament. Many amendments have been proposed and made in the Bill and the updated new draft was introduced by the Rajya Sabha in 2014. Because of the some loopholes in the Information Technology Act, initiatives have been made to bring a new legislation in order to cope up those loopholes. After this, in July 2017 the Ministry of Electronics and Information Technology framed a nine member committee of experts for making another draft on this issue. The Committee was headed by Justice B.N. Srikrishna which is to analyse and study various data protection issues in India and proposed a draft Bill in that regard. The main purpose of setting up of this committee was:

ensure growth of the digital economy while keeping personal data of citizens secure and protected.

Thereafter, the Committee presented its draft Bill on July 27, 2018 and has submitted the draft for further recommendations.

JURISPRUDENTIAL NOTION

The Indian judiciary has been a working very hard in order to cope up with one's right to privacy whether it relates to biomedical information or any other information. The protection of biomedical information rests within the domain of right to privacy. The court has once went on by saying that 'we have, therefore, no hesitation in holding that right to privacy is a part of right to life and personal liberty enshrined under Article 21 of the Constitution and once the facts in each case constitute a right to privacy under Article 21 is attracted, the said right cannot be curtailed, except according to procedure established by law' (Hidayathullah, 1984). It makes it crystal clear from this decision of the court that the right to privacy is not an absolute right in nature and can be, therefore, retrained, limited and restricted through lawful means for the prevention of crime, disorder or protection of health or moral or protection of rights or freedom of others (Janab k. Abdul Rahmin vs. The Divisional Electircal AIR, 2002).

The question was very much highlighted in the initial years of 1950's that whether the right to privacy is a fundamental right. It was decided in the case of *M.P. Sharma v. Satish Chandra, District Magistrate Delhi (1954),* where an investigation was to be made by the Union Government under the provisions of Companies Act to peep into the affairs of the company, which was in the process of liquidation on the ground that it had made an attempt to misappropriate and embezzle the funds as well as it had concealed the actual state of affairs of the company from the company's stakeholders. The allegations made were that the company had indulged in fraudulent transactions and had falsified all its records. Hence, the court reiterated in this decision as there exists no right to privacy under Article 20(3) of the Constitution of India, for the reason, of the absence of any provision analogous to the Fourth Amendment to the US Constitution. In *Gobind v. State of Madhya Pradesh (1992),* the Apex Court had held that right to privacy was to be understood as the part and parcel of Article 19 and 21 of the Constitution of India, as the right originates from these two provisions of the Constitution itself. The Apex court in *Sunil Batra v. Delhi Administration (1997),* observed that a minimal infringement of a prisoner's privacy is unavoidable as the officers have an obligation to keep a watch and ensure that their other human rights are being duly observed. In the case of *Indian Express v. Union of India (1981),* it was held that 'public interest in freedom of discussion of which freedom of the press' is considered to be one of the aspects that stems from the requirement from the members of a democratic society. The members in the society should be sufficiently informed so that they may influence intelligently and the decisions which may affect themselves. Elaborating upon the notion of right to privacy, the court in another landmark judgment (Ms. X vs Mr. Z, 2002). A stated that telephonic conversations made between people are the private conversations. Hence if any telephone tapping is done until and unless it is conducted through a procedure established by law, would amount to infringing the right to privacy and therefore unconstitutional.

There was a striking and conflicting opinion that arose in *S.P. Gupta v. Union of India (2003).* The Supreme Court held that a balance needs to be struck between the right to information and right to privacy. The court reiterated the point that a right to privacy is not an absolute and can be infringed to serve a serious public concern. There have different views given by Court with respect to right to privacy. It happened in 2002 when a matter came up before Delhi High Court. The matter was with regard to the person suffering from AIDS as his claim for maintaining right to privacy under the ambit of Article 21 of the Constitution of India. The Delhi High Court held that when a person is suffering from such a dreadful disease which might affect the life of another person, then such sufferer (former person) cannot claim his right to privacy. Hence the court decided that such persons cannot maintain the right of secrecy against his proposed bride and laboratory which tested his blood (Surjit Singh Thind vs. Kanwaljit Kaur,

2003). However, later this decision was once again reiterated by the Supreme Court in *Mr. X v. Hospital Z (2004)*. In this particular case, wife wanted to have full fledge knowledge about her husband health and if the doctor in this regard disclosed anything to the wife, that cannot be said to be an infringement of the right to privacy. Therefore, the court stated that the wife of a husband has the unequivocal and full right to have every knowledge and awareness about her husband's health. The doctor also is obliged to give proper information and is found to be under the legal authority to provide her with the correct information of the same. While protecting the wife's interest in this manner, the court in another case of *Surjit Singh Thind v. Kanwaljeet Kaur (2003)* also protected the interest of a lady in other aspect. In this case the court held that compelling or forcing a lady to undergo medical examination for checking her virginity or getting any biomedical information about her would be considered to be a flagrant violation of her right to privacy. In *Ajit Kapur v. Union of India (2007),* Delhi High Court reiterated that no one can be compelled to undergo any medical test againt her or her wishes, who is a party to the proceedings, otherwise that too would amount to violating of right to privacy. In all these exceptional cases, the court opined that it is no bars that women cannot be send for medical examination for this purpose, but however this would only be permissible under the conditions which patently *prima facie* require the matter to go through this procedure. In a very precisely stated judgment (Mishra et al, 2017), the Patna High Court held that citizens of India have the full right to enjoy drinks and liquor within their places or houses and in a behavioural manner and the same has been evolved from right to privacy under Article 21 of the Constitution of India. Latestly in 2017 itself another landmark pronouncement of *Shaikh Zahid Mukhtar v. State of Maharashtra (2011)*, turned up wherein Bombay High Court has struck down Section 5D of the Maharashtra Animal Preservation Act, 1976 on the ground that it is violating right to privacy of an individual. It makes it very clear that how the Indian judiciary has time and again reinterpreting the Article 21 of the Constitution and covering within its ambit various aspects of right to privacy and now even covering the privacy, security and confidentiality of biomedical information.

RIGHT TO INFORMATION AND BIOMEDICAL PRIVACY

As we all know that privacy is a matter of great concern when it comes to disclosing one's personal biomedical information to someone else. This is so because this component of privacy has its practical as well as fundamental context to make it more viable. In healthcare aspects, patient's confidentiality is to be well maintained, and then only the person will feel comfortable in deliberating his private information whether relating to physical or sexual activity, any bodily conduct and other medical function of the body. So such information should not be wanted by the patient to be discussed and disclosed to anyone otherwise it may lead to have negative consequences. Sometimes, the health issues are such which are stigmatising to the person and if disclosed, might cause embarrassment to the concerned person. Therefore, regarding the person's healthcare information, all the health centres should take a note that they should not reveal the information without the consensus of the patient. All the medical practitioners and medical professionals should be duty bound as not to disclose their patient's information without seeking their permission or unless it is required by law. There is a Medical Council of India which in its Code of Ethics Regulations states:

the physician shall not disclose the secrets of a patient that have been learnt in the exercise of his/her professions except in a court of law under orders of the Presiding Judge; in circumstances where there is a serious and identified risk to a specific person and/or community [or in case of] notifiable diseases (Mishra et al,, 2017)

Right to Information Act 2005 allows the citizens information (including biomedical information) to be given to other under some sort of government control. It might be viewed as threatening or endangering the privacy of patients or subjects of research, especially the ones which are there in the government departments or institutions (Mishra et al, 2017). However, it should be understood and kept in mind by all the clinicians as well as patients that Right to Information 2005 does not actually allows the disclosure of anyone's information to any of the third party but in fact allows it to be disclosed only in the exceptional situations and circumstances wherein the interest of larger public is involved. It happens most of the times when patient's information is asked to be disclosed to someone else on the agitation of latter's right to information. Nevertheless, it can be articulated that the provisions of Right to Information Act 2005 never go against the 'right to privacy' and is read in consonance with this right.

With the coming up of Right to Information Act 2005, people started wondering that the provisions made therein might start to infringe person's right to privacy. For instance, any private biomedical information, disclosed by a person, while getting his treatment done from a government hospital, might feel insecure about its privacy. So this has been enunciated in the Act itself that even such information is not to be disclosed without person's consent.

The Right to Information Act 2000 talks about inspection of words, books or any other document. It also encompasses so as to cover any notes, extracts, certified copies of the same etc. Under this Act, the term 'information' has been given a wider notion to include all records, documents, emails, any sort of memos, orders, circulars, advices etc., be it in any of the form which is held offline or through online mode or any other information of the person which can be made easily accessible to public authority under the law for time being in force (Mishra et al,, 2017). Now articulating upon these provisions, there arise numbers of questions in mind as to whether such sort of information also includes biomedical information which is generated in hospitals, both private and government? Whether right to information applies in this case also or not? The Information Technology Act 2000 was designed to ensure more transparency in the process. So however, it does not permit the intrusion by anyone into life of any person who is a participant in government aided research. This Act guarantees to maintain the confidentiality of Doctor – Patient relationship or even the researcher – subject relationship. The Act itself under the provision of Section 8 specifies that the following types of information are exempted from disclosure:

(1)(e) information available to a person in his fiduciary relationship such as the relationship of a physician or researcher with a patient or subject should not be disclosed unless a competent authority is satisfied that the larger public interest warrants the disclosure of such information. (Mishra et al,, 2017)

It implies that such information shall remain totally private and all the elements of confidentiality and secrecy are attached to it. There can be some situations when such information needs to be disclosed. But as it is not a routine matter or does not happen in daily circumstances, so the competent authority cannot allow such disclosure without hearing the affected party. Therefore, law of natural justice requires the competent authority to grant an opportunity of hearing to the person who had imparted such information in fiduciary relationship. Only after hearing such person, the decision regarding disclosure of such information could be taken. For example, if a doctor has to disclose any information given to him under fiduciary relationship by a patient, the doctor must hear the patient on this, even if it has to be disclosed in public interest. In *Central Board of Secondary Education and another* v. *Aditya Andhopadhyay and others [27]*, the Supreme Court held that the term 'fiduciary relationship' is used to describe a situation of transaction where one person (beneficiary) places a complete confidence in another person (fiduciary) in regard to its affairs, business or transactions. The person who is a 'fiduciary' is expected to act in full confidence and must be working for the benefit and advantage of the beneficiary.

(1)(j) information which relates to personal information the disclosure of which has no relationship to any public activity or interest, or which would cause unwarranted invasion of the privacy of the individual unless the Public Information Officer or the appellate authority, as the case may be, is satisfied that the larger interest justifies the disclosure of such information. (Mishra et al,, 2017)

It speaks of the information which is extremely confidential and private for the person. This information is deemed to have strictly personal elements in it and must not be disclosed to anyone under the provisions of this Act in its normal course of business. This sub-section guards purely private information against any unwarranted invasion in his private life until and unless some public interest is attached to the disclosure of any such information. this, however, implies that the individual privacy is not a purely personal affair but is also to some extent attached to social contract. If we have a look in our daily lives, we can come across so many things which are restricted to one's private life but still such things cannot be isolated from the domain of public.

It is pertinent to mention here that in a judgment by Central Information Commission (CIC) in 2007, it was clearly enunciated that any information regarding the results coming from the medical testing were totally exempted from disclosure under the provisions of Right to Information Act, for the reason, that the personal information whose disclosure is not at all related to any public activity or interest will ultimately lead to invasion of one's privacy [28]. Furthermore, the Chief Information Commission held that any information made available to the doctor in a fiduciary relationship cannot be seek on a ground of 'right to know or right to seek' as it would amount to violation of privacy. Therefore, Chief Information Commission was appropriate in deciding as to what amounts to public interest and what not. But on the other side, it cannot be seen valid as keeping any medical information confidential which may harm the larger public. For example informing about patient's communicable disease or reporting someone that the patient is unfit for particular kind of job because of his medical condition cannot be said as to infringing his privacy [29]. This is so because it might become troublesome for the society as a whole, if the information is not disclosed to the appropriate authority at an appropriate time and the person cannot be said to have his right to privacy being infringed.

AADHAAR: BIOMETRIC INFORMATION

While highlighting upon right to privacy with respect to biomedical information, the deliberation of 'Aadhaar' cannot be felt to left upon. As of now, we know that right to privacy being a contentious issue under the domain of right to life and personal liberty, many judgments have been delivered by the court in order to justify the cause for it. But with the technicalities coming up, the question which has started turning up in the court was "whether right to privacy is a fundamental right or not, as far as the information linked with Adhaar is concerned?" The answer to such question has still remains unanswered. Undoubtedly, privacy has been understood as a part and parcel of right to life under Article 21 of the

Constitution of India, but the information obtained under 'aadhaar' i.e. biometric information is seen as violation of one's right to privacy with a total effect of infringing Article 21 of the Constitution of India. However, giving a different colour to this aspect, persons who claim for 'aadhaar' in the country justifies themselves by stating that right to privacy is not an absolute right and therefore reasonable restrictions can be imposed which the Constitution of India itself guarantees. Now finally this issue was brought up before the Supreme Court in 2017 that whether the information obtained under 'aadhaar' comes within reasonable restriction or it is sheer violation of right to privacy?

It was in 2015 only, when number of petitions were filed challenging the 'Aadhaar' Scheme of the government as an account of its being violative of right to privacy. The petitions filed in the court has basically questioned the Aadhaar card scheme along with its bio-metric registration procedure and entirely linked to all the primary and fundamental subsidies, thereby claiming it as violative of right to privacy as it tends to disclose the biometric information of the persons. The matter was then decided to be sorted out by the Constitution Bench of the Supreme Court and the then Chief Justice of India, H.L. Dattu began to rag this controversy in the light of people's right to privacy. The five-judge bench led by Chief Justice of India H.L. Dattu said that the purely voluntary nature of the use of the Adhaar card to access public service will continue till the court takes a final decision on whether Adhaar scheme is an invasion into right to privacy of the citizen or not (Mishra et al,, 2017). In order to deal with this particular issues, there were many primary issues that needs to be sorted out and worked upon first. The nine judge bench was set up to peep into the matter. The first issue that popped out was that whether right to privacy is a fundamental right as well as basic structure of the Constitution or not? Once it was decided that it is a fundamental right, then another bunch of petitions came up challenging the constitutionality of Aadhaar card project, basically whether the project that mandates the parting of biometric information of its citizens amounts to violation of the right to privacy or not. The matter was discussed, analysed and deliberated by all senior judges in order to cull out the appropriate solution for the same.

There then came up number of arguments from both sides. The government started heating up and stated that right to privacy cannot be deemed as a fundamental right under Article 21 of the Constitution of India. Their contention was in support of the intention of the framers so as to justify that had the framers been intended to include right to privacy under right to life then they would have done it then and there only. They focussed more upon the originalistic content of the Constitution thereby giving prior regard to be intentionalism as well as textualism. On the other side, petitioners claimed right to privacy is a fundamental right under right to life and personal liberty. The petitioners tried to give a living interpretation to the Constitution of India thereby bringing right to privacy under Article 21. They agitated that no doubt right to privacy is not expressly stated in the Constitution but it does not imply that the right does not exist at all. Framers of the Constitution never wanted the Constitution of India to be a dead one rather they always wanted to inculcate in it the norms of vibrancy and dynamism. Petitioners argues that there have number of cases in past few decades enunciating upon right to privacy and hence, privacy means to let the person set free from external issues and no interruption at all of any such kind. As these counter arguments were hitting each other in the Court, it made the judges feel to rethink upon the two earlier decisions i.e. *Kharak Singh v. State of Uttar Pradesh (1962)* and *M.P.Sharma v. Satish Chandra, District Magistrate Delhi (1962),* wherein, it was firmly stated that right to privacy is not a fundamental right. The question of 'aadhaar' was left to be discussed later but in fact this issue became the priority. Hence finally it was decided that a bench of nine judges would hear and conclude these petitions. The Bench comprised of Chief Justice J.S. Khehar and Justices J. Chelameswar, S.A. Bobde,

R.K. Agrawal, Rohinton Nariman, A.M. Sapre, D.Y. Chandrachud, Sanjay Kishan Kaul and S. Abdul Nazeer. The judges while hearing of these many petitions made the decision in these terms: the decision in M.P. Sharma that privacy is not a fundamental right stands overruled; the decision in Kharak Singh that privacy is not a fundamental right stands overruled; right to privacy is protected as intrinsic part of right to life and liberty and all decisions subsequent to Kharak Singh make the position clear and will hold the field. All the nine judges gave their own opinion as to the privacy concern with respect to 'aadhaar' and biometric information. Following is their notion in this regard (Kharak Singh vs. The sate of U. P. and Others, 1962):

Justice Khehar:

Right to privacy, an inherent right, be unequivocally a fundamental right embedded in Part III of the Constitution of India, but subject to restrictions specified, relatable to that part. Hence, this is the call of today.

Justice Chelameswar:

No legal right can be absolute. Every right has limitations. This aspect of the matter is conceded at the bar. Therefore, even a fundamental right to privacy has limitations. The limitations are to be identified on case to case basis depending upon the nature of the privacy interest claimed.

Justice Chandrachud:

Life and personal liberty are inalienable rights. These are rights which are inseparable from a dignified human existence. The dignity of the individual, equality between human beings and the quest for liberty are the foundational pillars of the Indian Constitution. Privacy includes at its core the preservation of personal intimacies, the sanctity of family life, marriage, procreation, the home and sexual orientation but limitations can be imposed the right to privacy as well.

Justice Nariman:

It is clear that Article 21 would, therefore, not be the sole repository of these human rights but only reflect the fact that they were 'inalienable'. On this score, it is clear that the right to privacy is an inalienable human right which inheres in every person by virtue of the fact that he or she is a human being.

Justice Sapre:

I do not find any difficulty in tracing that the 'right to privacy' emanates from Preamble (liberty of thought, expression, belief, faith and worship as well as fraternity and dignity of the individual); Article 19(1)(a), Article 19(1)(d) and lastly Article 21. Right to privacy is a part of fundamental right of a citizen guaranteed under Part III of the Constitution. However, it is not an absolute right but is subject to certain reasonable restrictions, which the State is entitled to impose on the basis of social, moral and compelling public interest in accordance with law.

Justice Kaul:

Every individual should have a right to be able to exercise control over his/her own life and image as portrayed to the world and to control commercial use of his/her identity. This also means that an individual may be permitted to prevent others from using his image, name and other aspects of his/her personal life and identity for commercial purposes without his/her consent. Aside from the economic justifications for such a right, it is also justified as protecting individual autonomy and personal dignity. The right protects an individual's free, personal conception of the 'self.' The right of publicity implicates a person's interest in autonomous self-definition, which prevents others from interfering with the meanings and values that the public associates with her.

Justice Nazeer:

Like other rights which form part of the fundamental freedoms protected by Part III, including the right to life and personal liberty under Article 21, privacy is not an absolute right. A law which encroaches upon privacy will have to withstand the touchstone of permissible restrictions on fundamental rights. In the context of Article 21 an invasion of privacy must be justified on the basis of a law which stipulates a procedure which is fair, just and reasonable. The law must also be valid with reference to the encroachment on life and personal liberty under Article 21. An invasion of life or personal liberty must meet the three-fold requirement of (i) legality, which postulates the existence of law; (ii) need, defined in terms of a legitimate state aim; and (iii) proportionality which ensures a rational nexus between the objects and the means adopted to achieve them.

Justive Bobde:

The right to privacy is inextricably bound up with all exercises of human liberty – both as it is specifically enumerated across Part III and as it is guaranteed in the residue under Article 21. Any interference with privacy by an entity covered by Article 12's description of the 'state' must satisfy the tests applicable to whichever one or more of the Part III freedoms the interference affects. If a man has to die with dignity, he has to have some privacy.

Justice Agrawal:

Judicial recognition of the existence of a constitutional right of privacy is not an exercise in the nature of amending the Constitution nor is the court embarking on a constitutional function of that nature which is entrusted to Parliament. Privacy is the constitutional core of human dignity. Privacy has both a normative and descriptive function. At a normative level, privacy sub serves those eternal values upon which the guarantees of life, liberty and freedom are founded. At a descriptive level, privacy postulates a bundle of entitlements and interests which lie at the foundation of ordered liberty.

Therefore, all the nine judges of the Apex Court perceived a unanimous decision in this regard and went on to pronounce a landmark judgment in the case of *Justice K.S. Puttuswamy (Retd.) v. Union of India (2017)*, thereby stating that privacy is a constitutionally safeguarded fundamental right that has its genesis from Article 21 of the Constitution of India. It, therefore, implies that this judgment of the Supreme Court has undermined the expression as stated in the previous judgments (*Kharak Singh Case (1962)* and *M.P. Sharma Case (1954)*) relating to right to privacy. The judiciary has tried to maintain the doctrinal concept of the right to privacy even by considering the fact that the Constitution of India does not expressly grants this particular right. This view was taken the judges because it is a well known fact that all the fundamental rights are not being carved out from each other but in fact they do overlap and are hidden in each other in one or the other form.

CONCLUSION AND SUGGESTION

Privacy and confidentiality of an individual are most significant and influential values which is linked to person's autonomy and is considered to be highly prized in a country like India which has a democratic as well as republican set up. No doubt the data storage has become more convenient these days with the assistance of recoding the same on computers, thereby shifting from paper based health records to electronic health records (EHRs). But it had hampered one's secrecy from oneself. These EHRs provide for larger benefits in contrast to paper based recording system like: decrease in cost, improved standardisation, mobility in record maintenance, consistencies of security policies and many more. But however, the security and privacy through these electronic health records (EHRs) are tremendously threatened and attacked by various hackers, worms and different viruses. it makes it more clear that with respect to this, modern medicinal or biomedical information is facing complex issues. These issues are emerging in market under the medical identity theft and it is because of the advent of recording the information electronically as to why such offences are being committed. The bringing up of biometric program in India was basically done to end corruption. The government of India in 2016 onwards is trying to build up a nation as 'Digital India' in order to modernise this country. The government has even promoted for cashless transactions. It was, thus, the reason that 'Aadhaar' scheme was initiated as an identification program which is to gather each citizen's information such as fingerprints and eye scan in order to link it up with the person's voter identity cards, permanent account numbers (PAN), filing of income tax returns etc with an intensity to curb and cull out corruption in India. But such program is accelerating in a big troublesome situation in the country, posing threat to privacy and security issues. The fact remains that such scheme of the government is working 'for the country' but however it is not to be forgotten that such scheme may work 'against the country' as well. On one side people are relying on the government by giving their biometric information and on the other side, the common masses are not aware as to what may happen to their such information. The government needs to take some protective measures in order to assure the confidentiality and security of such information given by the people of the country to government, else time is not far when situation will come when all people will lose their trust and confidence in any government working for the country. Even the International Monetary Fund (IMF) said that India should definitely take some pro active and mandatory measures to secure privacy and confidentiality of various identification programs. The IMF also once stated that India's present digital government is trying to bring more digitalization for stronger governance all over thereby allowing more public transparency and awareness but these electronic modes of saving information has resulted in more leakages and privacy issues in India. Moreover, while dealing with the provisions of Right to Information Act in exceptional cases, it requires balancing of the situations as to maintain a line between right to privacy and right to know especially on medical grounds to understand feasibly the notion of public and private interest (Mishra et al, 2017). Hence the Act should be construed conservatively so as to make the situations at par including confidentiality on one side and intrusion to confidentiality on the other side.

REFERENCES

Ahmed, S., & Sengar, S. (2016). Right to privacy- Is Uidai a violation of an individual's 'fundamental right'? *The World Journal on Juristic Polity*. Retrieved from http://jurip.org/wp-content/uploads/2016/12/Sabreen-Ahmed.pdf

Ajit Kapur v. Union of India. (2017) 2 ABR 140 (India).

Appari & Johnson. (2010). Information Security and Privacy in Healthcare: Current State of Research. *Int. J. Internet and Enterprise Management*. Retrieved from www.ists.dartmouth.edu

Confederation of Indian Alcoholic Beverages Companies v. State of Bihar, 2016 (4) PLJR 369 (India).

Gobind v. State of Madhya Pradesh (July 27, 1992). India.

Hidayatullah, H. M. (1984). Constitutional law of India. New Delhi: Bar Council of India Trust.

Indian Express v. Union of India. AIR 1981 SC 365.

Janab K. Abdul Rahim vs The Divisional Electrical AIR 1954 SC 1077 (December 16, 2002).AIR 1975 SC 148.

Justice K. S. Puttaswamy (Retd.) and Anr. vs Union Of India And Ors. (24 August 2017)

Kharak Singh vs The State Of U. P. & Others on (18 December, 1962)

Luo, Y., & Bradley-Schmieg, P. (2018). *China Issues New Personal Information Protection Standard.* Retrieved from www.insideprivacy.com/international/china/china-issues-new-personal-information-protection-standard/

M. P. Sharma And Others vs Satish Chandra. (15 March, 1954)

Medical Informatics and Telemedicine. (n.d.). Retrieved from https://medicalinformatics.healthconferences.org/events-list/medical-informatics-and-biomedical-informatics

Mishra, N. M., Parker, L., & Deshpande, S. (2017). Privacy and the Right to Information Act, 2005. *Indian Journal of Medical Ethics*. Retrieved from https://www.ncbi.nlm.nih.gov/pmc/articles/PMC5473905/

Mr. X v. Hospital. AIR 2004 Del. 203 (India).

Ms. X vs Mr. Z. AIR 2002 Del 217 (India).

Mukhtar v. State of Maharashtra 2011 (2) ID 101 (SC).

Munn v. Illinois, 94 U.S. 113 (1876)

Office of Australian Information Commissioner. (n.d.). *Health Information and Medical Research.* Retrieved from https://www.oaic.gov.au/privacy-law/privacy-act/health-and-medical-research

P. Sharma v. Satish Chandra, District Magistrate Delhi on 30 August, 1954 SCC 494 (India).

Rajagopal, K. (2018, January 9). *Right to privacy verdict: A timeline of SC hearings.* Retrieved from https://www.thehindubusinessline.com/news/national/right-to-privacy-verdict-a-timeline-of-sc-hearings/article9829124.ece

Samira Kohli vs Dr. Prabha Manchanda & Anr (January 16, 2018)

S.P. Gupta v. Union of India (2003) 1 SCC 500 (India).

Srinivas, N., & Biswas, A. (2012). *Protecting Patient Information in India: Data Privacy Law and its Challenges.* Retrieved from www.docs.manupatra.in/newsline/articles/Upload/B3C7F081-838F-489F-9F77-AF1E209C26F8.pdf

Sunil Batra v. Delhi Administration, (1997) SC 568 (India).

Surjit Singh Thind vs Kanwaljit Kaur. AIR 2003 P&H 353 (India).

Chapter 5
A Review of Different Techniques for Biomedical Data Security

Harminder Kaur
Dr. B. R. Ambedkar National Institute of Technology, India

Sharvan Kumar Pahuja
Dr. B. R. Ambedkar National Institute of Technology, India

ABSTRACT

The aging population is vulnerable to various illnesses and health conditions because with increase in age the people suffer from chronic disease. Quite often, they are partially handicapped due to their restricted mobility and their reduced mental abilities. To resolve these problems, health monitoring systems are designed for real-time monitoring of patients. WBAN use medical sensors for acquiring patient physiological data with wireless technologies to send data to healthcare providers. Due to wireless transmission, the chances of attacking and occurring security issues in the data are more. So, the security of the system is the main concern because the system consists of patient privacy concerns. Due to these reasons there is need of designing security algorithms to prevent data from being stolen by attackers. The aim of this chapter is to present a review of different attacks that occurred during transmission of data and security issues related to data. The chapter also describes different algorithms to prevent data from being stolen through various attacks and security issues.

INTRODUCTION

In the developing countries like India, the poor medical facilities are the major concern especially in rural and remote areas. The population of India is assorted. As per National Rural Health Mission (NRHM) report 700 million people live in 636000 Indian villages where people don't have direct access to hospitals ("National Health Mission Report", 2014) which can be leads to death due to the poor doctor to patient ratio. In order to increase the patient care effectiveness there is a need of designing the effective health care monitoring systems (Alaa, 2017). These health care monitoring systems are used to acquire,

DOI: 10.4018/978-1-5225-7952-6.ch005

record, display and transmit the patient's physiological signals from patient's body to any other locations so the doctor can diagnose the patient condition. These healthcare monitoring systems can also be used to provide the medical help to the aged and disable people because with increase in age senior people losses their ability to take care of themselves due to chronic diseases, physical or mental disabilities (Marco, 2008). With designing of these health applications, one can easily know the health status of the elder and disable people. Various applications are designed based on wireless sensor network technology and IoT (Internet of Things) for e-health applications that are based on the daily living activities i.e. tracking of location, intake of medicine and other health status like monitoring of physiological signals Blood pressure, heart rate etc. of the elder or disable people (Magana-Espinoza, 2014). To design the e-health monitoring system there are basic requirements which have to keep in mind that are described below (Lopez-Nores, 2008):

- **Reliability**: The system should be reliable which can prevent duplication of information during the transmission of the data and provide the efficient Quality of Service.
- **Routing**: Choosing of greatest communication protocol which provides scalability, best route for send the information among others.
- **Mobility of Node**: Wireless nodes move freely in network. The wireless nodes should maintain their connectivity when they are moving in the defined network.
- **Security**: When the data is sent through the cloud or through internet the proper security mechanism should be used so that the patient data can be secure.

As mentioned above the medical data of the patient is transferred to the concerned person wirelessly if person is not available along with patient. During the wireless communication many types of attacks can affect the patient information which can be harmful for diagnose the disease. To provide suitable information to the doctor there is a need of proper security of the data. Many of techniques are introduced in passing years for the proper security of medical data. So the main aim of this book chapter is to provide the review of different attacks, security issues and available techniques of to remove security issues in biomedical data. The chapter also includes the advantages and disadvantages of available security techniques. The motivation behind this chapter to aware the bioengineers to provide the information regarding the available security techniques and security issues in medical data transmission so they can overcome the different issues occurred in data transmission and can provide the best solutions for more security of data. Figure 1 shows the workflow of this chapter.

USE OF WIRELESS SENSOR NETWORKS (WSN) AND INTERNET OF THINGS (IOT) IN BIOMEDICAL APPLICATIONS

WSN and IoT plays main role for designing home care applications. In WSN sensor nodes are distributed in home which provide patient information to user in different environment (Keshavarz, 2016). When wireless sensor networks are used for designing medical healthcare applications called as Wireless Medical Sensor Networks. Wireless medical sensor networks (WMSN) give the significant improvements for healthcare in 21st century (Meingast, 2006). Wireless medical sensors are placed on the patient body and record physiological data of patient like temperature, blood pressure, heart rate, oxygen saturation etc. and transmit that recorded data to some remote location without human interference and concerned

Figure 1. Work flow

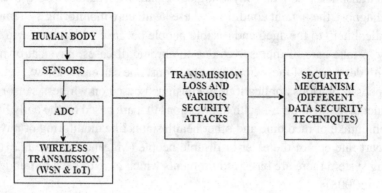

person or doctor can interpret the physiological data to assess patient's condition. So, with this patient's condition can be monitored continuously after discharging from the hospital. WMSN should support high mobility so the patient can carry device and provide high data rates with consistent communication. IoT is dynamic global network infrastructure which is used to collect object data and send it to the cloud (Shaikh, 2006). The coupling of biosensors with a wireless infrastructure enables real-time monitoring of an individual's health and related behaviors (Minaie, 2013).

The main benefit of using wireless networking in biomedical applications is that it allows the user to monitor patient situation within range and it increases the efficiency of treatment inside hospital. The wired biosensors are attached on the patient body which will attach patient to machine and gives vital readings. After recognizing the patient physiological readings, the data is sent to doctor or concerned person through cloud by using different wireless technologies which can improve data quality and data resolution. These readings can be helpful for diagnose the diseases and for patient treatment.

WSN is group of wireless-capable sensor nodes are working together to complete a mutual objective (Baker, 2007). WSN has one or more base stations which are used to collect data from the sensor devices and these base stations interface the WSN with the outer world for the communication (Stankovic, 2009). The basic principle of WSN is to perform networked sensing using a huge number of comparatively unsophisticated sensors instead of probable approach of developing a few expensive and sophisticated sensing modules and advantage of networked recognizing over conservative approach, can be concise as greater coverage, precision and dependability at a possibly lower cost (Li, 2008). When WSNs are used for designing the medical healthcare applications called as Wireless Medical Sensor Networks (WMSNs). WMSN give significant improvements for healthcare in 21st century (Meingast, 2006). Wireless medical sensors are placed on patient body and used to gather physiological data of the patient like temperature, blood pressure, heart rate, oxygen saturation etc. and transmit that collected data to some remote location without human interference. And concerned person can understand these sensor readings to assess patient's condition. So, with this patient condition can be monitored continuously within range after discharging from hospital. WMSNs are different from traditional WSNs. Traditional WSNs are automatic and self-determining and can be operate in large-scale networks in either fixed or distributed networks while on the other side WMSNs can be deployed in small scale; they have direct human connection with doctors, patient, nurse other providers etc. Wireless medical sensor network (WMSN) should support high mobility so the patient can carry the device and offer the high data rates with consistent communication. According to above requirements different health care systems are designed based on WSNs. WiSPH is a system based on (Magana, 2014) WSN technology which have capability of monitoring of heart rate and motion rate of elder within home. This system has capability of notifying caretaker or doctor about any physiological changes in patient health by a smartphone. The system uses the 128-bit AES encryption algorithm to protect transmitted data and for the security purpose so transmitted information does not segment with other network nodes which are not part of the network (Kumar, 2011). WiSPH is based on IEEE 802.15.4 Zigbee wireless technology which anticipates use of mobile nodes that form network setup. The infrastructure nodes switch Received Signal Strength Indication to proactively create the network and mobile nodes sends data when event will occur i.e. fluctuations in heart rate or a fall. Cost, Reliability and Power consumption are main application parameters in the WSN. A low system had been designed by (Stroulia, 2009) which offers low price, low power consumption and more reliability than other designed systems. The system detects the fall and movement of the patient for inside environments. The accelerometer offers most precise and reasonable way for detecting fall and position of user is calculated by employing RSSI measurements between user and network of wireless nodes deployed in environment.

Location based services are a support of universal computing and situation awareness. Location based services provides valuable services for detecting the location of the person based on GPS and GSM. Different positioning algorithms are designed for location purposes. ZUPS (Zigbee and Ultrasound Positioning System) is a system which had been designed for location detection of aged and disabled people (Marco, 2008). The system uses Zigbee and ultrasound to fulfill the application requirements differing from all others existing systems. A positioning algorithm had been designed based on passive positioning which detects the position of elder people to provide healthcare at chief care center and residential home (Yan, 2008).

GiraffPlus system is based on WSN infrastructure which is designed for monitoring of regular activities of seniors within their homes (Palumbo, 2014). The system had capability to monitor the physiological parameters like temperature, BP, glucose and environmental parameters like rate of motion etc. the alarm is generated if sudden problems happened.

Medication intake applications are designed for monitoring the intake of the patient's drugs. iCabi-NET gives solution that services a smart medicine manager that alert patients via a message or audio alarm at home to intake the medicine at time (Lopez, 2008). Additional medication intake application is iPackage consist of medication wrappers with RFID tags which are detected by RFID sensor at moment of ingestion and allowing authorized persons to monitor whether patient is following instructions or not (Pang, 2009).

Health care monitoring systems collects medical parameters like temperature, HR, glucose level, pulse rate etc. which explains current-state diagnose of patient and provide information to authorized person i.e. any family member or doctor about condition whether it is normal or not. If any abnormality occurs it can be immediately informed to authorized person through message or alarm. AlarmNet is a system, which monitors physical variables of patient, designed for assisted living and residential monitoring to detect physical abnormalities (Wood, 2008). Different applications are designed for monitoring physical parameters of neonates. Baby Glove is an application which measures dynamic signs of newborn baby or neonates. Data is collected by baby's romper and transmitted wirelessly which continuously measures variables and alert caretaker (Baker, 2007).

Heart diseases are one of major health problems which is leading causes of death in the world. According to World Health Report 2000, in each year 7 million people in which 13% of male deaths and 12% of female deaths are due to heart diseases. It is compulsory to develop self-organized wireless heart disease monitoring system which are based on hardware/software systems. MASN (Medical Ad Hoc Sensor Networks) is a system based on Adhoc Sensor networks which collects patient's ECG data through wireless medium (Hu, 2008). Another Home ECG monitoring system is designed which uses 3-electrode and system is combined to Wi-Fi Lan or Bluetooth for transmission attained data and to interconnect with doctor for immediate guidance. System uses the wet electrodes for acquiring the ECG signal and it is tested on different age group (20-25, 40-45, 50-55) people for the efficiency. SMART (Scalable Medical Alert and Response Technology) is a WSN based system introduced (Curtis, 2008) in 2008 for monitoring SpO2, ECG and situation of the patient. The data is sent wirelessly to central computer which assembles data and analyze that collected data. If any abnormality occurs in patient situation it will alert to doctor or any authorized person.

IoT is network infrastructure which is mixture of numerous technologies with diverse applications. IoT connects home appliances, physical devices and other devices with sensors etc. which permits these devices to connect and interchange data ("An Introduction to What is IoT", 2017). 'Things' in IoT refers to various devices like monitoring devices, sensors, biochip transponders etc. ("Introduction to Internet of Things", 2017). IoT plays vital role in remote health care monitoring. (Alaa, 2017) presented review of different smart home applications based on IoT. The data set had been collected from three databases i.e. IEEE Explore, Science Direct and Web of Sciences related to smart homes, app and IoT. Telemedicine provides quality of healthcare in remote areas by using various wireless technologies along with IoT. A model had been proposed based on IoT Health Prescription Assistant which helps patient to follow doctor instructions appropriately (Abideen, 2017) .A security system had also proposed for user authentication based on OpenID standard. A Security Access Token which is recognized as authorization ticket is allotted to user after authentication.

Due to availability of various communication technologies and smart devices the health problems can be looked after. Based on this a healthy healthcare model had been introduced for continuous monitoring of health status of patient during travelling by using various IoT sensors which is connected on human body and data is send to server through patient's smart phone(Carletti, 2017). This strong healthcare model consists of five layers named as IoT devices layer, network layer, internet layer, server layer and stackholder layer which perform different task like collecting, analyzing, storing and transferring of the data. According to WHO, falls are the second foremost reason of accidentally injury death after road traffic grievances. The largest possibility of falls occurs in aged people and disabled persons. So, in recent years research in analyzing of fall detection systems are increased. On the basis of this a fall detection system has been designed based on smart phone technology. The system is portable which is placed in the trouser pocket and self organising maps are used to distinguish between the ordinary happenings and falls of the patient because smart phones has the battery problem.

IoT enable to diagnose and monitor mobility and health status anywhere like home and while travelling etc. So there is a need of such type of smart technology within the IoT and has ability walk defines large aspects of quality of life in a wide range of health and disease conditions (Eskofier, 2017). Smart shoes have capability of sustenance prevention, analytic work-up and disease monitoring with a constant gait and mobility. Smart shoes can be intended to help as prevalent wearable computing schemes that permit advanced resolutions and services for the upgradation of well living and the revolution of health care.

M2M technology is a part of data communication which includes one and more things that do not essentially need user interaction while communication. It is a most ubiquitous application of IoT which is used in numerous fields. Based on this technology work had been done based on wireless technology in combine with WSN and IoT using M2M communication technology for smart home and security system (Jiang, 2015). The system is divided into two networks i.e. external network based in Time Division-Synchronization CDMA and The Home Network. The home gateway is used to interconnect these two networks.

WSNs are used to connect things to the internet through gateways and various routing protocols. There is a need of systems based on Zig-bee using internet of things. System is divided into scenarios i.e. remote access in which user is connected to server and internet access that is implemented to the smart home that provides internet access to the remote access (Khali, 2014). A technical architecture called SMMC (Sensors, Microcontroller, Machine to machine Protocols and Cloud) had been presented which measures the weight of the user (Ma, 2017). Data of user is collected by IoT sensors, processed by microcontroller and send to cloud. M2M protocols provide the algorithm to generate feedback and alert originating from cloud. The two-way communication occurs between microcontroller and cloud. The Thingspeak is used to collect, store, analyze, visualize and act of the data collected from the IoT sensors and this data that is sent to the Thingspeak is send through the arduino, Raspberry Pi and other hardware's.

COMPARISON OF WIRELESS BODY AREA NETWORKS (WBAN) AND WSN

WBAN is a wireless network of the wearable computing devices in which the devices are embedded inside human body or on surface of human body for recognizing physical activities of the human. On the other side WSN is a wireless network in which group of sensors are spatially spread for monitoring and controlling the physical conditions of environment and uniting collected data at some chief location. In recent years most of the research is done on WBAN, their designs, communication protocols etc. Table 1 represents the comparison between WSN and WBAN on the basis of different metrics.

Table 1. Comparison between WSN and WBAN (Kurs, 2007)

	WSN	WBAN
Deployment	WSN nodes are deployed in the places that are not easily accessible by the operators.	In WBAN, the sensor nodes are placed on the surface of the human body or embedded inside the human body.
Data Rate	WSN is based on event monitoring when events are occurred nodes will notify and the events are occurred at irregular time so data rate is irregular.	On the other side WBAN monitors human physiological activities continuously which provides high data rates.
Energy Consumption	There is a need of maximize the battery life of the WSN nodes because nodes are unreachable after deployment which provides the higher energy consumption.	Replacement of batteries in WBANs are easy so the energy consumption may be less in WBAN than WSNs.
Mobility	Wireless sensor nodes are considered as stationary.	BAN users can be move around so ban nodes share same mobility pattern.
Applications	Used for event and environment-based monitoring.	Used for continuous monitoring of human physiological activities.

ISSUES IN USING WBSN IN BIOMEDICAL FIELD

WBANs use different wireless technologies like Zigbee, Bluetooth etc. collected data from sensors is send to concerned person through cloud by using these wireless technologies. So, WBANs play a vital role for universal computing. But there are some issues occurs during designing WBANs which are described below:

Sensor Devices

The main issues in designing WBAN is selection of appropriate sensor devices. The sensors should be comfortable to wear: not invasive and not prominent. To attain this enhanced schemes should use the suitable circuit design, signal processing, signal extraction and communication techniques to minimize overall power consumption and size of sensor. It should also reduce harmful effect introduced by human skin on low-power radio signals.

Synchronization and Standardization of Biomedical Sensors

Synchronization and standardization of biomedical sensors is also a major concern for research which has too kept in mind while designing the BAN. Basically, in WSN sensor nodes are distributed so all nodes are not sharing the common battery source so the accurate calibration should be done between sensor nodes. And on other side the time synchronization is also needed between two or more sensor nodes for delay measurement which includes the two clocks. If the synchronization makes properly the system will gives the high accuracy and low delay between the packets.

Power Supply Issues

In BAN, biomedical sensor nodes are used to collect human physiological data, processing of that acquired data and transmission of acquired data to concerned person: for all these activities BAN devices need a battery source. So, there is a need of suitable battery devices for biomedical communication. As we know that all BAN devices need a battery source for operation: so, these battery sources may not be replaceable in cases when these are entrenched on human body. Such types of techniques should be used like remote battery charging and energy harvesting (Wang, 2006) which will not affect to operation of BAN devices.

Security, Data Authentication and Privacy Issues

In health care monitoring systems, the patient's data is sent to authorize person wirelessly. During transmission, hacker or attacker can misuse that data. So, data should be highly secured during transmission. Security is major concern in wireless transmission of data. Multimodal authentication systems based on human faces, hand features, and EEG signals, are being dynamically established in both academia and manufacturing. Complex but different human body features provide a perfect way for confirming users, but they also make other challenges like protective the confidentiality of the operators.

Standardization

The research had been done into interoperability of desktop telemedicine systems and bedside devices, e.g., development of Health Level 7 and ISO/IEEE 11073 standards (Kavitha, 2010). However, smart monitoring and behavioral systems retaining BANs have to follow standardized rules for ambulatory environments during communication. It provides point-of-care irrespective of user's location, while protecting patient's confidentiality. Interoperability protocols at application or domain level, e.g., sample rate, data accuracy should all be addressed by vendor-independent qualities, and homogenous user interfaces should be made.

SECURITY THREATS IN WBAN

WBANs are based on WSN and wireless data transmission so these networks are susceptible to enormous number of attacks and threats. Wireless body area networks are endangered to security attacks and threats due to broadcast nature of communication medium. Another reason of security issues in WSN is that nodes are freely placed in environment where they are not physically protected. The attacks in WBANs can be divided into different parts described below (Shi, 2004).

VARIOUS SECURITY ATTACKS BASED ON CAPABILITY OF ATTACKER

Node Concession Attacks and Passive vs. Dynamic Attacks

These attacks are also known as the foreigner and insider attacks. The foreigner attacks are defined as attacks which are not belong to WBAN while on the other side the insider attacks are occurred inside the wireless body area network (Zia, 2006). The insider attacks are occurred when authorized nodes of WBSN behave in unplanned ways. Passive attacks are occurred when network nodes exchange information within WBSN while dynamic attacks are arisen due to some modifications of data steam or creation of false stream.

Various Security Attacks Based on Transit Information

In BAN, various sensors are attached on human body non-invasively or invasively for physiological monitoring of patient. The sensors measure specific parameters and report to descend according to necessity. When data is transferred from sensor nodes to descend transit data can be attacked for providing wrong information to BS or sink nodes. The attacks occurred in transit information are described below (Akyildiz, 2002):

Intrusion Attack

In IA, communication link between sensor and sink node or from SN to destination node can be broken so data can be lost. This situation can harm service accessibility.

Interception

In WBAN, sensor network has been negotiated by a competitor where attacker gains the unauthorized access to nodes or data in network. These types of attacks can threaten data confidentiality. The main aim is to snoop on information carried in data packets.

Repeating of Existing Messages

In these types of attacks attacker will harm information carried by data packet. This action will threaten message cleanness. In this process the attacker can replace the original message and repeat the message again and again. The aim of the attacker is to confuse or mislead the both parties which are involved during the communication.

Security Attacks Based on the Protocol Stack

In wireless communication during the exchange of the information from source to destination the user has to follow communication rules which are known as the protocols. The communication in network are based on the OSI model which consist of the 7 different layers. The layers use different protocols for information processing. Similarly, in WBAN patient data is send from one location to another location wirelessly so layer architecture is also followed in medical data communication. The data will process through different layers. This section will explain the various attacks in WBSN layer architecture (Shaikh, 2006).

Physical Layer Attacks

Physical layer is responsible for bit to bit transmission of data between various devices using the electrical medium. The various attacks in the physical layer are jamming or congestion, radio intrusion and tempering or destruction. Jamming is the one of DoS attack which occurs in physical layer due to overflowing of data. Jamming attacks in wireless body area networks are classified into three types i.e. continuous, dishonest, random and volatile. In continuous jamming attacks the packets will get corrupted when they are transmitted, in dishonest or deceptive attacks, attacker will send stream of bits which will added in actual data and data will look like genuine traffic. On the other side in random jamming attacks information will arbitrarily substitutes between sleep and jamming to save energy. The volatile jamming attack will add a jam signal in data when it senses traffic. To overcome these types of attacks spread spectrum techniques are used to avoid collision and jamming. In these types of techniques, jammed area is mapped in network and routing area (Raymond, 2008). The techniques are CDMA and CDMA-CA.

In radio interference challenger either produces large amount of interference irregularly. This interference can harm entire data packet. To overcome this issue a symmetric key algorithm is designed in which revelation of keys is delayed by some time interval (Saxena, 2007).

When attacker gets the physical access to information present at the physical layer the attacker can also extract the important information in the data packet like cryptographic keys and other available data which can be defined as node tempering and destruction in data.

Data Link Layer Attacks

Data link layer is responsible for reduction of transmission error and provide well defined interface to network layer. The data link layer receives continuous transmission of signal data delivered by physical layer. The data link layer has to give continuous channel access to user which may leads to exhaustion. A malicious node interrupts MAC protocol, by unceasingly requesting over transmission channel which will leads to starvation for nodes participating in network. To overcome these types of errors or attacks in the network a TDM can be used in which a time slot will give to each node in network so node can transmit its information in given time slot.

In FDM technique a particular frequency band has been allotted to each node. But sometimes nodes try to transmit information at similar frequency bands instantaneously which can be led to the collision in network. Due to this when the packets will collide a change will occur in data packet which is not a reliable communication. Because at destination end mismatch will occurs. This transmitted data will not be considered at receiver end in body sensor networks. Repeated applications of these collapse and collision based medium access control layer attacks can lead to injustice. This type of attacks are the fractional DoS attacks which are responsible for system performance degradation.

Sybil Attacks is very much prominent attack in link layer. First type of Sybil attack is data aggregation in which single malicious node acts as Sybil nodes to give negative supports to make combined message a false message. Second type of Sybil attack is voting. In Data Link Layer different MAC protocols initialize voting technique to find better and cheaper way of information transmission from available paths. Here the attacker can use the stuff of election box by which the attacker can know outcome of voting and off course attacker can use it for wrong purpose (Sarma, 2006).

Network Layer Attacks

The network is responsible for data routing in the network. The different routing protocols are used to route data from one station to another station. Routing is main part in communication as well as in the WBAN. Because data of patient should be route properly from source to destination. So, many number of attacks will occur in network layer to harm routing information.

Sinkhole attack basically works on network layer by making the cooperated node adjacent network node with respect to routing algorithms. This attack makes an adversary node around that nodes which will provide the high-quality path to base stations. Because routing protocols continuously tries to verify quality of path with end-to-end acknowledgments. So, depending on routing protocols, a sinkhole attack tries to trap nearly all the network traffic on the way to the cooperated node by creating a symbolic sinkhole with rival at center (Pathan, 2006).

WBAN use the Multihop routing technique same as that of WSN. In Multihop routing technique network used multiple hops to send data from source to destination hence nodes who are participating in Multihop process will send message faithfully. The malicious nodes will refuse to forward packet or may drop it or destroy it. If malicious nodes continuously drop all packets through them it is called a Blackhole Attack. Sometimes if some of nodes forward the packets it is called selective forwarding. To overcome this type of attack Multi path routing can be used as the grouping with arbitrary selection of paths from source to destination (Shi, 2004).

Figure 2. Wormhole attack

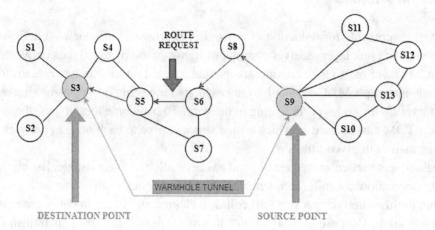

The wormhole nodes make a false shorter route than novel one within network which will confuse routing protocols based on shorter route's acknowledgements. The malicious node will capture original packet from one location to transmit to another location which are distributed in neighborhood. To overcome this type of attack data traffic should route to BS along with path which should be physically shortest or use very constricted time management among nodes which is infeasible in practical surroundings.

The nodes in wireless network, however they are in WBANs or WSNs, send hello packets to their neighbors to confirm that they are part of network and range of sender. A laptop-class rival can send hello packets to all network nodes so that they have confidence in attacker node is belongs to their network. This will cause whole network because if network nodes accept the packets from the attacker node they will also revert back to attacker node. With this attacker can know personal information of nodes and can get authentication key to decrypt packet.

The routing algorithms used in sensor networks requires acknowledgements from receiver top confirm that message has been received. The attacker node can takeoff that acknowledgements of packets to destine neighbor nodes to deliver wrong information to that neighbor nodes. The solution of this problem is to authenticate packets via encryption methods along with packet header.

The packets use that path which requires less time to deliver packets from source to destination. For this purpose, the nodes use multihopping technique in which message go through the different hops to reach at destination. The attacker node will try to participate in Multihop process to misdirect packet and to provide false information to its neighbor nodes (Pathan, 2006). The main aim of attacker present in network is to attack routing information present in routing protocol when it is exchanged in between neighboring nodes. The attacker can spoof, interchange or replay routing information to disturb traffic in network. These disturbances include the creation of routing loops again and again, increase the routing paths, to generate fake errors and increasing of end-to-end expectation. The efficient authentication and encryption keys are solution to overcome these types of attacks.

Transport Layer Attacks

TL is responsible for the end to end communication of the network, error correction, provide superiority and consistency to end user. This layer allows the host to refer and accept error corrected data, packets or messages over a network and is network module that permits multiplexing. The attacks in TL are the flooding and De-synchronization.

The main aim of TL is to send error free data in network. On the basis of this attacker can repeatedly generate correction requests until resources reach maximum limit. This will exhaust network traffic and can produce simple resource limitations for genuine nodes. The proposed solution of this type of attack is that each client should validate its commitment to connection by resolving puzzle. To defense from attack a limit should be set for number of connections (Sarma, 2006).

In De-synchronization attack, rival will continuously establish packet to both end to end points which request to nodes for retransmission of missed packets. When these missed packets are retransmitted to end nodes the rival node will maintain the proper timing to exchange any useful information. It will cause damage of energy of genuine nodes in whole network because nodes have to send the packets again and again which will be a wastage of energy. The proposed solution to overcome this type of attacks is to require verification of all packets including control fields communicated between hosts and full packet should be validate to defeat this type of attacks.

Application Layer Attacks

Application layer provides process to process communication and helps network to communicate with outsider world. The application layer includes following attacks;

The overpower attack enables the attacker to attempt overpower to the network nodes with sensor incentives which will cause network to forward large number of traffic to BS. To handle large number of traffic nodes should need extra power, extra bandwidth and node energy. To overcome this type of attack we have to adjust sensor nodes carefully so that only specified incentives can activate that nodes.

The overflow attack includes network programming. If network programming is not secure attacker can seizure this process and effect the network reprogramming and attacker can take large portion of network. The solution of this types of attack is to use authentication streams to secure overflow process.

The Path-based DOS attack involves inoculation of repeated packets in network at sprig nodes. This type of attack can starve network genuine traffic because it consumes large number of resources on path to the BS thus it will affect other nodes to send and receive data. The solution of this type of attacks is that packet authentication should be provided by combining packets.

PRIVACY ISSUES

As that of information security privacy is also a major concern in WBSNs. The data which is related to health should be always isolated in nature so external environment does not affect patient information (Meingast, 2006). Privacy in wireless body area networks defines the information secretion that authorized person has only secretion key to decrypt data. Because in WBAN, patient data send through wireless medium in which there are chances of occurrence of privacy threats in environment.

The many question related to privacy of information has been raised by the many authors. Like authors in (Dimitriou, 2008) raised a question that where the data of patient should be store and who can authorize patient data. There is another question that to whom this patient information has been revealed to without patient agreement and who will be responsible for maintaining patient data if any problem arises. These are the several issues regarding patient information privacy that should be resolved for privacy as well as for data security.

In addition of above mentioned other privacy measures includes that all communication over wireless medium should require to be encrypted for data privacy. Only authorized users have access to decrypt that information when there is a need. One another privacy measures is public awareness. Public should be aware about data privacy and data security. This will be beneficial if people are educated regarding security and privacy issues and their effect on communication. Because common person does not know about various new technologies. As a result, he/she does not able to manage if there will be any error or issue will be occurred. So, educating the common people will help to resolve the security and privacy issues in communication.

SECURITY SOLUTIONS IN WIRELESS BODY AREA NETWORKS

An example of BAN is patient health monitoring systems which are used to monitor real-time physiological data of patient remotely. With the help of wireless communication this monitored data can be forward to authorize person who is far away from patient. The WSN sensors made the wireless body area network cost-effective and medical sensors nodes to create a network for monitoring physiological data of patient. The wireless communication deals with many types of communication threats and security issues during information exchange which will harm the patient information. To overcome these threats and security issues different solutions are provided from recent years. Like for security of data different encryption and decryption algorithms are used. Encryption is process of converting plain text into cipher text in order to provide security to transferring data. On the other side decryption is process of converting cipher text into plain text to dichepher key data.

Data Encryption Standard Algorithm (DES)

Data Encryption Algorithm is one of data encryption and decryption algorithm in which source and destination shares same private key for encrypt and decrypt data. This algorithm uses 64-bit plaintext data for encryption process at transmitter side and convert into 64-bit cipher data for decryption process at receiver side. DES algorithm uses permutation process including 16 rounds of key calculation and reverse permutation. The 16 rounds of key calculation will be drawn into 16*16 matrix table as shown in fig 3. During 1st step of key calculation message will be divides into two parts left and right parts. The next step includes Replacement box, Extension Table and Key Generation part. After completing the 16 rounds of key generation last step executes which will be inverse permutation for generation cipher text. Each round uses different 48-bit round key generated from cipher key according to algorithm. The cipher text is designed from early permutation that is followed by 16 rounds of private key and substitution of 32-bit. The advantage of DES algorithm is that it is one of simple security solution of data security which can be used for short level communication.

3 DES Algorithm

The 3 DES algorithm is same as DES algorithm but it uses 3 times private key for encryption and decryption for providing more security. The private key of 3DES algorithm is 192-bits with block size of 64-bit.

BLOWFISH Algorithm

Blowfish algorithm is a security algorithm which uses 64-bit block size. Blowfish algorithm is divided into two categories i.e. key expansion and data encryption (Ahmad, 2013). Each key expansion is divided into P-array and S-boxes with utilization of may sub keys which requires initial permutation before encryption and decryption process. P-array keys consist of different sub keys which are of 32-bits. In BLOWFISH algorithm total 448 bits are converted into different array sub keys so total sub array size is 4168 bytes.

Firstly, P-array is initialized by four s-boxes in which each box containing 32-bit sub key. Then first 32-bit S-box is XORing with P1 and second 32-bit S-box is XORing with P2 and so on until key bits are up to P14. This cycle will continue until entire P-array has been XORed to key bits. Then BLOW-FISH algorithm is used to encrypt all zero-string retaining sub keys in above steps. Then P1 and P2 are replaced with output of zero-string retaining of sub keys. Then similarly output of zero retaining of sub keys of P1 and P2 is replaced P3 and P4. The process is continued to replace all elements of P-array that are followed by S-boxes. The output of process will be changed after every iteration.

BLOWFISH data encryption algorithm originates with 64-bit block element of plaintext which is converted into 64-bit cipher text. Firstly, 64-bit block element is converted into two parts for XOR operation. XOR operation is carried out between first segment of 32-bit block that is referred as L and first P-array. After XORing process output of process is fed to F-function which permutes data into 32-bit block segment. This 32-bit block segment is then XORed with second segment of 32-bit block which can be say as R. L and R will be interchanges for future repetitions of BLOWFISH algorithm. Figure 4

Figure 3. DES algorithm

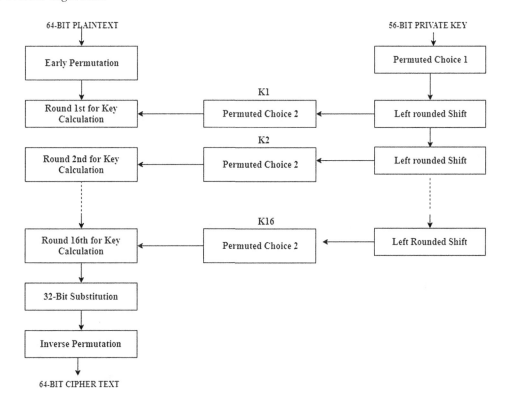

Figure 4. BLOWFISH algorithm
(Ahmad, 2013)

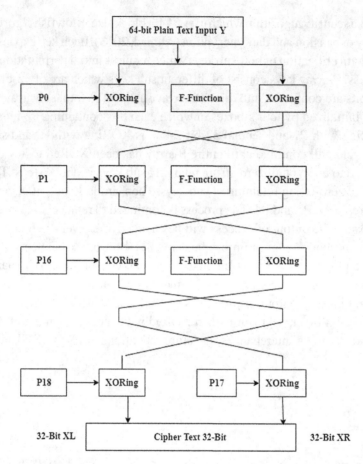

is showing function of the BLOWFISH algorithm with 16 rounds of the private key. The input of 64-bit plaintext is given which is denoted as the Y. The input Y is divided into two parts i.e. YL and YR which is of 32-bit each.

As shown in the Figure 4 output of XORing operation of P-array and 32-bit plaintext data is fed to F-function. The F-function is complex part of BLOWFISH algorithm. F-function consist of S-boxes which accepts 32-bit stream of data. In S-boxes the data is divided into four equal parts of 8-bits. Then this 8-bit box is changed into 32-bit data stream using equivalent of each portion S-box. The 32-bit data that is attained is XOR-ed or combined to give a final 32-bit value for permutations of BLOWFISH algorithm. The working of the F-function is given in Figure 5.

RC4 Security Algorithm

RC4 security algorithm is a stream cipher algorithm which shares the same key for encryption and decryption process. The plaintext data is XORed with the generated key sequence with the block size of 32, 64 and 128 bits. The variable key length in the RC4 security algorithm is of 256 bits which prepares the 256-bit state table. This state table is used to generate the pseudo-random bits and pseudo-random

Figure 5. Architecture of F-function
(Singh, 2013)

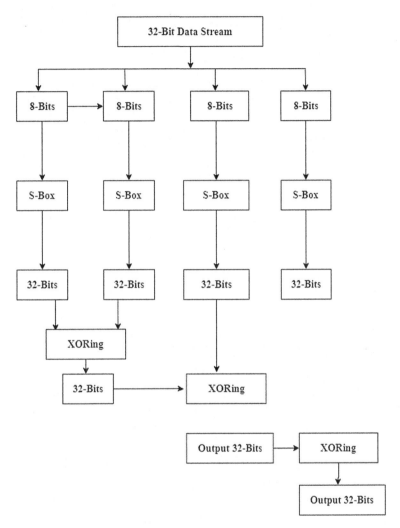

stream of the data which is then XORed with the input plaintext data for generation of cipher data. The operation of RC4 algorithm can be divided into two parts i.e. initialization and action (Mousa, 2006) In first stage when the 256-bit state table has been set up the S-box block will continue to be modified in steady state pattern for encryption of data. After encryption of data swapping of numbers started (locations of the number 0-255) which are given in state table. This will complete initialization process. After completion of first stage algorithm will generate pseudo random values of data stream. Then each bit of plaintext data is XORed with each bit of the pseudo-random data stream bits which will generate cipher data.

Figure 6. RC4 algorithm
(Kumar, 2011)

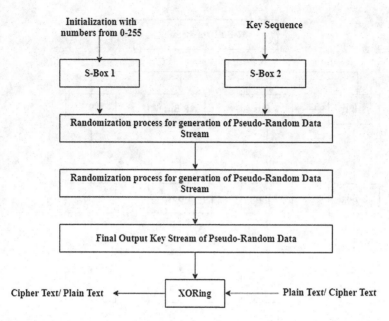

RSA (Rivest-Shamir-Adleman) Security Algorithm

RSA algorithm is designed by the Ron Rivest, Adi Shamir and Leonard Adleman in 1978 for security of communication data from timing attack. RSA algorithm uses two keys i.e. private and public key for encryption and decryption process. Private Key can be defined as the symmetrical key in which both sender and receiver shares same key for encrypt and decrypt data. On the other side public key is an asymmetrical key in which sender and receiver uses two keys i.e. private as well as public. The receiver public key is used to encrypt data before sending this data to receiver. When receiver receives this message, it will decrypt by using private key of receiver. The sender has not public key. When receiver sends the acknowledgement or want to send message then sender will act as a receiver and can use public key. This process will be one-way communication. Similarly, RSA algorithm is an asymmetrical algorithm which uses two keys in which the sender encrypts message by using receiver public key and receiver will decrypt this message by using its own private key (Kumar, 2011). RSA algorithm operation can be divides into 3 parts i.e. key generation, encryption and decryption. In key generation process two random numbers are selected i.e. p and q in which p should not equal to q. Then these two numbers are multiplied p*q for public key generation denoted as n. Then calculate: phi (n) = (p-1) (q-1) and choose an integer which will 1<e<phi (n). Compute d to satisfy correspondence relation d × e = 1 mod phi (n); d is kept as private key exponent. The public key is (n, e) and private key is (n, d). The values d, p, q and phi should be kept secret. In encryption process plaintext should be P<n cipher text will be $C=P^e$ mod n. and in decryption process cipher text will be C and plaintext will be $P= C^d$ mod n (Singh, 2011).

AES (Advanced Encryption Standard) Security Algorithm

AES algorithm is introduced by NIST to replace DES security algorithm for security of data. The AES algorithm uses 128-bit, 192-bit and 256-bit key length. In AES encryption process system will go through 10 rounds for 128-bit key, 12 rounds for 192-bit key and 14 rounds for 256-bit key to convert plaintext into cipher text and vice versa (Cho, 2014). In AES -128-bit key length whole operation is divided into 4 parts or blocks which consist of array of bytes and make the 4*4 matrix. The process of encryption and decryption process is beginning with add round key in every stage. The system will go through nine rounds before reaching to 10th round (Figure7). Each round performs 4 main operations i.e. Sub-bytes, Shift rows, Mix-columns and Add Round Key. In final round there will be no mix-column operation will take place. This is whole process of encryption of data in AES algorithm and decryption process will be reverse of encryption process. In AES-128, system contains data block of 128-bit i.e. each data block has 16 bytes. In sub-byte transformation of AES process each byte will be transformed into another block by using 8-bit substitution box which is donated as S-box. In shift row process last 3 rows of 4*4 matrix will be shifted according to their location. The shift will be circular shift. For the 2nd row of column 1-byte circular shift will be done. Similarly, for 3rd and 4th row 2-byte and 3-byte circular shift will be done respectively. The mix-column state contains multiplication of vector column and with fixed matrix. The XOR operation will be carried out in add round stage key. This operation will be performed between round generated key and current state (Singh, 2011).

TINYSEC Security Solution for Biomedical Data

TinySec security solution is designed for data link layer security in wireless biomedical body sensor networks (Zhou, 2011). It is an architecture for WSN which generates security packets by encrypting information packets. In TinySec security solution sender and receiver sensor nodes shared group key including MAC address of packet in header file. This security solution uses one encryption key which has been apply on sensor nodes before deployment. This solution does not work on node capture attacks. It is weakest point of this solution. If any of the attacker node will learn the encryption key it can get the access of whole network and can get useful information or harm it.

Biometric Method for Data Security

Biometric method for biomedical data security supports use of the human body itself for handling the encryption keys for the symmetric cryptography (Cherukuri, 2003). The biomedical sensors which are attached on human body will generate pseudo-random number by using measured physiological value if they are able to measure previously agreed physiological value instantaneously. When same number will be generating then this number will use for encrypt and decrypt symmetric key. The main task in this type of method is to select the physiological key which should be time discrepancy and arbitrary.

Figure 7. AES algorithm

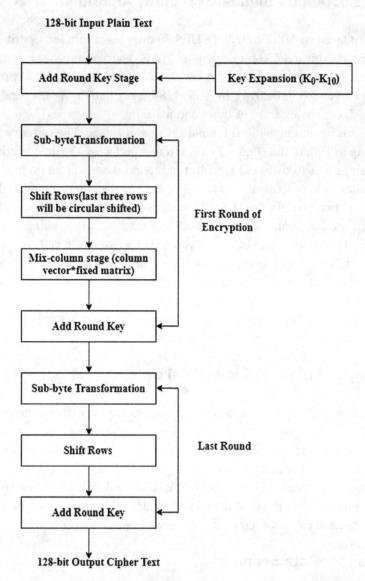

ADVANTAGES AND DISADVANTAGES OF PRESENT SECURITY TECHNIQUES

The above sections explained various security issues, security attacks and security solutions for the medical data. The different security solutions are introduced in recent years. The advantages are of these solutions are:

The advantage of DES algorithm is that it is one of simple security solution of data security which can be used for short level communication. The 3DES algorithm provides the 3 times more security to data. 192-bit security key is used to cipher data which is not easy to decipher without knowing private key. BLOWFISH algorithm uses 64-bit element and converted into 64-bit cipher text with XORing process. Blowfish algorithm is in the public domain, allowing it to be freely used for any purpose. The biometric method provides the high security as of other methods because if the previous values are matched with present value then only the data will transmitted.

The disadvantage of DES algorithm is that it provides only 32-bit key which will take huge time to provide security to huge data of patient. The key schedule in Blowfish is moderately time-consuming (corresponding to encryption of about 4 KB of data). However, this can be an advantage in some circumstances as protection against brute-force attacks. The small block size of Blowfish (64 bits) is more vulnerable to centennial attacks than the 128 bits used by AES.

CONCLUSION

The advances in wireless sensor network have been empowered to monitoring of the patient data remotely. The recent technologies in the wireless communication as well as in the field of wireless sensor network are mostly used for designing the health monitoring systems. This chapter presented the use of the wireless sensor networks in designing healthcare applications and currently available health monitoring systems. The chapter has also been presented the review of the different attacks occurred during the wireless transmission of the data and different security issues occurred in the wireless data transmission. The different security solution is given by different authors with time to time. The chapter also reviewed these available security solutions for the wireless biomedical data. The more research can be done on basis of present security techniques. As the available techniques are time consuming. The complexity of the techniques should be reduced.

REFERENCES

Abideen, Z. U., & Shah, M. A. (2017). An IoT based robust healthcare model for continuous health monitoring. In *Proceedings of Automation and Computing (ICAC), 2017 23rd International Conference on* (pp. 1-6). IEEE.

Ahmad, F., & Mahmod, R. (2013). Security Analysis of Blowfish Algorithm. *Informatics and Applications (ICIA), Second International Conference.*

Akyildiz, I. F., Su, W., Sankarasubramaniam, Y., & Cayirci, E. (2002). Wireless sensor networks: A survey. *Computer Networks*, *38*(4), 393–422. doi:10.1016/S1389-1286(01)00302-4

Al Ameen, M., Liu, J., & Kwak, K. (2012). Security and privacy issues in wireless sensor networks for healthcare applications. *Journal of Medical Systems*, *36*(1), 93–101. doi:10.100710916-010-9449-4 PMID:20703745

Alaa, M., Zaidan, A. A., Zaidan, B. B., Talal, M., & Kiah, M. L. M. (2017). A review of smart home applications based on Internet of Things. *Journal of Network and Computer Applications*, *97*, 48–65. doi:10.1016/j.jnca.2017.08.017

Alabaichi, A., Ahmad, F., & Mahmod, R. (2013, September). Security analysis of blowfish algorithm. In *Informatics and Applications (ICIA), 2013 Second International Conference on* (pp. 12-18). IEEE. 10.1109/ICoIA.2013.6650222

An Introduction to what is Internet of Things. (2017, August 31). Retrieved from https://www.eduonix. com/blog/internet-of-things/introduction-internet-things-iot/

Baker, C. R., Armijo, K., Belka, S., Benhabib, M., Bhargava, V., Burkhart, N., ... Ho, C. (2007, May). Wireless sensor networks for home health care. In *21st International Conference on Advanced Information Networking and Applications Workshops (AINAW'07)* (Vol. 2, pp. 832-837). IEEE. 10.1109/ AINAW.2007.376

Carletti, V., Greco, A., Saggese, A., & Vento, M. (2017, September). A Smartphone-Based System for Detecting Falls Using Anomaly Detection. In *International Conference on Image Analysis and Processing* (pp. 490-499). Springer. 10.1007/978-3-319-68548-9_45

Chen, M., Gonzalez, S., Vasilakos, A., Cao, H., & Leung, V. C. (2011). Body area networks: A survey. *Mobile Networks and Applications*, *16*(2), 171–193. doi:10.100711036-010-0260-8

Cherukuri, S., Venkatasubramanian, K. K., & Gupta, S. K. (2003, October). Biosec: A biometric based approach for securing communication in wireless networks of biosensors implanted in the human body. In *Parallel Processing Workshops, 2003. Proceedings. 2003 International Conference on* (pp. 432-439). IEEE. 10.1109/ICPPW.2003.1240399

Cho, Y. B., Lee, S. H., & Woo, S. H. (2014, June). Security Issues Using Remote Medical Treatment in Health Care Information. In International Conference on Future Information & Communication Engineering (Vol. 6, No. 1, pp. 193-196). Academic Press.

Curtis, D., Shih, E., Waterman, J., Guttag, J., Bailey, J., Stair, T., . . . Ohno-Machado, L. (2008, March). Physiological signal monitoring in the waiting areas of an emergency room. In *Proceedings of the ICST 3rd international conference on Body area networks* (p. 5). ICST (Institute for Computer Sciences, Social-Informatics and Telecommunications Engineering). Available online on: http:// Minnie.tuhs .org/ NetSec/Slides

Dimitriou, T., & Ioannis, K. (2008, October). Security issues in biomedical wireless sensor networks. In *Applied Sciences on Biomedical and Communication Technologies, 2008. ISABEL'08. First International Symposium on* (pp. 1-5). IEEE. 10.1109/ISABEL.2008.4712577

Eskofier, B., Lee, S., Baron, M., Simon, A., Martindale, C., Gaßner, H., & Klucken, J. (2017). An overview of smart shoes in the internet of health things: Gait and mobility assessment in health promotion and disease monitoring. *Applied Sciences*, *7*(10), 986. doi:10.3390/app7100986

Hossain, M., Islam, S. R., Ali, F., Kwak, K. S., & Hasan, R. (2018). An Internet of Things-based health prescription assistant and its security system design. *Future Generation Computer Systems*, *82*, 422–439. doi:10.1016/j.future.2017.11.020

Hu, F., Jiang, M., Celentano, L., & Xiao, Y. (2008). Robust medical ad hoc sensor networks (MASN) with wavelet-based ECG data mining. *Ad Hoc Networks*, *6*(7), 986–1012. doi:10.1016/j.adhoc.2007.09.002

Introduction to Internet of Things. (2016, March 17). Retrieved from https://www.slideshare.net/Blackvard/introduction-to-internet-of-things-iot

Jiang, T., Yang, M., & Zhang, Y. (2015). Research and implementation of M2M smart home and security system. *Security and Communication Networks, 8*(16), 2704–2711. doi:10.1002ec.569

Jiang, Y., Liu, X., & Lian, S. (2016). Design and implementation of smart-home monitoring system with the Internet of Things technology. In *Wireless Communications, Networking and Applications* (pp. 473–484). New Delhi: Springer. doi:10.1007/978-81-322-2580-5_43

Kavitha, T., &Sridharan, D. (2010). Security vulnerabilities in wireless sensor networks: A survey. *Journal of information Assurance and Security, 5*(1), 31-44.

Keshavarz, A., Tabar, A. M., & Aghajan, H. (2006, October). Distributed vision-based reasoning for smart home care. *Proc. of ACM SenSys Workshop on DSC.*

Khalil, N., Abid, M. R., Benhaddou, D., & Gerndt, M. (2014, April). Wireless sensors networks for Internet of Things. In *2014 IEEE ninth international conference on Intelligent sensors, sensor networks and information processing (ISSNIP)* (pp. 1-6). IEEE. 10.1109/ISSNIP.2014.6827681

Kumar, A., Jakhar, D. S., & Makkar, M. S. (2012). Comparative Analysis between DES and RSA Algorithm's. *International Journal of Advanced Research in Computer Science and Software Engineering, 2*(7), 386–391.

Kumar, P., & Lee, H. J. (2011). Security issues in healthcare applications using wireless medical sensor networks: A survey. *Sensors (Basel), 12*(1), 55–91. doi:10.3390120100055 PMID:22368458

Kurs, A., Karalis, A., Moffatt, R., Joannopoulos, J. D., Fisher, P., & Soljačić, M. (2007). Wireless power transfer via strongly coupled magnetic resonances. *Science, 317*(5834), 83-86.

Li, Y., & Thai, M. T. (Eds.). (2008). *Wireless sensor networks and applications.* Springer Science & Business Media. doi:10.1007/978-0-387-49592-7

Lopez-Nores, M., Pazos-Arias, J. J., Garcia-Duque, J., & Blanco-Fernandez, Y. (2008, January). Monitoring medicine intake in the networked home: The iCabiNET solution. In *Pervasive Computing Technologies for Healthcare, 2008. PervasiveHealth 2008. Second International Conference on* (pp. 116-117). IEEE.

Lu, C. H., & Fu, L. C. (2009). Robust location-aware activity recognition using wireless sensor network in an attentive home. *IEEE Transactions on Automation Science and Engineering, 6*(4), 598–609. doi:10.1109/TASE.2009.2021981

Ma, J., Nguyen, H., Mirza, F., & Neuland, O. (2017). Two way architecture between IoT sensors and cloud computing for remote health care monitoring applications. *Twenty-Fifth European Conference on Information Systems (ECIS),* 2834–2841.

Magaña-Espinoza, P., Aquino-Santos, R., Cárdenas-Benítez, N., Aguilar-Velasco, J., Buenrostro-Segura, C., Edwards-Block, A., & Medina-Cass, A. (2014). Wisph: A wireless sensor network-based home care monitoring system. *Sensors (Basel), 14*(4), 7096–7119. doi:10.3390140407096 PMID:24759112

Marco, A., Casas, R., Falco, J., Gracia, H., Artigas, J. I., & Roy, A. (2008). Location-based services for elderly and disabled people. *Computer Communications, 31*(6), 1055–1066. doi:10.1016/j.comcom.2007.12.031

Meingast, M., Roosta, T., & Sastry, S. (2006, August). Security and privacy issues with health are information technology. In *Engineering in Medicine and Biology Society, 2006. EMBS'06. 28th Annual International Conference of the IEEE* (pp. 5453-5458). IEEE. 10.1109/IEMBS.2006.260060

Minaie, A., Sanati-Mehrizy, A., Sanati-Mehrizy, P., &Sanati-Mehrizy, R. (2013). Application of wireless sensor networks in health care system. *Age, 23*(1).

Mitra, U., Emken, B. A., Lee, S., Li, M., Rozgic, V., Thatte, G., & Levorato, M. (2012). KNOWME: A case study in wireless body area sensor network design. *IEEE Communications Magazine, 50*(5), 116–125. doi:10.1109/MCOM.2012.6194391

Mousa, A., & Hamad, A. (2006). Evaluation of the RC4 algorithm for data encryption. *IJCSA, 3*(2), 44–56.

National Health Mission Report. (2018, August 14). Retrieved from http://nhm.gov.in/nrhm-components/rmnch-a/child-health-immunization/child-health/annual-report.html

Palumbo, F., Ullberg, J., Štimec, A., Furfari, F., Karlsson, L., & Coradeschi, S. (2014). Sensor network infrastructure for a home care monitoring system. *Sensors (Basel), 14*(3), 3833–3860. doi:10.3390140303833 PMID:24573309

Pang, Z., Chen, Q., & Zheng, L. (2009, November). A pervasive and preventive healthcare solution for medication noncompliance and daily monitoring. In *Applied Sciences in Biomedical and Communication Technologies, 2009. ISABEL 2009. 2nd International Symposium on* (pp. 1-6). IEEE. 10.1109/ISABEL.2009.5373681

Pathan, A. S. K., Lee, H. W., & Hong, C. S. (2006, February). Security in wireless sensor networks: issues and challenges. In *Advanced Communication Technology, 2006. ICACT 2006. The 8th International Conference* (Vol. 2, pp. 6-pp). IEEE. 10.1109/ICACT.2006.206151

Pragnya, K. R., Harshini, G. S., &Chaitanya, J. K. (2013). Wireless home monitoring for senior citizens using ZigBee network. *Advance in Electronic and Electric Engineering*.

Raymond, D. R., & Midkiff, S. F. (2008). Denial-of-service in wireless sensor networks: Attacks and defenses. *IEEE Pervasive Computing, 7*(1), 74–81. doi:10.1109/MPRV.2008.6

Sarma, H. K. D., & Kar, A. (2006, October). Security threats in wireless sensor networks. In *Carnahan Conferences Security Technology, Proceedings 2006 40th Annual IEEE International* (pp. 243-251). IEEE.

Saxena, M. (2007). *Security in wireless sensor networks-a layer based classification*. Department of Computer Science, Purdue University.

Shaikh, R. A., Lee, S., Song, Y. J., & Zhung, Y. (2006, June). Securing distributed wireless sensor networks: Issues and guidelines. In *Sensor Networks, Ubiquitous, and Trustworthy Computing, 2006. IEEE International Conference on* (Vol. 2, pp. 226-231). IEEE.

Shi, E., & Perrig, A. (2004). Designing secure sensor networks. *IEEE Wireless Communications, 11*(6), 38–43. doi:10.1109/MWC.2004.1368895

Shi, G., & Ming, Y. (2016). Wireless Communications. *Networking and Applications*, 1269-1278.

Singh, G. (2013). A study of encryption algorithms (RSA, DES, 3DES and AES) for information security. *International Journal of Computers and Applications, 67*(19).

Singh, M. G., Singla, M. A., & Sandha, M. K. (2011). Cryptography algorithm comparison for security enhancement in wireless intrusion detection system. *International Journal of Multidisciplinary Research, 1*(4), 143–151.

Stankovic, J. A., Cao, Q., Doan, T., Fang, L., He, Z., Kiran, R., . . . Wood, A. (2005, June). Wireless sensor networks for in-home healthcare: Potential and challenges. In High confidence medical device software and systems (HCMDSS) workshop (Vol. 2005). Academic Press.

Stroulia, E., Chodos, D., Boers, N. M., Huang, J., Gburzynski, P., & Nikolaidis, I. (2009, May). Software engineering for health education and care delivery systems: The Smart Condo project. In *Software Engineering in Health Care, 2009. SEHC'09. ICSE Workshop on* (pp. 20-28). IEEE.

Tabar, A. M., Keshavarz, A., & Aghajan, H. (2006, October). Smart home care network using sensor fusion and distributed vision-based reasoning. In *Proceedings of the 4th ACM international workshop on Video surveillance and sensor networks* (pp. 145-154). ACM. 10.1145/1178782.1178804

Wang, Y., Attebury, G., & Ramamurthy, B. (2006). *A survey of security issues in wireless sensor networks.* Academic Press.

Warren, S., & Jovanov, E. (2006, January). The need for rules of engagement applied to wireless body area networks. *Proc. of the IEEE consumer communications and networking conference, CCNC.* 10.1109/CCNC.2006.1593184

Wood, A. D., Stankovic, J. A., Virone, G., Selavo, L., He, Z., Cao, Q., ... Stoleru, R. (2008). Context-aware wireless sensor networks for assisted living and residential monitoring. *IEEE Network, 22*(4), 26–33. doi:10.1109/MNET.2008.4579768

Yan, H., Xu, Y., Gidlund, M., & Nohr, R. (2008, August). An experimental study on home-wireless passive positioning. In *Sensor Technologies and Applications, 2008. SENSORCOMM'08. Second International Conference on* (pp. 223-228). IEEE.

Zhou, X., & Tang, X. (2011, August). Research and implementation of RSA algorithm for encryption and decryption. *Strategic Technology (IFOST), 2011 6th International Forum on, 2,* 1118–1121.

Zia, T., & Zomaya, A. (2006, October). Security issues in wireless sensor networks. In Null (p. 40). IEEE. doi:10.1109/ICSNC.2006.66

Chapter 6
Medical Data Security Tools and Techniques in E–Health Applications

Anukul Pandey
https://orcid.org/0000-0003-2737-112X
Dumka Engineering College, India

Butta Singh
Guru Nanak Dev University, India

Barjinder Singh Saini
Dr. B. R. Ambedkar National Institute of Technology, India

Neetu Sood
Dr. B. R. Ambedkar National Institute of Technology, India

ABSTRACT

The primary objective of this chapter is to analyze the existing tools and techniques for medical data security. Typically, medical data includes either medical signals such as electrocardiogram, electro-encephalogram, electromyography, or medical imaging like digital imaging and communications in medicine, joint photographic experts group format. The medical data are sensitive, subject to privacy preservation, and data access rights. Security in e-health field is an integrated concept which includes robust combination of confidentiality, integrity, and availability of medical data. Confidentiality ensures the data is inaccessible to unauthorized access. Integrity restricts the alteration in data by the unauthorized user. Whereas availability provides the readiness of the data when needed by the authorized user. Additionally, confidentiality, integrity and availability, accountability parameter records the back action list which answers the why, when, what, and whom data is accessed. The selected tools and techniques used in medical data security in e-health applications is discussed.

DOI: 10.4018/978-1-5225-7952-6.ch006

INTRODUCTION

With the progressions in information and communication technologies (ICT) has unlocked fresher prospects for telemedicine(Ingenerf, 1999; Pattichis et al., 2002) by enabling medical data accessibility across geographical boundaries through Internet, mobile links, and other wireless/wired communication channels and thus covering rural/remote areas, accident sites, ambulance, and hospitals for e-health applications(Silva, Rodrigues, Canelo, Lopes, & Lloret, 2014). The histrionic expansion of contemporary communication technologies, the security of medical information has become an essential topic when it is transferred or deposited over open channels(Society, 1996).

Medical Data Security

Medical data attributes to the health-pertained information in association with the clinical trial program either in form of reports/signal/image(Hossain & Chellappan, 2014; Lu, Wu, Liu, Chen, & Guo, 2013; Yachana, Kaur, & Sood, 2017). Medical data also referred to as personal health information, commonly refers to geographic information, medical antiquities, assessment and laboratory results, mental/physical health situations, insurance information, and other data that a healthcare specialized gathers to classify an individual and govern suitable care. Medical data security is needed in e-health management framework due to essentially i) Medical data is having the capacity to reveal identity information, ii) prevent medical data tempering, which may mislead clinical diagnosis(A. Pandey, Saini, Singh, & Sood, 2017; Anukul Pandey, Saini, Singh, & Sood, 2018; Anukul Pandey, Singh, Saini, & Sood, 2016).

A patient privacy protection scheme for medical information system (Lu et al., 2013) is explored for the construction of the index of privacy data, and translation into a new query over the corresponding index for a query operation over privacy data so that it can be performed at the server side instantly. Prior to database storage at the server side of a medical information system, patient's privacy data being first encrypted to prevent the leakage of patient's private information caused internal staff. Based on millions of tuples of privacy fields experimental evaluation validate the effectiveness of patient privacy protection scheme.

MEDICAL DATA SECURITY TOOLS

FireHost

Texas-based FireHost is a cloud based Compliance as a Service (CaaS). The FireHost supplies CaaS with safeguarding the secret data and guaranteeing the necessities as documented in HIPAA. The multiple security yields are reduced by the FireHost (Chris Paoli, 2014).

FireLayers

FireLayers prevent unauthorized access with its new security access application for apps running in the cloud that offers surplus protection and monitoring. The FireLayers app security includes a dominant console with administrators control over guidelines, authorizations and admittance. FireLayers demonstrations recognized threats and employ rules to kiosk them and reports the precise limitations (Chris Paoli, 2014).

NetApp Storage Tool

Data security can be enhanced by storing the PHI at the known location. For doing so, NetApp storage tool offers monitoring tools in which PHI can be tracked based on the movement observed in PHI. This storage management tool observes massive amounts of unclassified information and keep it constant with identical security levels extended to confidential enterprise information. Automatic encoding and access management capabilities restrict unauthorized access and information leak. The NetApp Storage incorporates geo-distributed abrasion cryptography, in which information is fragmented and encoded with tautological information items and keep over multiple datacenters, guaranteeing that if there's a rupture, information can keep protected (Chris Paoli, 2014).

CloudFlare

CloudFlare providing denial-of-service attacks to the Websites hosted in its service. CloudFlare, offers keyless secure sockets sayer feature permits firms to permit their encrypted information to travel through the CloudFlare network while not redeeming the keys to the information. keyless SSL is presently solely offered through the CloudFlare net protection service (Chris Paoli, 2014).

SharePlan for Enterprises Code 42 Software Inc.

SharePlan for projects/industry/enterprise keep documents related data protected and encrypted while enabling for comfortable data access, whether on-premises or cloud (Chris Paoli, 2014).

MEDICAL DATA SECURITY TECHNIQUES

Efficient medical information access in electronic arrangement is vital in improving the superiority and efficacy of healthcare establishment. Health-care services in distant regions by communication network needs the patient information security. As the communication network is an open platform for transmission and reception of the information which is vulnerable to unauthorized accessed. Consequently, privacy or security to the information can be enabled by the several encryption and steganography techniques.

Medical Data Encryption

Medical encryption is an crucial contrivance to keep the secret patient data safe. Pseudorandom permutation image encryption algorithm (Yoon & Kim, 2010) is combinatorial generated from small permutation matrices based on chaotic plots. The random-like nature of chaos is effectively spread into encrypted images by using the permutation matrix. The proposed method used the security measures such as histogram and correlation coefficients for comparison with Baker chaotic map and Logistic chaotic map based encryption mechanism.

Compression and encryption of ECG signal using wavelet and chaotically huffman code (Raeiat-ibanadkooki, Quchani, KhalilZade, & Bahaadinbeigy, 2016) pre-process to remove the noise and detect the ECG features, then ECG signal is compressed. At compression stage, wavelet transform and thresholding are used. Afterwards, Huffman coding with chaos is further used for compression and encryption of the ECG signal.

Chaos based crossover and mutation for securing DICOM image is proposed (Ravichandran, Praveenkumar, Balaguru Rayappan, & Amirtharajan, 2016) to ensure the safe storage and transmission of medical images. This approach utilized the chao-cryptic system that confuse and diffuse the DICOM image pixels by employing crossover and mutation. This approach achieved DICOM cryptosystem with desirable amount of protection for medical image security applications.

ECG data encryption then compression using singular value decomposition(Liu, Lin, & Wu, 2017) protect ECG data privacy and provide the good quality of the reconstructed signals without losing the compression efficacy compared to unencrypted ECG data compressions.

Medical Data Steganography

Hiding patients confidential data in the ECG signal via transform-domain quantization scheme(Chen et al., 2014) shows that watermarking technique based on three transform domains, DWT,DCT, and DFT are adopted. the proposed watermarking scheme is blind due to the change in the ECG features PQRST complexes and amplitude is very small.

chaotic map & sample value difference method for electrocardiogram steganography (A. Pandey et al., 2017) The sample value difference approach successfully hides the patient's confidential data in ECG sample pairs at the chaotically defined locations. The chaotic map creates these predefined locations through the use of selective control parameters.

ECG steganography using curvelet transform (Edward Jero, Ramu, & Ramakrishnan, 2015) provides adaptive selection of watermark location and a new threshold selection algorithm.

Binary-block embedding for reversible data hiding (Shuang & Zhou, 2017) embed binary bits in lower bit-planes of the original image into its higher bit-planes. A bit-level scrambling process after secret data embedding to spread embedded secret data to the entire marked encrypted image to avert secret data loss. Security analysis has demonstrated the robustness of binary-block embedding approach in contrast to various attacks.

IMPROVISE THE MEDICAL DATA SECURITY

Assessment of Security Risk

As per requirement of the Health Insurance Portability and Accountability Act (HIPAA) security precept, security prospect assessments must be conducted annually to suffice the principles of the significant use Electronic Health Records (EHR) stimulus program. Exercises might have to purchase software to enhance their EHR's security mechanisms, which may comprise only some aspects of medical data security ("10 ways to improve patient data security," 2017).

Medical Data Encryption

Under the HIPAA security precept, inpatient data should be encrypted whenever viable. Any prevailing certified EHR can accomplish this job. encryption is essential practices should not rely on this strategy solely or on different technological predicaments such as antivirus and firewalls to shield the secrecy and preservation of secret information. The limitation of encryption methodologies is that it relies on shielding admittance to the system. The stolen passwords can access secret data irrespective of the encryption mechanism. Several practices would steal Protected Health Information (PHI), they could unconsciously inject malware.

Control Access

Access control is a fundamental ingredient of medical data security appropriates distinct configurations depending on a practice's network and how its EHR and patients information administration system are treated. EHR merchants configure the security characteristics for their efficient medical data management to have access control. If personage takes a password, or if malware activated on the network, then medical data security is in danger of unauthorized control access.

Users Authentication

A login ID and a password based EHRs authentication of users are common practice in healthcare management system. Frequent change in passwords may improvise the medical data security eco system which protects unauthorized access to preserve PHI. To withstand the brute force attack two-stage authentication perform better by use of coupling the password with biometric identification or enabled by one-time password responded through users mobile.

Secure Remote Access

Healthcare service providers may require remote access to patient medical information to process the work. Possible malware contamination of medical data access computer is being coupled with a robust firewall and secure antivirus and intrusion detection software will support to keep secret remote access. Cybercriminals can, however, withdraw data during remote user access sessions with the insecure communication network. To counteract this, virtual private network that encrypts the information in transition and leaves after initiated session completion. A virtual private network is a protected, temporary association but need somebody with subtle technical skill to construct and use.

Access Role

EHRs enabled healthcare management practices to configure their software to limit different levels of access role control of the system to representatives that require to use a particular portion of the statement and inspect and analyze the connected data. This strategy helps preserve secrecy and restrict the use of PHI to perpetrate impostor. In addition, if a healthcare management's password is taken and that representative has limited access to the EHR, which restricts the damage.

Restricted Data Storage on Local Devices

But ingesting so executes the secret information further exposed to hackers. Therefore, Restricted data storage on local devices of PHI on the local storage unit. Centralized accommodation of PHI on a server is competent, with proper educated and trained staff handle this server. If the representatives aren't conscious of the consequence of PHI which is being incorporated, then there is possible leaking of the PHI. Erase medical information on those devices after used locally with have a copy on the centralized server.

Audit Logs Usage and Scanning

All health care management system must have audit logs which register users medically related transactions with time logs. Yet, health care management usually doesn't scan those audit logs on or configure them accurately. Activation and configuration of audit logs should be carried out frequently by healthcare management system by use of automatic scanning of audit logs and detection of irregularities which indicate possible a cyber attack, unauthorized user logging.

Back Up for Security Purposes

Practices that use a client-server scheme should have onsite backup, such as a mirrored server that can replace the main server any failure happens. Furthermore, each module must have proper backups for security purposes. A cloud-based EHR vendor should have back up EHR data. Practices that have client-server systems should back up their data on offline storage device and daily move it to offsite. It's vital to keep these backups offline in a circumstance on hacker takes control over the network. Also, backups should be encrypted. Else, a lost backup storage device is reflected a security gap under HIPAA.

STRENGTH AND WEAKNESS OF THE STUDY

The strength of the present chapter is it reports essential Medical Data Security Tools: *FireHost, FireLayers, NetApp* Storage GRID Webscale, *CloudFlare and Code 42 Software* and Techniques Encryption and steganography. Whereas, the chapter weakness is that the presented tools and techniques perhaps could not sustenance real time-bound amenities.

CONCLUSION

In this chapter, medical data security tools and techniques in e-health applications is being discussed. The medical data security tools such as *FireHost, FireLayers, NetApp* Storage GRID Webscale, *CloudFlare and Code 42 Software* provide promising solutions. The medical data security techniques including medical data encryption and steganography reports the state-of-art methods to secure the medical data. Furthermore, this chapter includes the main ways to improve medical data security norms by use of encryption, use of control system access, authenticate users periodically, provide remote access securely, adopt role-based access, Don't store data on user devices, Use and scan audit logs, and Back up data off site.

REFERENCES

Chen, S.-T. T., Guo, Y.-J. J., Huang, H.-N. N., Kung, W.-M. M., Tseng, K.-K. K., & Tu, S.-Y. Y. (2014). Hiding patients confidential data in the ECG signal viaa transform-domain quantization scheme. *Journal of Medical Systems*, *38*(6), 54. doi:10.100710916-014-0054-9 PMID:24832688

Edward Jero, S., Ramu, P., & Ramakrishnan, S. (2015). ECG steganography using curvelet transform. *Biomedical Signal Processing and Control*, *22*, 161–169. doi:10.1016/j.bspc.2015.07.004

Hossain, I., & Chellappan, K. (2014). Collaborative Compressed I-Cloud Medical Image Storage with Decompress Viewer. *Procedia Computer Science*, *42*, 114–121. doi:10.1016/j.procs.2014.11.041

Ingenerf, J. (1999). Telemedicine and Terminology. *Different Needs of Context Information*, *3*(2), 92–100. PMID:10719490

Liu, T. Y., Lin, K. J., & Wu, H. C. (2017). ECG data encryption then compression using singular value decomposition. *IEEE Journal of Biomedical and Health Informatics*, *22*(3), 707–713. doi:10.1109/JBHI.2017.2698498 PMID:28463208

Lu, C., Wu, Z., Liu, M., Chen, W., & Guo, J. (2013). A patient privacy protection scheme for medical information system. *Journal of Medical Systems*, *37*(6), 1–10. doi:10.100710916-013-9982-z PMID:24166018

Pandey, A., Saini, B. S., Singh, B., & Sood, N. (2017). An integrated approach using chaotic map & sample value difference method for electrocardiogram steganography and OFDM based secured patient information transmission. *Journal of Medical Systems*, *41*(12), 1–20. doi:10.100710916-017-0830-4 PMID:29043502

Pandey, A., Saini, B. S., Singh, B., & Sood, N. (2018). Complexity sorting and coupled chaotic map based on 2D ECG data compression-then-encryption and its OFDM transmission with impair sample correction. *Multimedia Tools and Applications*. doi:10.100711042-018-6681-2

Pandey, A., Singh, B., Saini, B. S., & Sood, N. (2016). A joint application of optimal threshold based discrete cosine transform and ASCII encoding for ECG data compression with its inherent encryption. *Australasian Physical & Engineering Sciences in Medicine*, *39*(4), 833–855. doi:10.100713246-016-0476-4 PMID:27613706

Paoli, C. (2014). 6 Security Tools To Protect Enterprise Data. *Redmond Magazine*. Retrieved November 19, 2018, from https://redmondmag.com/articles/2014/11/01/security-tools.aspx

Pattichis, C. S., Kyriacou, E., Voskarides, S., Pattichis, M. S., Istepanian, R., & Schizas, C. N. (2002). Wireless telemedicine systems: An overview. *IEEE Antennas & Propagation Magazine*, *44*(2), 143–153. doi:10.1109/MAP.2002.1003651

Raeiatibanadkooki, M., Quchani, S. R., KhalilZade, M. M., & Bahaadinbeigy, K. (2016). Compression and encryption of ECG signal using wavelet and chaotically huffman code in telemedicine application. *Journal of Medical Systems*, *40*(3), 1–8. doi:10.100710916-016-0433-5 PMID:26779641

Ravichandran, D., Praveenkumar, P., Balaguru Rayappan, J. B., & Amirtharajan, R. (2016). Chaos based crossover and mutation for securing DICOM image. *Computers in Biology and Medicine, 72*, 170–184. doi:10.1016/j.compbiomed.2016.03.020 PMID:27046666

Shuang, Y., & Zhou, Y. (2017). Binary-block embedding for reversible data hiding in encrypted images. *Signal Processing, 133*, 40–51. doi:10.1007/SpringerReference_24796

Silva, B. M. C., Rodrigues, J. J. P. C., Canelo, F., Lopes, I. M. C., & Lloret, J. (2014). Towards a cooperative security system for mobile-health applications. *Electronic Commerce Research*, (1). doi:10.100710660-014-9171-2

Society, B. (1996). *IEEE Standard for Medical Device Communications — Overview and Framework.* IEEE.

10 . ways to improve patient data security. (2017). *Medical Economics.* Retrieved October 12, 2018, from http://www.medicaleconomics.com/e-h-r/10-ways-improve-patient-data-security

Yachana, K. N., & Sood, S. K. (2017). A trustworthy system for secure access to patient centric sensitive information. *Telematics and Informatics.* doi:10.1016/j.tele.2017.09.008

Yoon, J. W., & Kim, H. (2010). An image encryption scheme with a pseudorandom permutation based on chaotic maps. *Communications in Nonlinear Science and Numerical Simulation, 15*(12), 3998–4006. doi:10.1016/j.cnsns.2010.01.041

KEY TERMS AND DEFINITIONS

Cryptography: The transformation of secret data into codes for transmission over a communication network to restrain unauthorized access.

Data Accountability: The ability to identify all the amendments made to the data.

Data Availability: The ability to ensure the data readiness when needed.

Data Confidentiality: The ability to ensure that data is accessible to the authorized user only.

Data Encryption: It is a process of scrambling the data prior to the secret communication to ensure that it is not being intercepted by an unauthorized user.

Data Integrity: The ability to restrain the data from being altered by unauthorized user.

Data Privacy: The control or authority of what information related to data can be disclosed by whom and to whom it can be disclosed.

Data Security: It is the combination of procedure, processes, and systems used to attain the fulfilment of data confidentiality, accountability, integrity, and availability as needed.

Steganography: The hiding of a secret message within a cover data and the extraction of secret message at its terminus.

Telemedicine: The delivery of healthcare support systems at a distance using communication channels.

Chapter 7
Electrocardiogram Beat Classification Using BAT-Optimized Fuzzy KNN Classifier

Atul Kumar Verma
Dr. B. R. Ambedkar National Institute of Technology, India

Indu Saini
Dr. B. R. Ambedkar National Institute of Technology, India

Barjinder Singh Saini
Dr. B. R. Ambedkar National Institute of Technology, India

ABSTRACT

In this chapter, the BAT-optimized fuzzy k-nearest neighbor (FKNN-BAT) algorithm is proposed for discrimination of the electrocardiogram (ECG) beats. The five types of beats (i.e., normal [N], right bundle block branch [RBBB], left bundle block branch [LBBB], atrial premature contraction [APC], and premature ventricular contraction [PVC]) are taken from MIT-BIH arrhythmia database for the experimentation. Thereafter, the features are extracted from five type of beats and fed to the proposed BAT-tuned fuzzy KNN classifier. The proposed classifier achieves the overall accuracy of 99.88%.

INTRODUCTION

Electrocardiogram (ECG) provides detailed information of cardiac heart activities and important procedure to diagnose conduction dysfunction and cardiac arrhythmias. The feature extraction and classification steps are crucial in such diagnosis. The arrhythmic ECG signal contains different arrhythmic beats which can classify using the classification system. In the classification system, the segmented ECG beats are denoised, then features are extracted and finally classify them in the different classes. There are various methods for the classification of the ECG beats (Lagerholm et al. 2000; Prasad and Sahambi 2003; Osowski et al. 2004; Rodriguez et al. 2005; Alickovic and Subasi 2016). Many techniques are developed in the literature for the extraction of the ECG features (Prasad and Sahambi 2003; Alickovic

DOI: 10.4018/978-1-5225-7952-6.ch007

and Subasi 2016). However, the selection of the more robust and efficient classifier for the ECG beats discrimination is a still pending work. So, various classification techniques existing in the literature are concentrated on the classifier performance. The work by (Lagerholm et al. 2000) which uses the self-organizing neural networks with the hermite function encoding and the dynamic interval information as an extracted feature. The sixteen beats of arrhythmia taken from MIT-BIH are obtained an overall accuracy of 98.49%. In (Prasad and Sahambi 2003), the dynamic interval features with the wavelet transform are used as a input feature and fed to the neural network classifier. The experimentation is done on the thirteen MIT-BIH beats and achieves the overall accuracy of 96.77%. In (Osowski et al. 2004), the cumulants of the second, third, and fourth orders with the hermite function encoding are used a feature vector and fed the Support Vector Machine (SVM) classifier achieves an overall accuracy of 98.18%. In (Rodriguez et al. 2005), morphological features are fed to the decision tree for the characterization of the fourteen ECG beats and attain an overall accuracy of 96.13%. In (Alickovic and Subasi 2016), the statistical features for each wavelet coefficients are evaluated and combined with the ratio of the absolute mean values of adjacent sub-bands to fed on the random forest classifier for the characterization of Normal (N), Right Bundle Block Branch (RBBB), Left Bundle Block Branch (LBBB) Atrial Premature Contraction (APC), and Premature Ventricular Contraction (PVC) beats. The average accuracy is achieved as 99.30%. In (Melgani et al. 2008), the authors fed the combined morphological and temporal features to the particle swarm optimization (PSO) tuned SVM classifier for the ECG beat characterization. The kernel parameter γ, and regularization parameter C of the SVM classifier are tuned in such a manner to obtain the maximal discrimination of the beats. The experimentation is done on the six beat types, i.e., N, APC, PVC, RBBB, LBBB, paced beat and obtained an overall accuracy of 89.72%. In (Korurek and Dogan 2010), the authors fed the morphological features to the PSO tuned radial basis function (RBF) neural network for beats classification. The parameters of the RBFNN, i.e., bandwidth σ, center c of the neurons are tuned in such a manner that achieves the maximal discrimination of the heartbeats. The six beats such as N, APC, PVC, RBBB, Fusion of Ventricular and Normal beat, Fusion of Paced and normal beat are used for the experimentation and obtained an average sensitivity of 95.46%. In (Khazaee and Ebrahimzadeh 2010), the authors fed the power spectral, and timing features to the genetic algorithm (GA) tuned SVM classifier. The SVM parameters such as C, γ are optimized by the GA optimization algorithm to attain the maximum discrimination of the beats and obtained an overall accuracy of 96.00% when experimented on N, LBBB, RBBB, APC, and PVC beats.

The limitations of the above methods are that, these methods not effectively classify the beats due to which the classification performance measure not obtain optimal value and the designed methods are not optimal one which gives better characterization results. To overcome the limitation of the existing methods, a new beat classification method is proposed. The objective of the paper is to design a classification approach which utilizes the BAT tuned fuzzy k-nearest neighbor (FKNN) classifier for ECG arrhythmia characterization. In this work, the four RR interval features are extracted from the segmented heartbeats and then, obtained feature vector is fed to the designed FKNN-BAT classifier for the discrimination of the ECG heartbeats. In the designed FKNN-BAT classifier, the overall classification accuracy is depending on the two FKNN tuning parameters which are the number of nearest neighbor (k), and constant parameter (m). To achieve beat characterization of the ECG beats, the two FKNN parameters are optimized using the BAT optimization algorithm.

The rest of the chapter is organized as: Section 2 describes the mathematical background behind the designing of the proposed classification system. The analysis and comparison of the proposed method with the existing methods of the literature is explained in Section 3. Finally, Section 4 ends with the conclusion.

MATHEMATICAL BACKGROUND

Fuzzy k-Nearest Neighbor (FKNN)

The fuzzy *k*-nearest neighbor algorithm (Keller et al. 1985) assigns class membership to a sample vector rather than assigning the vector to a particular class. The values of the membership should provide a level of assurance to accompany the resultant classification. The FKNN algorithm is to assign membership as a function of the vector distance from its *k*-NN and those neighbors memberships in the possible classes. Let $S = \{x_1, x_2, x_3, \ldots x_m\}$ be the vector of *m* labeled samples and $u_i(x)$ is the membership of the vector *x*. The membership of the ith class of the jth vector of the labeled sample set. The fuzzy membership function $u_i(x)$ is mathematically defined as (Keller et al. 1985):

$$u_i(x) = \frac{\sum_{j=1}^{k} u_{i,j}\left(1/\left\|x - x_j\right\|^{2/(m-1)}\right)}{\sum_{j=1}^{k}\left(1/\left\|x - x_j\right\|^{2/(m-1)}\right)} \tag{1}$$

where, *k* is the number of nearest neighbor, and *m* is a constant parameter which determines the weight of each nearest neighbor in the computation of the fuzzy membership. The fuzzy membership of *x* is affected by the inverse of the distance from the nearest neighbors and their class membership. The inverse of the distance is used to weight the vector of the membership. The pseudo code of the FKNN algorithm follows as (Keller et al. 1985):

```
BEGIN
Input x, of the unknown classification
Set k, 1 ≤ k ≤ n
Initialize i=1.
DO UNTIL (k-nearest neighbors to x found)
Evaluate distance from x to xᵢ
IF (i ≤ k) THEN
Include xᵢ in the set of k-NNs
ELSE IF (xᵢ closer to x than any previous nearest neighbor) THEN
Delete the farthest of the k- nearest neighbors
Include xᵢ in the set of k-nearest neighbors
END IF
END DO UNTIL
Initialize i=1
```

```
DO UNTIL (x assigned membership in all classes)
Compute  u_i(x) from (1)
Increment i
END DO UNTIL
END
```

BAT Algorithm

A metaheuristic optimization algorithm was named as BAT which was a bat-inspired algorithm developed by Yang (Yang 2010). The BAT algorithm is based on the echolocation of micro-bats. The echolocation characteristics of bats are estimated as rules given in (Yang 2010). The velocity v_i^{t-1} and position x_i^{t-1} for each bats (assume *i*) are updated on the basis of the movement of the bats in d -dimensional search space. The updated instantaneous frequency f_i, position x_i^t, and velocity v_i^t at time step *t* are mathematically written as

$$f_i = f_{min} + (f_{max} - f_{min})\alpha \qquad (2)$$

$$x_i^t = x_i^{t-1} + v_i^t \qquad (3)$$

$$v_i^t = v_i^{t-1} + (x_i^t - x^*)f_i \qquad (4)$$

here, $\alpha \in [0,1]$ is a random vector drawn from a uniform distribution, $x*$ is the current global best location obtained after comparing all the solutions among all the *n* bats at the current iteration and the frequencies f_{min}, f_{max} are depends on the domain size of the problem of interest. After the selection of the current best solution from the local search part, a new solution for each bat is generated locally using random walk. The new position, pulse rate, and loudness are denoted by x_{new}, r_i, A_i respectively updated as,

$$x_{new} = x_{old} + \varepsilon A^t \qquad (5)$$

$$A_i^{t+1} = \beta A_i^t \qquad (6)$$

$$r_i^{t+1} = r_i^0[1 - \exp(-\gamma t)] \qquad (7)$$

where $\varepsilon \in [-1,1]$ is a random number, A^t is the average loudness of all the bats at time step t, β is the pulse frequency increasing coefficient (typically $0 < \beta < 1$), γ is the pulse amplitude attenuation coefficient ($\gamma > 0$), r_i^0 is the initial emission rate (typically from 0 to 1), and x_{old} is the solution in the current optimization solution set. When the bats are moving towards the optimal solution the emission rates and loudness (4), (6) and (7) are then updated. The BAT initialized values as population size=30, loudness=0.2, emitting sound pulse rate=0.4, minimum frequency=0, maximum frequency=2, and no. of generation of bats=10.

ANALYSIS AND COMPARISON

The ECG signals contains various types of noises (Khaing, A. S., & Naing 2011) such as electrode movements, muscle contraction, power-line interference, and baseline noises which can disturb the fiducial point detection of the ECG signal. To overcome this, the artifacts by the noise is reduced. The ECG filtering is crucial to reduce various noises, such as artifacts due to baseline using wavelet-based denoising technique (Singh and Tiwari 2006), (Addison 2005). After that, the heartbeat segmentation which normally needs peak position of the R wave. The peak positions of heartbeat segments are obtained by utilizing the annotations of beat positions given in the MIT-BIH arrhythmia database which is most prominent for the heartbeat segmentation. After obtaining the R peak positions, the heartbeats are fragments by taking the average of the RR intervals. Thereafter, the four RR-interval features explained in subsection 3.1 are extracted from the segmented heartbeats. A MIT-BIH arrhythmia records used in this work. The five types of beats which are N, RBBB, LBBB, APC and PVC are used in this study and the training as well as testing beats are presented in *Table 1*.

Feature Extraction

In this study, the RR-interval feature is computed to gather the dynamic characteristic of the cardiac heartbeats. The four RR interval are calculated that correspond to the pattern of cardiac signals which are listed below as:

Table 1. MIT-BIH records beat types with the testing and training samples are used in this study

Type of Beat	MIT-BIH Arrhythmia Data	Training Beats	Testing Beats	Total Beats
N	100, 101, 103, 105, 108, 113, 115, 117, 121, 123	5828	5827	11655
RBBB	118, 124, 212, 231	500	500	1000
LBBB	109, 111, 207, 214	500	500	1000
APC	118, 207, 220, 222, 232	718	718	1436
PVC	106, 114, 116, 119, 124, 201, 203, 214, 215, 219, 221, 228	1504	1504	3008
Total		9050	9049	18099

1. Previous RR (Pre_RR): It is defined as the distance between a given beat location and the previous beat location given as (Jung and Lee 2017),

$$Pre\_RR = R_i - R_{i-1} \tag{8}$$

2. Post RR ($Post\_RR$): It is the distance between a given beat location and the following beat location as (Jung and Lee 2017),

$$Post\_RR = R_{i+1} - R_i \tag{9}$$

3. Ratio of Pre to Post RR (Pre_post_ratio): It is defined as the ratio of the Pre_RR and $Post\_RR$ intervals as (Jung and Lee 2017),

$$Pre\_post\_ratio = \frac{Pre\_RR}{Post\_RR} \tag{10}$$

4. Ratio of Post to Pre RR ($Post\_pre\_ratio$): It is defined as the ratio of the $Post\_RR$ and Pre_RR intervals (Jung and Lee 2017),

$$Post\_pre\_ratio = \frac{Post\_RR}{Pre\_RR} \tag{11}$$

The features explained in (8), (9), (10), and (11) are extracted from each of the heartbeat and combines to develop a new feature vector.

Classification

The new feature vector is used as an input to the FKNN classifier for the ECG heartbeat classification. The parameters k, m of the FKNN classifier needs to be optimized for the efficient classification of the five types of beats which are N, LBBB, RBBB, APC, and PVC. The BAT optimization algorithm is used in this study to optimized the parameters of the FKNN classifier. The performance of the classification approach can be evaluated by the performance measures which are Positive predictivity (Pp), Specificity (Sp), Sensitivity (Se), and overall Accuracy (Acc) can be defined as in [2]

$$Pp = \frac{TP}{TP + FP} \times 100 \tag{12}$$

$$Sp = \frac{TN}{TN + FP} \times 100 \tag{13}$$

$$Se = \frac{TP}{TP + FN} \times 100 \tag{14}$$

$$Acc = \frac{TP + TN}{TP + TN + FP + FN} \times 100 \tag{15}$$

where FN, FP, TN, and TP denote the false negative, false positive, true negative, and true positive respectively.

The confusion matrix for the five beats using the proposed classification approach with the optimized values of k, m of FKNN classifier are 3, and 30 respectively presented in *Table 2*.

The classification performance metrics are to be evaluated and presented in *Table 2*. The classification results are showed in terms of the classification performance measures and presented in *Table 3*.

The steps of proposed classification system are summarized as:

Step 1: The raw ECG data is taken from MIT-BIH arrhythmia database and denoised using wavelet approach.

Table 2. Confusion matrix of beats using the proposed classification technique

		Predicted Labels				
		N	LBBB	RBBB	APC	PVC
Reference	N	5827	0	0	0	0
	LBBB	0	500	0	0	0
	RBBB	0	0	500	0	0
	APC	0	0	0	717	10
	PVC	0	0	0	1	1494

Table 3. The results for classification of beats using proposed classification technique

Heartbeat Types	Test	Train	Total	TP	FP	FN	Se (%)	Pp (%)	Sp (%)
N	5827	5828	11655	5827	0	0	100	100	100
LBBB	500	500	1000	500	0	0	100	100	100
RBBB	500	500	1000	500	0	0	100	100	100
APC	718	718	1436	717	10	1	99.861	99.88	98.624
PVC	1504	1504	3008	1494	1	10	99.335	99.987	99.933
Total	9049	9050	18099				**99.878**	**99.878**	**99.97**

Step 2: After denoising, the data is segmented into the heartbeats by taking the average of the RR intervals.

Step 3: The four RR interval features are extracted from segmented ECG beats.

Step 4: The designed FKNN-BAT classifier in which the two tuning parameters, i.e., number of nearest neighbor (k), and constant parameter (m) of FKNN classifier are optimized by the BAT algorithm.

Step 5: The extracted feature vector set is fed to the proposed classifier for the efficient discrimination of the arrhythmia.

The flowchart of the proposed classification system is shown in *Fig.1*.

Comparison

In present work, the proposed ECG classification approach efficiently discriminate the five types of beats. The MIT-BIH arrhythmia database used in the present work. The new feature vector contains four RR interval features are computed from each of the segmented heartbeats. Thereafter, the new feature vector is fed to the proposed FKNN classifier which provides maximum classification accuracy compared to the other classification approaches in the literature tabulated in *Table 4*. The comparative results of the classification accuracy using the existing and the proposed classification approach are presented in *Table 4*.

Figure 1. Flowchart of the proposed classification system

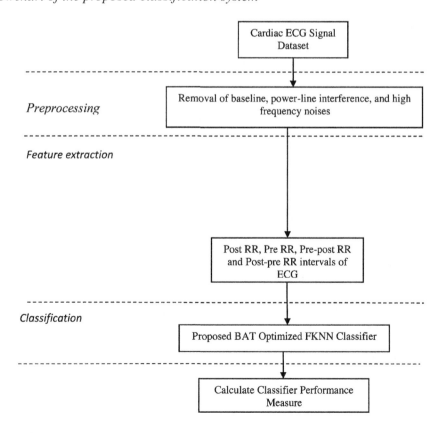

Table 4. Comparative results of classifier accuracy for existing and proposed classification technique

Reference	No. of Beats	Techniques	Acc (%)	Computational Time Required (s)
(Elhaj et al. 2016)	5	WT + PCA	98.91	-
(Martis et al. 2011)	5	PCA + SVM	93.48	-
(Li et al. 2014)	5	Features + SVM	98.60	-
(Li, H., Liang, H., Miao, C., Cao, L., Feng, X., Tang, C., & Li 2016)	5	PCA-KICA features + LIBSVM-GA	97.78	-
(Khazaee and Ebrahimzadeh 2010)	5	Power spectral features + SVM-GA	96.00	19321
Proposed	**5**	**Dynamic time domain features + FKNN-BAT**	**99.88**	**14210**

CONCLUSION

The present chapter motivated to design a BAT tuned FKNN classifier for discrimination of the arrhythmic beats. The four dynamic time domain features are evaluated from the segmented ECG heartbeat and then fed to the FKNN-BAT optimized classifier. The experimental results demonstrate that the designed ECG beats characterization method is superior as compared with the other existing techniques for the beats classification.

REFERENCES

Addison, P. S. (2005). Wavelet transforms and the ECG: A review. *Physiological Measurement*, *26*(5), R155–R199. doi:10.1088/0967-3334/26/5/R01 PMID:16088052

Alickovic, E., & Subasi, A. (2016). Medical decision support system for diagnosis of heart arrhythmia using DWT and random forests classifier. *Journal of Medical Systems*, *40*(4), 108. doi:10.100710916-016-0467-8 PMID:26922592

Elhaj, F. A., Salim, N., Harris, A. R., Swee, T. T., & Ahmed, T. (2016). Arrhythmia recognition and classification using combined linear and nonlinear features of ECG signals. *Computer Methods and Programs in Biomedicine*, *127*, 52–63. doi:10.1016/j.cmpb.2015.12.024 PMID:27000289

Jung, W-H., & Lee, S-G. (2017). *An Arrhythmia Classification Method in Utilizing the Weighted KNN and the Fitness Rule*. Academic Press.

Keller, J. M., Gray, M. R., & Givens, J. A. (1985). A fuzzy k-nearest neighbor algorithm. *IEEE Transactions on Systems, Man, and Cybernetics*, *SMC-15*(4), 580–585. doi:10.1109/TSMC.1985.6313426

Khaing, A. S., & Naing, Z. M. (2011). Quantitative Investigation of Digital Filters in Electrocardiogram with Simulated Noises. *Int J Inf Electron Eng*, *1*, 210.

Khazaee, A., & Ebrahimzadeh, A. (2010). Classification of electrocardiogram signals with support vector machines and genetic algorithms using power spectral features. *Biomedical Signal Processing and Control*, *5*(4), 252–263. doi:10.1016/j.bspc.2010.07.006

Korurek, M., & Dogan, B. (2010). ECG beat classification using particle swarm optimization and radial basis function neural network. *Expert Systems with Applications*, *37*(12), 7563–7569. doi:10.1016/j.eswa.2010.04.087

Lagerholm, M., Peterson, C., Braccini, G., Edenbrandt, L., & Sornmo, L. (2000). Clustering ECG complexes using Hermite functions and self-organizing maps. *IEEE Transactions on Biomedical Engineering*, *47*(7), 838–848. doi:10.1109/10.846677 PMID:10916254

Li, H., Liang, H., Miao, C., Cao, L., Feng, X., Tang, C., & Li, E. (2016). Novel ECG Signal Classification Based on KICA Nonlinear Feature Extraction. *Circuits, Systems, and Signal Processing*, *35*(4), 1187–1197. doi:10.100700034-015-0108-3

Li, Q., Rajagopalan, C., & Clifford, G. D. (2014). A machine learning approach to multi-level ECG signal quality classification. *Computer Methods and Programs in Biomedicine*, *117*(3), 435–447. doi:10.1016/j.cmpb.2014.09.002 PMID:25306242

Martis, R. J., Acharya, U. R., Ray, A. K., & Chakraborty, C. (2011). Application of higher order cumulants to ECG signals for the cardiac health diagnosis. Engineering in medicine and biology society, 1697–1700. doi:10.1109/IEMBS.2011.6090487

Melgani, F., Member, S., & Bazi, Y. (2008). Classification of Electrocardiogram Signals With Support Vector Machines and Particle Swarm Optimization. *IEEE Transactions on Information Technology in Biomedicine*, *12*(5), 667–677. doi:10.1109/TITB.2008.923147 PMID:18779082

Osowski, S., Hoai, L. T., & Markiewicz, T. (2004). Support vector machine-based expert system for reliable heartbeat recognition. *IEEE Transactions on Biomedical Engineering*, *51*(4), 582–589. doi:10.1109/TBME.2004.824138 PMID:15072212

Prasad, G. K., & Sahambi, J. S. (2003). Classification of ECG arrhythmias using multi-resolution analysis and neural networks. *TENCON 2003. Conference on Convergent Technologies for the Asia-Pacific Region*, 227–231. 10.1109/TENCON.2003.1273320

Rodriguez, J., Goni, A., & Illarramendi, A. (2005). Real-time classification of ECGs on a PDA. *IEEE Transactions on Information Technology in Biomedicine*, *9*(1), 23–34. doi:10.1109/TITB.2004.838369 PMID:15787004

Singh, B. N., & Tiwari, A. K. (2006). Optimal selection of wavelet basis function applied to ECG signal denoising. *Digital Signal Processing*, *16*(3), 275–287. doi:10.1016/j.dsp.2005.12.003

Yang, X. S. (2010). A new metaheuristic bat-inspired algorithm. In *Nature inspired cooperative strategies for optimization* (pp. 65–74). Springer. doi:10.1007/978-3-642-12538-6_6

Chapter 8
Medical Data Are Safe:
An Encrypted Quantum Approach

Padmapriya Praveenkumar
Shanmugha Arts, Science, Technology, and Research Academy (Deemed), India

Santhiyadevi R.
Shanmugha Arts, Science, Technology, and Research Academy (Deemed), India

Amirtharajan R.
Shanmugha Arts, Science, Technology, and Research Academy (Deemed), India

ABSTRACT

In this internet era, transferring and preservation of medical diagnostic reports and images across the globe have become inevitable for the collaborative tele-diagnosis and tele-surgery. Consequently, it is of prime importance to protect it from unauthorized users and to confirm integrity and privacy of the user. Quantum image processing (QIP) paves a way by integrating security algorithms in protecting and safeguarding medical images. This chapter proposes a quantum-assisted encryption scheme by making use of quantum gates, chaotic maps, and hash function to provide reversibility, ergodicity, and integrity, respectively. The first step in any quantum-related image communication is the representation of the classical image into quantum. It has been carried out using novel enhanced quantum representation (NEQR) format, where it uses two entangled qubit sequences to hoard the location and its pixel values of an image. The second step is performing transformations like confusion, diffusion, and permutation to provide an uncorrelated encrypted image.

INTRODUCTION

The proliferation of telemedicine applications forces a massive requirement on the security and accurateness of the medical data transmission through communication channels. HealthInsurance Portability and Accountability Act (HIPAA) states that over 17 crores of medical data have been breached("Healthcare Data Breach Statistics"). IBM security and Ponemon Institute stated that the average cost of stolen record is increased to 4.8%(*Global Overview*, 2018). 20% of the victims received wrong diagnosis or delayed

DOI: 10.4018/978-1-5225-7952-6.ch008

treatment due to the illegal use of healthcare information("MIFA Shares Industry Wisdom on Medical Identity Theft and Fraud").The medical report includes personal details, health insurance policy number and healthcare history. Using this vast information, forged insurance can be claimed. The challenges in any medical system are that the number of images handled by the unit is substantial; also the size of the imagesis bulky. In contrast to the normal images, medical images have more redundant data. As a result, it is essential to devise encryption methods to process these medical images, so as to reduce the computational complexity. To manage this situation in classical image processing; the concept of quantum-based computation has been integrated with image encryption algorithms to achieve high computation speed and to provide parallelism and minimal storage requirements.

BACKGROUND

A good encryption scheme should possess Confidentiality, Integrity and Authentication (CIA). The first one indicates that the data is kept private from unauthorised disclosure. Integrity is offered by constructing the data that has not been transformed or tampered. Finally, authentication is the method of data recognition by the sender and receiver.

Undeniably, a well-devised healthcare security system should fulfil two conditions: confusion and diffusion to accomplish CIA in any security system. The chaotic equations are induced for achieving the above-said conditions, due to its aperiodic nature and susceptible to the primary condition. The first chaotic system-based encryption was proposed by Fridrich J(Fridrich, 1998). Since then, a variety of chaotic system-based encryption algorithms were framed. Further to prevail over the weakness like small key space and to eliminate the discontinuous range of chaotic behaviour, Zhou *et al.*(Zhou, Bao, & Chen, 2014) proposed a new chaotic system, by integrating the existing chaotic maps.

For the bulky medical data, conventional encryption algorithms like Advanced Encryption Standard (AES), Data Encryption Standard (DES)and s-box permutation matrix are incapable of surviving against various brute force, statistical and differential attacks. Therefore, a number of encryption algorithms have been developed based on DeoxyriboNucleic Acid (DNA), watermarking and hash algorithms to provide privacy and to ensure the integrity of the medical images used across the globe. Transmitting the entire bulky medical data tends to overload the traffic across communication channels. To evade this scenario, partial encryption and integrity check algorithms were proposed recently by many researchers (Ravichandran *et al*, 2017).

Classical image encryption algorithms are naturally extended to the quantum scenario due to the breakthrough of quantum information and quantum computation. Quantum computation has become an innovative tool for meeting with the real-time computational requirements. In an information storage and parallel computing, it has numerous exclusive computational qualities such as superposition of quantum state, quantum coherence and entanglement which makes quantum computing greater to its classical counterpart. In (Feynman, 1982), Feynman framed the initiative for the quantum computer, which comprises a physical machine which accepts input states as a superposition of many inputs (Deutsch, 1985).

In a quantum-enabled computer, the quantum image is an edition of the classical image. A variety of methods have been projected to signify the importance of quantum images and quantum image processing algorithms. Various quantum representation schemes were evolved to store the quantum image; few of them were Novel Enhanced Quantum Representation (NEQR), Entangled, Real ket, Multi-Channel Representation of Quantum Image (MCRQI), Flexible Representation of Quantum Images (FRQI) and log-polar (Latorre, 2005; Sang, Wang, & Niu, 2016; S. E. Venegas-Andraca & Ball, 2010; Salvador E. Venegas-Andraca & Bose, 2003; Y. Zhang, Lu, Gao, & Xu, 2013). In NEQR format, two entangled qubit sequences are used for hoarding both the location and its pixel values of an image. The advantages of using NEQR are the time required for preparing the Quantum image representation is less, image retrieval is accurate, and a range of image operations can be done expediently as compared to other quantum image formats.

Most of the encryption algorithm uses quantum gates for encrypting the images due to its reversible properties (Tofoli, 1980). Heidari*et al.*(Heidari& Naseri, 2016), proposed a quantum m-bit embedding and watermarking procedures utilising NEQR format. Watermarking procedure by utilizing Quantum Wavelet Transform (QWT) is proposed by Song *et al.*(Song, Wang, Liu, Abd El-Latif, & Niu, 2013). However, the cover image cannot be retrieved in these quantum watermark algorithms. Image encryption algorithms assisted with quantum principle employing scrambling and diffusion operations is proposed by Beheri *et al.* (Beheri, Amin, Song, & El-latif, 2016). A novel quantum encryption algorithm is framed which utilises quantum gates and quantum gray code to provide uncorrelated cipher output (Abd El-Latif, Abd-El-Atty, & Talha, 2017).However, these proposed frameworks were unable to meet the optimum condition in terms of security analysis. Also researchers have validated their proposed algorithms using metrics like Number of Pixel Change Rate (NPCR), Unified Average Change in Intensity (UACI), (Wu*et al*, 2011),entropy, correlation and chi-square tests (Fu et al., 2013; Fu, Zhang, Bian, Lei, & Ma, 2014; Helmy, El-Rabaie, Eldokany, & El-Samie, 2017; Li, Wang, Yan, & Liu, 2016; Praveenkumar et al., 2015; Ravichandran *et al.*, 2016; X. Wang & Liu, 2017; S. Zhang, Gao, & Gao, 2014).

By examining numerous quantum encryption methodologies in the available literature, this chapter concentrates the following aspects in preserving and transferring the medical images:

- Proposes an image encryption algorithm employing quantum concepts, quantum gates and a hash function for integrity check and to protect the medical images.
- The proposed methodology utilizes Quantum SWAP, CNOT gates and Secure Hash Algorithm-512 (SHA-512).
- It can be implemented in both selective and complete image encryption applications.

PRELIMINARIES

Novel Enhanced Quantum Representation (NEQR)

By operating NEQR, the classical image can be represented in quantum representation. NEQR is preferred over FRQI because the time required to prepare NEQR quantum image reveals a rough quadratic drop and additional image operations can be carried out. NEQR uses two-qubit sequences for storing both the pixel and its position values. Therefore, it requires q+2n qubits for storing the pixel value of an image. NEQR of the colorDigital Imaging and Communication in Medicine (DICOM) image can be represented as,

$$|I\rangle = \frac{1}{2^n}\sum_{Y=0}^{2^n-1}\sum_{X=0}^{2^n-1}|C_{YX}\rangle|YX\rangle \tag{1}$$

Figure 1. NEQR representation for a 2×2 colour images

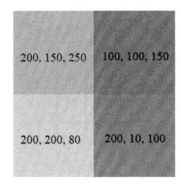

$|I\rangle = \frac{1}{2}$ ($|11001000, 10010110, 11111010\rangle \otimes |00\rangle +$
$|01100100, 01100100, 10010110\rangle \otimes |01\rangle +$
$|11001000, 11001000, 01010000\rangle \otimes |10\rangle +$
$|11001000, 00001010, 01100100\rangle \otimes |11\rangle$).

$$C_{YX} = C_{YX}^{0R} .... C_{YX}^{7R} C_{YX}^{0G} .... C_{YX}^{7G} C_{YX}^{0B} .... C_{YX}^{7B}$$
$$= C_{YX}^{0} .... C_{YX}^{7} C_{YX}^{8} .... C_{YX}^{15} C_{YX}^{16} .... C_{YX}^{23}, C_{YX}^{k} \in \{0,1\}, C_{YX} \in [0, 2^q - 1] \tag{2}$$

Therefore, equation (1) can be rewritten as,

$$\left| I \right\rangle = \frac{1}{2^n} \sum_{YX=0}^{2^{2n}-1} \otimes_{i=0}^{23} \left| C_{YX}^i \right\rangle \otimes \left| YX \right\rangle \tag{3}$$

Figure 1 illustrates the NEQR paradigm for a 2×2 RGB (R-Red, G- Green, B-Blue) DICOM image, where g (0,0) = (200, 150, 250) i.e. R=200, G=150, B=250. Then, the basis state can be denoted as $|11001000, 10010110, 11111010\rangle \otimes |00\rangle$.

CONTROLLED-NOT (CNOT Gate)

CNOT is a type of two input quantum gate. Circuit diagram of CNOT gate and its wire diagram are shown in Figures. 2 and 3 respectively. It has the mapping of (a, b) to (a'=a, b'=a⊕b), where a and b represents control and the target qubits respectively. ⊕symbol in the mapping is used to represent the CNOT operation. If the control qubit is $|1\rangle$ then the target qubit is flipped else the target remains unaffected.

Figure 2. The CNOT gate

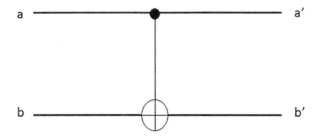

Figure 3. Wire diagram of CNOT gate

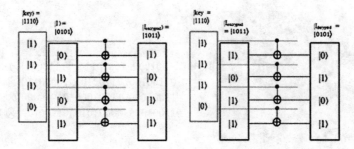

SWAP Gate

SWAP gate is yet another type of two-input quantum gate. The circuit diagram and its wire diagram are illustrated in Figures. 4 and 5 respectively. It maps (x,y) to (x'=y, y'=x).

Bit Planes

A bit-plane comprises of a collection of bits mapping to the bit position of the given image. The RGB DICOM image will have the range from [0 - 255] for all the three (R, G and B) planes. The Least Significant Bit (LSB)is hoarded in the first-bit plane, and Most Significant Bit (MSB) of all pixel values

Figure 4. The SWAP gate

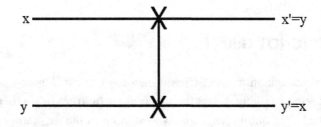

Figure 5. Wire diagram of SWAP gate

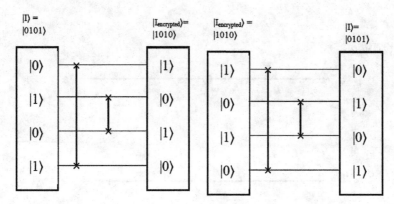

Figure 6. Bit planes of the R component of original image 1

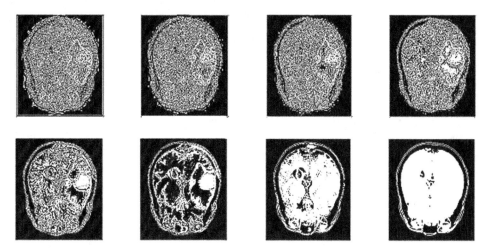

will be kept in the eighth-bit plane and so on. Figure. 6 illustrates bit plane representation of the Red channel of the original image 1.

Fingerprint and Hash

The fingerprint image is normally used for ensuring the integrity of the image. Both the sender and receiver will have the fingerprint image, which acts as a key input to the hash algorithm. It is a one-way function if x is given, then calculating h(x)=y is trivial. But given y, it is difficult to compute $h^{-1}(y)=x$. Here, the SHA-512 algorithm is used which takes variable length image as input and produces 512-bit hash value output. Both the sender and the receiver estimate the hash value with the fingerprint image. These 512-bits are converted into an 8×8 matrix, and this hash value is incorporated in the image for verification, if there is any alteration in the cipher image during transit, then the original image cannot be retrieved at the receiver end.

QUANTUM ENCRYPTION AND INTEGRITY CHECK ALGORITHM

Medical image encryption algorithm utilising quantum concepts along with SHA-512, quantum bit planes and quantum gates are detailed in this section. Further, the proposed algorithm is integrated with fused Logistic, Tent and Sine maps. Figure 7 portraits the block diagram of the proposed methodology.

Initially, the hash value is produced from the fingerprint image by utilising the SHA-512 algorithm. Then the Region of Interest (ROI) and Region of Non-Interest (RONI)are separated from the original DICOM image. Further ROI and RONI image, chaotic map and the hash values are converted into quantum image format. The quantum ROI image is subjected to the 1st stage of encryption by utilising the swap gate, between the quantum bit-planes and diffused by employing the CNOT gate. The 2nd stage of encryption is attained by exploiting the row and column shuffling. Additionally, it is diffused by applying the circular shift operation. Between the two encryption stages, the hash value is employed by

Figure 7. Block representation of the projected encryption scheme

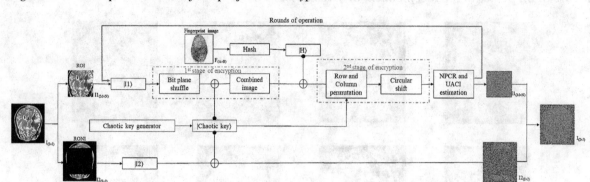

operating the CNOT gate. At the end of two encryption stages, NPCR and UACI values are estimated and updated by the rounds of operation.

The Integrated Logistic-Tent (ILT) and Integrated Logistic-Sine (ILS) maps are specified in equations (4) and (5) respectively.

$$x_{n+1} = \begin{cases} \left[\mu x_n \left(1-x_n\right) + \dfrac{\left(4-\mu\right)x_n}{2} \right] \mathrm{mod}\,1; x_n < 0.5 \\ \left[\mu x_n \left(1-x_n\right) + \dfrac{\left(4-\mu\right)\left(1-x_n\right)}{2} \right] \mathrm{mod}\,1; x_n \geq 0.5 \end{cases} \tag{4}$$

$$y_{n+1} = \left[r y_n \left(1-y_n\right) + \left(4-r\right)\sin\left(\pi y_n\right)/4 \right] \mathrm{mod}\,1 \tag{5}$$

where (μ, r) are control parameters and (μ, r) $\in$ (0,4], (x_n, y_n) are initial parameters and (x_n, y_n) $\in$ [0,1].

Encryption Algorithm

Input: Original RGB DICOM image.
Output: RGB DICOM ROI image, RBG DICOM RONI image.
Step 1: Dividethe DICOM image ($I_{(I \times J)}$) into ROI ($I_{1(M \times N)}$) and RONI ($I_{2(I \times J)}$). The initial point ($I_{1(M1, N1)}$), height and width of ROI is taken as the key (kc1, kc2, kc3, kc4) for separating ROI at the decryption stage.The procedure to separate ROI and RONIis given below:

ROI and RONI Separation Procedure

Crop ROI ($I_{1(M \times N)}$) from the DICOM image as ($I_{(I \times J)}$) and the left-over part is considered as RONI ($I_{2(I \times J)}$).

The initial point ($I_{1(M1, N1)}$), height and width of ROI is taken as keys (kc1 (M1), kc2 (N1), kc3, kc4) for separating ROI at the decryption stage.

ROI Encryption Process

Input: RGB DICOM ROI image.

Output: Interlinked image.

Step 2: Split the ROI DICOM image into red, green and blue planes.

Step 3: Transform the ROI red plane into NEQR quantum bit-plane representation (6) and convert the red plane into an array. Interlink the image pixels by operating equation (vii) on the array. Figure. 8 shows the pixel interlinking procedure using (7). Further, the obtained array is converted into the matrix, according to the size of ROI planes.

$$\left| I_{red} \right\rangle = \frac{1}{2^n} \sum_{Y=0}^{2^n-1} \sum_{X=0}^{2^n-1} \otimes_{i=0}^{8} \left| C_{YX}^i \right\rangle \left| YX \right\rangle \tag{6}$$

$$\left| A_{red} \right\rangle = CNOT\left(I_{red}\left(i, j-1 \right), I_{red}\left(i, j \right) \right) \tag{7}$$

Step 4: Choose 'μ' and 'x_n'(K_1) and iterate ILS map for 's' times and neglect first 't' iterations for avoiding the transient effect. Choose the chaotic sequence X= {x_{t+1}, x_{t+2}, ... x_s}, where the size of X should be equal to M × N and operate equation (6) on 'X' and represent it as a quantum bit-plane image to get the sequence |X⟩ and operate equation (viii) on |X⟩ to get |X'⟩.

Figure 8. Example of pixel interlink

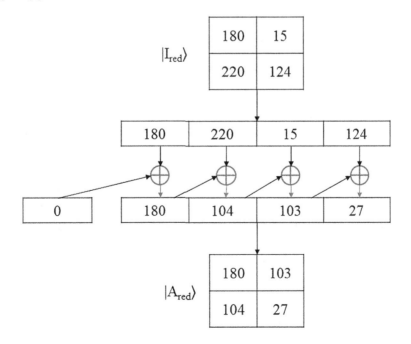

$$|X'\rangle = floor\left(\mathrm{mod}\left(\|X\rangle \times 10^{17}\right), 256\right) \tag{8}$$

Phase One: 1st Stage of Encryption

Input: Interlinked image, key-$|X'\rangle$.

Output: Diffused image.

Step 5: By operating the SWAP gate, bit-planes of $|A_{red}\rangle$ are shuffled to get $|A_{\_red}\rangle$.

Step 6: Operate CNOT gate on $|A_{\_red}\rangle$ and $|X'\rangle$ to get $|I_{CNOT}(i)\rangle$ where i = 1 to 8 (no. of bit planes), $|X'\rangle$ is the control bit, and $|A_{\_red}\rangle$ is the target bit. Finally, combine all the eight planes of $|I_{CNOT}\rangle$.

Figure 9 (a and b) shows the wire diagram of the proposed encryption and decryption modules.

Phase Two: Hash ValueImplementation

Input : Diffused image, Hash values.

Output: Hash image.

Step 7: The fingerprint image of size A × B is given as input to the SHA-512 algorithm (Chai, Zheng, Gan, Han, & Chen, 2018), (M. Wang, Wang, Zhang, & Gao, 2018) and the output 512-bits are converted to decimal and reshaped into the 8×8 matrix. Transform the hash matrix into NEQR as

$$|H = \frac{1}{2^n} \sum_{Y=0}^{2^n-12^n-1} \sum_{X=0} \otimes_{i=0}^8 \left|C_{YX}^i\right| YX \tag{9}$$

Step 8: Consider $|H\rangle$ as control bit and $|I_{CNOT}\rangle$ as target bit and execute CNOT operation to obtain the output $|H'\rangle$. The CNOT gate is applied to the first 8×8 matrix of $|I_{CNOT}\rangle$.

Phase Three: 2nd Stage of Encryption

Input: Hash image, Key-K_2, K_3.

Output: Encrypted ROI DICOM image.

Step 9: Choose 'r' and 'y_n' (K_2) and iterate ILT map for 's' times. To avoid transient effect, neglect the first 1000 iterations. Choose the chaotic sequence I_Row = {I_Row$_{1001}$, I_Row$_{1002}$, ...I_Row$_s$} and sort I_Row to obtain the sorted index value as Row$_{sorted}$= {R$_1$, R$_2$, ... R$_s$}. Shuffle the rows of $|H'\rangle$ using Row$_{sorted}$to get $|I\_row\rangle$.

Step 10: Choose different 'r' and 'y_n' (K_3) values and iterate ILT map for 's' times. To avoid transient effect, neglect the first 1000 iterations. Choose the chaotic sequence Column = {Column$_{1001}$, Column$_{1002}$, ... Column$_s$} and sort Column either in ascending or descending order to get the sorted index value as Column$_{sorted}$= {C$_1$, C$_2$, ... C$_s$}. Shuffle the columns of $|I\_row\rangle$ using Column $_{sorted}$ to get $|I'\rangle$. Figure.10 shows the example of row and column shuffle.

Step 11: Convert each row of $|I'\rangle$ into its binary equivalent vector as,

Figure 9. (a and b) Wire diagram of proposed encryption (a) and decryption (b) algorithm

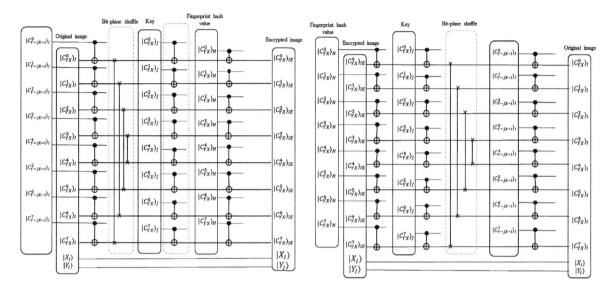

Figure 10. Row and Column Shuffled image

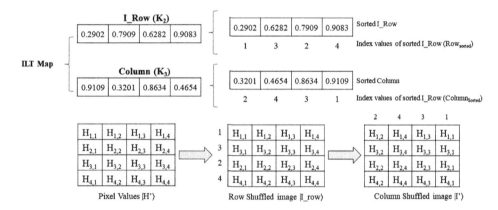

$$\left| Row\left(i \right) \right\rangle = de2bi\left(\left| I' \right\rangle, 8 \right) \tag{10}$$

where i =M (no. of rows in the image).

Step 12: Calculate the number of one's in |Row⟩ and let it be |N⟩.

Step 13: Compute |D⟩ using equation (xi), if |D⟩=0, then |Row⟩ is right circular shifted by |N⟩ times and if |D⟩=1, then it is left circular shifted by |N⟩ times and the resultant matrix be |Row'⟩.

$$\left| D \right\rangle = \mathrm{mod}\left(\left| N \right\rangle, 2 \right) \tag{11}$$

Step 14: Convert each row of binary values into its decimal equivalent by using equation (xii), to get the encrypted image.

$$\left| I\_1_{encrypt} \right\rangle = bi2de\left(\left| Row' \right\rangle, 8 \right) \tag{12}$$

Step 15: The final encrypted red plane ROI image is $|I\_1_{encrypt}\rangle$. The encrypted green and blue planes of ROI image are obtained by repeating steps 3 to 14 with the same key, and the final encrypted ROI is attained by concatenating the encrypted red, green and blue ROI planes.

RONI Encryption Process

Input: RGB DICOM RONI image.
Output: Encrypted RONI DICOM image.
Step 16: Split the RGB RONI DICOM image of the size I × J × 3 into red, green and blue planes.
Step 17: Transform the red plane of RONI image into NEQR quantum bit-plane representation as (13)

$$\left| RONI_{red} = \frac{1}{2^n} \sum_{Y=0}^{2^n-12^n-1} \sum_{X=0} \otimes_{i=0}^{8} \left| C_{YX}^i \right| YX \tag{13}$$

Step 18: Repeat step 4 for ILT map (K_4) and transform it into NEQR quantum bit-plane representation. Operate CNOT gate by considering |Key⟩ as control bit and |RONI$_{red}$⟩ as target bit to get the encrypted RONI as |RONI$_{encrypt}$⟩.

$$\left| Key = \frac{1}{2^n} \sum_{Y=0}^{2^n-12^n-1} \sum_{X=0} \otimes_{i=0}^{8} \left| C_{YX}^i \right| YX \tag{14}$$

Step 19: Repeat steps 17 and 18 to get the encrypted green and blue RONI planes and the final encrypted RONI is attained by concatenating all the encrypted planes.
Step 20: Combine the encrypted ROI and RONI to get the encrypted image. The decryption procedure is the inverses of the encryption procedure as the qubits are invertible.

SIMULATION RESULTS AND ANALYSIS

The security of the projected scheme is demonstrated by using two 256×256 ROI RGB DICOM images as in Figure. 11 (a & d). The test images were taken from the web source (www.osirix-viewer.com) for various analysis. Owing to the deficiency of quantum computers, the proposed scheme is simulated in a personal laptop with Intel® Core™ i5 processor, 2.5GHz and 8GB RAM equipped with MATLAB R2016b. Further, the projected scheme is subjected to various attacks to prove that it is invulnerable to statistical, chosen plain text and differential attacks.

Figure 11 shows the different test images and their corresponding ROI and RONI images that are used in the proposed algorithm. Figure 12 (a-g) provides the various encryption stages output in ROI, Figure 13 (a-c) illustrates the output of RONI and Figure 14 (a-c) illustrates the output of the proposed algorithm.

EXHAUSTIVE ATTACK

KeyspaceAnalysis

Brute-force attack is also known as exhaustive attack. The hackers try to guess the key by checking all the possible keys. The proposed algorithm should have huge keyspace to counter-attack brute-force. In the proposed algorithm, for encrypting ROI, three sets of keys $Key_1 = \{K_1, K_2, K_3\}$ are used, and each

Figure 11. Test images. (a) original image 1, (b) ROI 1, (c) RONI 1, (d) original image 2, (e) ROI 2, (f) RONI 2

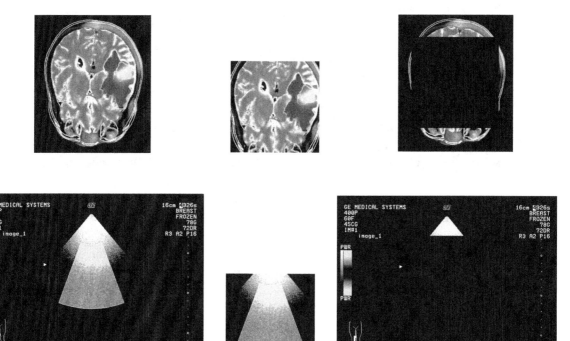

For a more accurate representation see the electronic version.

Figure 12. Output of the ROI encryption scheme. (a) ROI 1, (b) Bit-plane shuffled 1, (c) CNOT 1, (d) Row and column shuffle 1, (e) encrypted ROI 1, (f) decrypted ROI 1

For a more accurate representation see the electronic version.

Figure 13. Output of RONI encryption scheme. (a) Original RONI 1, (b) encrypted RONI 1, (c) decrypted RONI 1

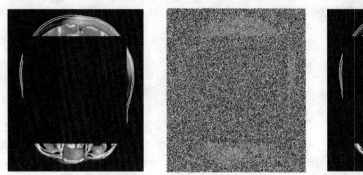

For a more accurate representation see the electronic version.

Figure 14. Output of the proposed encryption algorithm. (a) original image 1, (b) encrypted image 1, (c) decrypted image 1

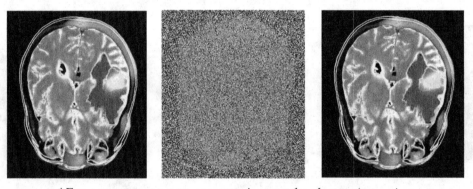

For a more accurate representation see the electronic version.

set contains two keys. Therefore, six secret keys are used for encrypting ROI. One set of keys (Key$_2$= {K$_4$}) is used for encrypting RONI. So, the proposed algorithm uses four pairs of keys totalling eight secret keys. The keyspace of the proposed algorithm is 10^{112}, by setting the precision of each key to -14. Keyspace of $10^{112}$is large enough to endure brute-force attack.

Key Sensitivity Analysis

The ILT and ILS maps are sensitive to the control parameters and the initial seed values. The sensitivity of ILT and ILS maps are tested by slightly differing one of the secret keys. Figure. 15prove that even if a single bit is altered in the original key, the proposed algorithm cannot retrieve the original image. Figure. 15 (a and b) shows the ROI image 1 and encrypted ROI image 1 respectively. Figure 15 (c-e) shows the decrypted image from (b) with {Key set 1, Key set 2, Key set 3} respectively. Table 1 gives the precise and incorrect key sets.

From this examination, it is clear that the proposed algorithm is susceptible to the key which means that the proposed algorithm can counterattack exhaustive attack.

Figure 15. Key sensitivity test. (a) ROI 1, (b) encrypted image with Key, (c) decrypted image with Key set 1, (d) decrypted image with Key set 2, (e) decrypted image with Key set 3, (f) decrypted image with Key

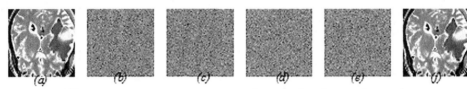

For a more accurate representation see the electronic version.

Table 1. Different keysets used for key sensitivity analysis

Values		Key	Key Set 1	Key Set 2	Key Set 3
K$_1$	μ1	3.67676767676767	3.67676767676767	3.67676767676767	3.67676767676766
	x1	0.76767676767676	0.76767676767677	0.76767676767676	0.76767676767676
K$_2$	r1	3.45645645645645	3.45645645645645	3.45645645645645	3.45645645645645
	y1	0.29029029029029	0.29029029029029	0.29029029029129	0.29029029029029
K$_3$	r2	3.87687687687687	3.87687687687687	3.87687687687687	3.87687687687687
	y2	0.91091091091091	0.91091091091091	0.91091091091091	0.91091091091091
K$_4$	r3	3.67676767676767	3.67676767676767	3.67676767676767	3.67676767676767
	y3	0.76767676767676	0.76767676767676	0.76767676767676	0.76767676767676

Statistical Attack

By analysing the statistical nature of the cipher image hacker tries to gain knowledge about the key and the encryption algorithm. To examine the statistical nature and strength of the proposed algorithm against statistical attack, the proposed algorithm is subjected to various analysis like histogram analysis, correlation analysis, entropy and chi-square test. Table 2 provides the calculation of the percentage of 1's in all the bit planes. A suitable encryption algorithm should encrypt the image not only in pixel level but also in bit level. From Table 2, it is well-defined that the proposed algorithm encrypts the image perfectly even in bit-level.

Histogram Analysis

The histogram is the graphical illustration of the Intensity level (x-axis) to the number of pixels (y-axis). Figure. 16 (a-c) gives the histogram of red, green and blue planes of ROI 1 images respectively. Figure. 16 (d-f) provides the histogram of red, green and blue planes of encrypted ROI 1 images respectively. From this, it is clear that the proposed algorithm produces a uniformly flat histogram for encrypted images even though the pixels are concentrated over the region in the original image.

Table 2. Percentage of 1's in ROI and encrypted ROI bit planes

Images/Planes			1	2	3	4	5	6	7	8
ROI 1	Original	R	51.7608	51.0635	50.8987	52.7862	48.5504	35.6445	73.7258	82.7377
		G	47.5402	47.3007	47.6409	46.5667	48.5046	45.4849	49.4171	34.6069
		B	60.5636	61.2762	62.4496	63.6978	66.9693	74.3133	77.5726	78.9047
	Encrypted	R	49.8413	49.6505	50.2655	50.2090	50.1770	49.8992	50.2166	50.0152
		G	50.2105	49.9877	50.1678	49.9282	50.2258	49.6673	49.8962	50.1831
		B	50.2105	49.9877	50.1678	49.9282	50.2258	49.6673	49.8962	50.1831
ROI 2	Original	R	61.4196	60.4522	59.9868	60.9954	65.9027	45.4910	44.0948	42.5308
		G	47.6516	49.9435	47.7279	47.9599	51.9470	33.6517	32.3196	28.5736
		B	27.8640	26.7303	26.3168	27.2430	31.7077	11.1007	9.6984	8.1344
	Encrypted	R	49.8992	49.9893	50.0991	50.2517	49.9054	50.1754	49.8855	50.2029
		G	49.3164	49.9054	49.9420	49.9694	50.1052	49.8489	49.9847	49.6414
		B	50.0503	49.8825	49.6749	49.9969	50.2533	50.1403	49.9954	50.0915

Figure 16. Histogram analysis. (a) histogram of red plane in ROI 1, (b) histogram of green plane in ROI 1, (c)histogram of blue plane in ROI 1, (d) histogram of red plane in encrypted ROI 1, (e) histogram of greenplane in encrypted ROI 1, (f) histogram of blueplane in encrypted ROI 1

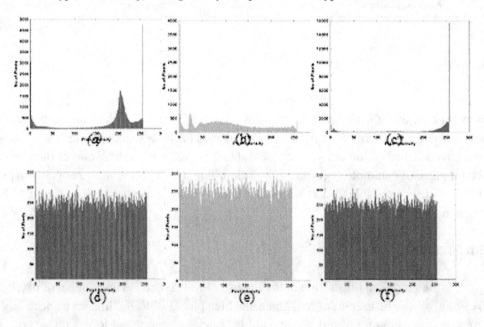

Chi-Square (X²) Test

The uniform distribution of pixels in cipher image can be statistically understood with this test, and this is calculated by using (15),

$$\chi^2 = \sum_{m=i}^{256} \frac{\left(observed_i - expected_i\right)^2}{expected_i} \qquad (15)$$

where i is the level of intensity and the expected value is 256 for 256×256 image (Praveenkumar et al., 2015; Ravichandran et al., 2016,). Observed$_i$ and expected$_i$ in the equation are the original and expected values of the pixel from the histogram. For 255 degree of freedom, the significant levels for 5% and 1% are 293.2478 and 310.457 respectively. From Table 3 it is clear that the hypothesis is accepted for the 5% and 1% significant level which signifies the pixels are randomly distributed.

Correlation Analysis

Correlation gives the amount of relationship between a pair of adjacent pixels in the image, and this is estimated using equation (16). It is evident that in the plain image the pixels have a strong relationship with neighbouring pixels, but in the cipher image, the statistical relationship between the adjacent pixels should be reduced to withstand statistical attack. Figure 17 (a-c) shows the correlation of ROI 1 and (d-f) shows the correlation of encrypted ROI 1. Table 4 gives the correlation analysis of the proposed algorithm in all the three (X, Y and Z) directions. The value of correlation indicates that the suggested algorithm can withstand statistical attack.

$$Correlation_{mn} = \frac{\text{cov}\left(m,n\right)}{\sqrt{D\left(m\right)}\sqrt{D\left(n\right)}} \qquad (16)$$

$$\text{cov}\left(m,n\right) = \frac{1}{N}\sum_{i=1}^{N}\left(m_i - E\left(m\right)\right)\left(n_i - E\left(n\right)\right), \ D\left(m\right) = \frac{1}{N}\sum_{i=1}^{N}\left(m_i - E\left(m\right)\right)^2 \ E\left(m\right) = \frac{1}{N}\sum_{i=1}^{N}m_i$$

Table 3. Chi-Square analysis

Images	ROI 1			ROI 2		
	R	**G**	**B**	**R**	**G**	**B**
χ^2 Value	287.1484	227.8984	228.1875	252.8984	281.7734	248.5313
Decision	Accept	Accept	Accept	Accept	Accept	Accept

Table 4. Correlation analysis of the proposed algorithm

Images			Horizontal	Vertical	Diagonal
ROI 1	Original	R	0.9399	0.9764	0.9262
		G	0.9264	0.9667	0.9029
		B	0.9595	0.9833	0.9472
	Diffused	R	0.0032	-0.0039	0.0048
		G	-0.0051	0.0035	0.0030
		B	-0.0087	0.0024	0.0050
ROI 2	Original	R	0.9868	0.9868	0.9808
		G	0.9683	0.9663	0.9543
		B	0.8939	0.8934	0.8574
	Diffused	R	0.0030	-0.0035	-0.0051
		G	-0.0045	-0.0015	-0.0016
		B	0.0048	0.0039	0.0042

Figure 17. Correlation analysis. (a) horizontal correlation of ROI 1, (b) vertical correlation of ROI 1, (c) diagonal correlation of ROI 1, (d) horizontal correlation of encrypted ROI 1, (e) vertical correlation of encrypted ROI 1, (f) diagonal correlation of encrypted ROI 1

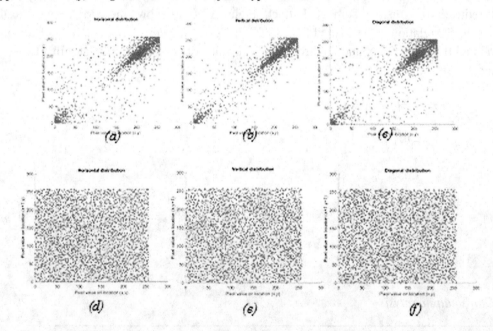

Entropy Analysis

Global Shannon entropy is used for evaluating the randomness of the information, and this can be calculated by (17),

$$Entropy(\alpha) = -\sum_{i=0}^{2^N-1} p(\alpha_i) \log_2 p(\alpha_i) \qquad (17)$$

p(α_i) is the probability of occurrence of symbol α. For a random image with 2^N symbols, the entropy should be close to N. For an RGB DICOM image, in each plane, the grayscale range will be 2^8 and if it is assumed that each level of gray is equiprobable and then the theoretical value of entropy will be 8. From the Table 5 and Table 6, it is evident that the calculated values are close to 1 and 8 in the bit planes and in the encrypted images respectively. The proposed algorithm can generate highly random cipher image and can withstand statistical attack.

Table 5. Entropy analysis of ROI image and encrypted ROI image in bit planes

Images/Planes			1	2	3	4	5	6	7	8
ROI 1	Original	R	0.9991	0.9996	0.9997	0.9977	0.9993	0.9396	0.8308	0.6636
		G	0.9982	0.9978	0.9983	0.9965	0.9993	0.9941	0.9999	0.9305
		B	0.9675	0.9629	0.9548	0.9451	0.9152	0.8219	0.7678	0.7433
	encrypted	R	0.9999	0.9999	0.9999	0.9999	0.9999	0.9999	0.9999	1.0000
		G	0.9999	1	0.9999	0.9999	0.9999	0.9999	0.9999	0.9999
		B	1	0.9999	0.9999	0.9999	0.9999	1	0.9999	0.9999
ROI 2	Original	R	0.9620	0.9682	0.9710	0.9648	0.9257	0.9941	0.9899	0.9838
		G	0.9984	0.9999	0.9985	0.9987	0.9989	0.9214	0.9078	0.8631
		B	0.8535	0.8375	0.8314	0.8449	0.9011	0.5029	0.4593	0.4068
	encrypted	R	0.9999	1	0.9999	0.9999	0.9999	0.9999	0.9999	0.9999
		G	0.9998	0.9999	0.9999	1	0.9999	0.9999	1	0.9999
		B	0.9999	0.9999	0.9999	1	0.9999	0.9999	1	0.9999

Table 6. Entropy analysis of original ROI and encrypted ROI images

Images/Directions	Original			Encrypted		
	R	G	B	R	G	B
ROI 1	6.7001	7.7369	6.1922	7.9968	7.9974	7.9974
ROI 2	4.8030	6.2290	4.4097	7.9972	7.9968	7.9972

Differential Attack

Number of pixel change rate (NPCR) and Unified Average Change in Intensity (UACI) gives the number of pixels transformed and the mean difference between two cipher images. A pair of cipher images is obtained from the original image after encryption and other one by changing a pixel value in the plain image. The proposed framework should produce different cipher images even if there is a single pixel change in the plain image. This is calculated by using (18) and (19),

$$NPCR = \frac{\sum_{mn} Image(m,n)}{H \times W} \times 100\% \tag{18}$$

$$UACI = \frac{1}{H \times W} \left(\frac{\left| Image_1(m,n) - Image_2(m,n) \right|}{255} \right) \times 100\% \tag{19}$$

$$Image(m,n) = \begin{cases} 0 \, if \, Image_1(m,n) = Image_2(m,n) \\ 0 \, if \, Image_1(m,n) \neq Image_2(m,n) \end{cases}$$

where H and W denote the column and row size of the image, $Image_1$ and $Image_2$ are the two cipher images before and after a pixel change in the plain image. The NPCR and UACI values are listed in Table 7 and 8and from this table, it is evident that both the values are in the optimum range. The values are compared with critical value as in (Wu et al., 2011), and from this, it can be decided that the proposed algorithm can endure differential attacks.

Performance Comparison Analysis

Table 9 provides a comparison analysis of the proposed algorithm with recent studies available in Literature.

Table 7. UACI values

Images		UACI (%)	UACI Critical Values		
			$U^{*-}_{0.05}$ = 33. 2824% $U^{*+}_{0.05}$ = 33. 6447%	$U^{*-}_{0.01}$ = 33. 2255% $U^{*+}_{0.01}$ = 33. 7016%	$U^{*-}_{0.001}$ = 33. 1594% $U^{*+}_{0.001}$ = 33. 7677%
ROI 1	R	33.4418	PASS	PASS	PASS
	G	33.4560	PASS	PASS	PASS
	B	33.4539	PASS	PASS	PASS
ROI 2	R	33.4393	PASS	PASS	PASS
	G	33.4669	PASS	PASS	PASS
	B	33.403	PASS	PASS	PASS

Table 8. NPCR values

Images		NPCR (%)	NPCR Critical Values		
			NPCR *0.05 = 99.5693%	NPCR *0.01 = 99.5527%	NPCR *0.001 = 99.5341%
ROI 1	R	99.5941	PASS	PASS	PASS
	G	99.5971	PASS	PASS	PASS
	B	99.5910	PASS	PASS	PASS
ROI 2	R	99.6093	PASS	PASS	PASS
	G	99.6017	PASS	PASS	PASS
	B	99.6048	PASS	PASS	PASS

Table 9. Performance Comparison Analyses

	Correlation			Entropy	UACI	NPCR
	Horizontal	Vertical	Diagonal			
(Abd El-Latif et al., 2017)	-0.0027	-0.0119	-0.0053	7.98913	33.5018	99.63
(Praveenkumar et al., 2015)	-0.0033	0.0033	0.0117	7.9975	33.45	99.62
(Ravichandran et al., 2016)	-0.0519	-0.0385	0.00046	7.9992	33.37	99.996
(Ravichandran et al., 2017)	-0.0025	-0.0016	0.0116	7.9972	33.4399	99.5982
(Fu et al., 2014)	NA	NA	NA	7.9992	33.48	99.60
(S. Zhang et al., 2014)	-0.0154	0.0193	0.0032	NA	NA	NA
(Fu et al., 2013)	-0.0061	0.0122	-0.0197	7.9993	NA	NA
(Li et al., 2016)	0.0043	0.0046	0.00315	7.9954	NA	NA
(X. Wang & Liu, 2017)	-0.0011	-0.0016	0.0012	7.9974	33.44	99.61
(Helmy et al., 2017)	0.00183	NA	NA	NA	NA	NA
Proposed	-0.0012	0.00014	0.0017	7.9971	33.4435	99.5997

Entropy, correlation, NPCR and UACI values of the proposed algorithm are compared with the existing algorithms. (Abd El-Latif et al., 2017; Fu et al., 2013, 2014; Helmy et al., 2017; Li et al., 2016; Praveenkumar et al., 2015; Ravichandran et al., 2016, 2017; X.-Y. Wang et al., 2015; S. Zhang et al., 2014). The values are provided in Table 7 and from these values, it is obvious that the proposed algorithm can withstand different attacks. Table 10provides the detailed description, advantages and disadvantages of the similar encryption schemes available in literature with the proposed methodology.

Table 10. Pros and Cons of the proposed scheme with the literature study

Title	Description	Advantages	Disadvantages
A Novel LSB Based Quantum Watermarking.(Heidari & Naseri, 2016)	Based on the m-bit embedding key, the watermark image is embedded in the LSB of the cover image.	No attacker can reach the watermarked secret image.	The cover image is not retrieved. In medical image watermarking, the cover image is required. Hence, this method is not applicable to medical images.
Adynamic watermarking scheme for quantum images using quantum wavelet transform.(Song et al., 2013)	The embedding capacity is controlled based on the dynamical diagonal vector which is based on the carrier and watermark images.	Max capacity is achieved.	The cover image is not retrieved. Therefore, this method cannot be utilised for medical systems.
Quantum image encryption based on Scrambling- Diffusion (SD) approach. (Beheri et al., 2016)	The image is confused by utilising the Arnold cat map and Fibonacci transformation and then diffused by gray-code.	Can be applied to all image formats.	The optimum values are not achieved.
Robust Encryption of Quantum Medical Images.(El-latif, Abd-el-atty, & Talha, 2017)	The medical image is confused by using the gray-code and then diffused by utilising the CNOT gate.	The proposed method is robust, and higher efficiency when compared to its classical counterpart.	The optimum values are not achieved.
Proposed methodology	Medical image encryption algorithm utilising quantum concepts together with SHA-512, quantum bit plane arrangements, gates and Integrated coupled Logistic maps using Tent and Sine maps.	• Can be used for all image formats • Can be implemented both in the selective and complete image regions	Lack of quantum computers.

FUTURE RESEARCH DIRECTIONS

The proposed encryption scheme can be extended by adopting a unitary matrix to preserve entropy. Also, Hadamatrix can be integrated to achieve image compression.

CONCLUSION

This chapter proposes a quantum assisted image encryption scheme to safeguard DICOM images when transmitted over public networks. The proposed scheme uses NEQR procedure to convert the classical DICOM into quantum image format. Further, to reduce the channel overload the quantum converted DICOM is divided into ROI and RONI. Further by applying the chaotic key generated by the combined Logistic Sine and Tent maps, permutation was carried out in the ROI image. Additionally, the integrity of the proposed work is upheld by adopting the hash mechanism in the permuted ROI. Finally, CNOT gate operation was carried out between the RONI and the generated chaotic key. Encrypted ROI and RONI were combined to produce the uncorrelated cipher image output. Encryption metrics were evaluated to validate confusion, permutation and diffusion operations in the proposed encryption scheme.

ACKNOWLEDGMENT

The authors wish to acknowledge SASTRA Deemed University, Thanjavur, India for extending infrastructural support to carry out this work.

REFERENCES

Abd El-Latif, A. A., Abd-El-Atty, B., & Talha, M. (2017). Robust Encryption of Quantum Medical Images. *IEEE Access: Practical Innovations, Open Solutions, 6*, 1073–1081. doi:10.1109/ACCESS.2017.2777869

Beheri, M. H., Amin, M., Song, X., & El-latif, A. A. A. (2016). Quantum image encryption based on Scrambling- Diffusion (SD) approach. *Frontiers of Signal Processing (ICFSP)*, (2), 43–47.

Chai, X., Zheng, X., Gan, Z., Han, D., & Chen, Y. (2018). An image encryption algorithm based on chaotic system and compressive sensing. *Signal Processing, 148*, 124–144. doi:10.1016/j.sigpro.2018.02.007

Deutsch, D. (1985). Quantum Theory, the Church-Turing Principle and the Universal Quantum Computer. *Proceedings of the Royal Society A: Mathematical, Physical and Engineering Sciences, 400*(1818), 97–117. 10.1098/rspa.1985.0070

El-latif, A. A. A., Abd-el-atty, B., & Talha, M. (2017). *Robust encryption of quantum medical images.* Academic Press.

Feynman, R. P. (1982). Simulating Physics With Computers By R P Feynman.pdf. *International Journal of Theoretical Physics, 21*(6–7), 467.

Fridrich, J. (1998). *Symmetric Ciphers Based on Two-Dimensional Chaotic Maps.* Academic Press.

Fu, C., Meng, W., Zhan, Y., Zhu, Z., Lau, F. C. M., Tse, C. K., & Ma, H. (2013). An efficient and secure medical image protection scheme based on chaotic maps. *Computers in Biology and Medicine, 43*(8), 1000–1010. doi:10.1016/j.compbiomed.2013.05.005 PMID:23816172

Fu, C., Zhang, G., Bian, O., Lei, W., & Ma, H. (2014). A Novel Medical Image Protection Scheme Using a 3-Dimensional Chaotic System. *PLoS One, 9*(12), e115773. doi:10.1371/journal.pone.0115773 PMID:25541941

Global Overview. (2018). Retrieved from https://public.dhe.ibm.com/common/ssi/ecm/55/en/55017055usen/2018-global-codb-report_06271811_55017055USEN.pdf

Healthcare Data Breach Statistics. (n.d.). Retrieved September 11, 2018, from https://www.hipaajournal.com/healthcare-data-breach-statistics/

Heidari, S., & Naseri, M. (2016). A Novel LSB Based Quantum Watermarking. *International Journal of Theoretical Physics, 55*(10), 4205–4218. doi:10.100710773-016-3046-3

Helmy, M., El-Rabaie, E.-S. M., Eldokany, I. M., & El-Samie, F. E. A. (2017). 3-D Image Encryption Based on Rubik's Cube and RC6 Algorithm. *3D Research, 8*(4), 38.

Latorre, J. I. (2005). *Image compression and entanglement*. Retrieved from http://arxiv.org/abs/quant-ph/0510031

Li, X., Wang, L., Yan, Y., & Liu, P. (2016). An improvement color image encryption algorithm based on DNA operations and real and complex chaotic systems. *Optik - International Journal for Light and Electron Optics, 127*(5), 2558–2565.

MIFA Shares Industry Wisdom on Medical Identity Theft and Fraud. (n.d.). Retrieved September 11, 2018, from https://www.hipaajournal.com/mifa-shares-industry-wisdom-on-medical-identity-theft-and-fraud-3657/

Osiri, X. DICOM Viewer | DICOM Image Library. (n.d.). Retrieved December 21, 2018, from http://www.osirix-viewer.com/resources/dicom-image-library/

Peres, A. (1985). Reversible logic and Quantum Computers. *Physical Review A., 32*(6), 3266–3276. doi:10.1103/PhysRevA.32.3266 PMID:9896493

Praveenkumar, P., Amirtharajan, R., Thenmozhi, K., & Balaguru Rayappan, J. B. (2015). Medical Data Sheet in Safe Havens - A Tri-layer Cryptic Solution. *Computers in Biology and Medicine, 62*(C), 264–276. doi:10.1016/j.compbiomed.2015.04.031 PMID:25966921

Ravichandran, D., Praveenkumar, P., Balaguru Rayappan, J. B., & Amirtharajan, R. (2016). Chaos based crossover and mutation for securing DICOM image. *Computers in Biology and Medicine, 72*, 170–184. doi:10.1016/j.compbiomed.2016.03.020 PMID:27046666

Ravichandran, D., Praveenkumar, P., Rayappan, J. B. B., & Amirtharajan, R. (2017). DNA Chaos Blend to Secure Medical Privacy. *IEEE Transactions on Nanobioscience, 16*(8), 850–858. doi:10.1109/TNB.2017.2780881 PMID:29364129

Sang, J., Wang, S., & Niu, X. (2016). Quantum realization of the nearest-neighbor interpolation method for FRQI and NEQR. *Quantum Information Processing, 15*(1), 37–64. doi:10.100711128-015-1135-5

Song, X. H., Wang, S., Liu, S., Abd El-Latif, A. A., & Niu, X. M. (2013). A dynamic watermarking scheme for quantum images using quantum wavelet transform. *Quantum Information Processing, 12*(12), 3689–3706. doi:10.100711128-013-0629-2

Toffoli, T. (1980). *Reversible computing*. Berlin: Springer. doi:10.21236/ADA082021

Venegas-Andraca, S. E., & Ball, J. L. (2010). Processing images in entangled quantum systems. *Quantum Information Processing, 9*(1), 1–11. doi:10.100711128-009-0123-z

Venegas-Andraca, S. E., & Bose, S. (2003). *Storing, processing, and retrieving an image using quantum mechanics*. Academic Press.

Wang, M., Wang, X., Zhang, Y., & Gao, Z. (2018). A novel chaotic encryption scheme based on image segmentation and multiple diffusion models. *Optics & Laser Technology, 108*, 558–573. doi:10.1016/j.optlastec.2018.07.052

Wang, X., & Liu, C. (2017). A novel and effective image encryption algorithm based on chaos and DNA encoding. *Multimedia Tools and Applications*, *76*(5), 6229–6245. doi:10.100711042-016-3311-8

Wang, X.-Y., Zhang, Y.-Q., & Bao, X.-M. (2015). A novel chaotic image encryption scheme using DNA sequence operations. *Optics and Lasers in Engineering*, *73*, 53–61. doi:10.1016/j.optlaseng.2015.03.022

Wu, Y., Member, S., Noonan, J. P., & Member, L. (2011, April). NPCR and UACI Randomness Tests for Image Encryption. *Cyber Journals: Multidisciplinary Journals in Science and Technology, Journal of Selected Areas in Telecommunications*, 31–38.

Zhang, S., Gao, T., & Gao, L. (2014). A Novel Encryption Frame for Medical Image with Watermark Based on Hyperchaotic System. *Mathematical Problems in Engineering*, *2014*, 1–11. doi:10.1155/2014/917147

Zhang, Y., Lu, K., Gao, Y., & Xu, K. (2013). A novel quantum representation for log-polar images. *Quantum Information Processing*, *12*(9), 3103–3126. doi:10.100711128-013-0587-8

Zhou, Y., Bao, L., & Chen, C. L. P. (2014). A new 1D chaotic system for image encryption. *Signal Processing*, *97*, 172–182. doi:10.1016/j.sigpro.2013.10.034

Chapter 9
Optimization Techniques for the Multilevel Thresholding of the Medical Images

Taranjit Kaur
Indian Institute of Technology Delhi, India

Barjinder Singh Saini
Dr. B. R. Ambedkar National Institute of Technology, India

Savita Gupta
Panjab University, India

ABSTRACT

Multilevel thresholding is segmenting the image into several distinct regions. Medical data like magnetic resonance images (MRI) contain important clinical information that is crucial for diagnosis. Hence, automatic segregation of tissue constituents is of key interest to clinician. In the chapter, standard entropies (i.e., Kapur and Tsallis) are explored for thresholding of brain MR images. The optimal thresholds are obtained by the maximization of these entropies using the particle swarm optimization (PSO) and the BAT optimization approach. The techniques are implemented for the segregation of various tissue constituents (i.e., cerebral spinal fluid [CSF], white matter [WM], and gray matter [GM]) from simulated images obtained from the brain web database. The efficacy of the thresholding technique is evaluated by the Dice coefficient (Dice). The results demonstrate that Tsallis' entropy is superior to the Kapur's entropy for the segmentation CSF and WM. Moreover, entropy maximization using BAT algorithm attains a higher Dice in contrast to PSO.

DOI: 10.4018/978-1-5225-7952-6.ch009

INTRODUCTION

Image segmentation is the process of extracting meaningful objects from the image. Computed tomography and MRI are the common imaging modalities that help physicians to non-invasively study the brain structures (Gondal and Khan, 2013). MRI is preferred modality of choice due to its higher soft tissue contrast and the availability of multispectral images. Upon careful analyzing these multiple images, a radiologist provides a decision about the lesion extent and the therapy treatment. Various tissue constituents in an MR image can be either manually marked by the radiologists (Georgiadis *et al.*, 2007, 2008; Zacharaki *et al.*, 2009) or they can make use of the semi-automatic or fully automatic computer-assisted approaches. Manual segmentation of MR image is both tedious and time-consuming due its 3D nature. Also, the outlined tissue constituent suffer from the effect of interobserver variability (Dou *et al.*, 2007; Corso *et al.*, 2008; Hemanth *et al.*, 2013). Though several segmentation methods have been presented in the past year's, thresholding is undoubtedly one of the most attractive technique due to its simplicity.

For the analysis of the medical images, many thresholding techniques have been developed in recent years which are either based on Kapur's entropy maximization (Kapur, Sahoo and Wong, 1985; Manikandan et al., 2014) or the cross entropy minimization (Kaur, Saini and Gupta, 2016). The entropy criteria proposed by Kapur's and Otsu's based between class variance approach has been widely used to find the optimal thresholds in the case of images with bimodal histogram but for images with multimodal histogram, these approaches suffer from the drawback of an exponential surge in the computational time (Manikandan et al., 2014). To overcome this problem heuristic based algorithms have been applied for dividing the image into several regions by obtaining the optimal set of threshold values.

Yin (Yin, 2007) presented a method that used particle swarm optimization (PSO) for finding of the optimal thresholds. The criteria employed for the multilevel thresholding was minimum cross entropy, and the efficacy of the method was validated by the measure of the computation time that was faster in than the exhaustive search methods. Nakib et al. (Nakib et al., 2007) devised two-dimensional survival exponential entropy criteria based on PSO for MR image segmentation. The results were compared with those obtained using 2D Shannon entropy as the objective function in terms of the misclassification error.

Djerou et al. (Djerou et al., 2009) proposed binary PSO for determining the optimum number and the corresponding values of the various thresholds. The Kapur's entropy and the Otsu's criteria were employed as objective function, uniformity measure, and computation time were used as a performance metric. The results illustrate that the Otsu's method was faster than the Kapur's method.

De et al. (De et al., 2010) performed the segmentation of diseased MRI using PSO based Shannon entropy criteria. The segmented region was post-processed by applying masking operation. The method was based on the conception that diseased area would have different intensity level in contrast to the normal regions. Firstly, the normalized image histogram was obtained and then the entropy maximization was used to find the range of gray values for the diseased region using PSO. After that, region growing in the form of masking was also done to attain the final segmented image.

Gao et al. (Gao et al., 2010) developed a multilevel thresholding technique based on quantum-behaved cooperative PSO (CQPSO). The proposed approach circumvented the problem of local trapping by preserving the fast convergence rate of basic PSO. The maximization of between class variance was used as an objective function. The experimental results indicate that, compared with the existing population-based thresholding methods, the CQPSO algorithm gets more effective and efficient results in terms of the objective function value and the computation time. Hongmei et al. (Hongmei et al., 2010) devised a multilevel threshold image segmentation based upon improved PSO. The modified PSO used random numbers for the acceleration coefficients instead of fixed values of two to counteract the problem of premature convergence present in the basic PSO. The improved PSO increases the exploration capabilities of basic PSO and thus increases the diversity. The Shannon entropy was used as fitness criteria, and the proficiency of the method was justified by its comparison with basic PSO using the metric of uniformity.

Sathya and Kayalvizhi (Sathya and Kayalvizhi, 2010) proposed a Bacterial Foraging optimization (BFO) based Tsallis entropy method for multilevel thresholding. The performance of BFO, PSO and Genetic Algorithm (GA) were explored on a set of natural images. The CPU time, peak signal to noise ratio (PSNR) and standard deviation were used to prove the efficiency of the proposed method. For the entire set of images, the BFO based Tsallis entropy method achieved higher value of objective function, and the PSNR value in contrast to the PSO and GA algorithms.

Agarwal et al. (Agrawal et al., 2013) performed multilevel image thresholding using Tsallis entropy computationally aided with the cuckoo search algorithm. Its application on a set of natural images demonstrated its effectiveness for image segmentation problem. The results obtained were compared with BFO, artificial bee colony (ABC), and GA algorithm. From the achieved results, it was concluded that cuckoo search algorithm outperforms other algorithms. The objective function value, structural similarity index (SSIM), PSNR, computational time and Feature similarity index (FSIM) higher than the other competing optimization algorithms.

Manikandan et al. (Manikandan et al., 2014) introduced real coded GA (RGA) with stimulated binary crossover for MRI brain image segmentation. The Kapur's entropy was used as an objective measure. Uniformity was employed as a performance measure, and the comparison with the other existing metaheuristic algorithms like PSO, BF and Adaptive Bacterial Foraging (ABF) demonstrated the superior performance of the RGA with stimulated binary crossover.

From the findings in the literature, it is seen that although Kapur's and Tsallis entropy has been used for the MR Image segmentation, the optimal thresholds for segregation have been mostly obtained using the PSO based algorithms only. The PSO algorithm although results in faster convergence but it tends to fall into local optima leading to local trapping or premature convergence. To circumvent this drawback, BAT algorithm was designed that uses an amalgamation of the major strengths of the PSO and the Harmony Search algorithm (Yang, 2010). Moreover, BAT algorithm has exhibited better performance than the GA, PSO, and the Harmony Search Algorithm (Yang, 2010).

The present chapter explores the performance of both Kapur's and Tsallis entropy for accurate segmentation of brain constituents using the PSO and the BAT algorithm. The MR images along with their ground truth were taken from the brain web database (http://brainweb.bic.mni.mcgill.ca/brainweb). The efficiency of both the optimization techniques have been explored using the metric of spatial overlap, i.e., Dice coefficient.

The structure of the remaining chapter is as follows, the next section presents the overview of the employed optimization techniques, i.e., PSO and the BAT algorithm. Section 3 describes about the employed fitness criteria and its application to the image segmentation process. Section 4 gives the results and discussion of the algorithm and finally conclusion is presented in the last section.

OVERVIEW OF THE OPTIMIZATION TECHNIQUES

During the past years, many swarm intelligence algorithms have evolved in literature. They comprise of GA (Staal et al., 2002), PSO (Kennedy and Eberhart, 1995), and Harmony Search Algorithm (Mahdavi,

Fesanghary and Damangir, 2007). The GA (Staal et al., 2002) is inspired by the genetic process of the biological organisms. The solution comprises of chromosomes encoded as the binary value of 0 and 1. In accordance with the fitness function, the merit of the chromosome is evaluated that subsequently undergoes cross-over and mutation to obtain the optimal solution. The limitation of the algorithm is that it is time-consuming (El Aziz and Hassanien, 2016). The PSO mimics the collective behavior of the bird flocks (Kennedy and Eberhart, 1995). It is based on a velocity and position update mechanism for finding the optimal solution. Although it has fewer parameters to fine tune, it has the drawback of premature convergence or local trapping due to which swarm diversity gets reduced (Lin and Hua, 2009). Harmony search algorithm (Mahdavi, Fesanghary and Damangir, 2007) represents the creativeness process of music players. The search ability of the algorithm is influenced by several parameters like harmony memory considering rate (HMCR), pitch adjusting rate (PAR), and distance bandwidth.

Apart from all these techniques, Bat Algorithm (BAT) introduced by Yang (Yang, 2010) is a recent metaheuristic algorithm inspired by the echolocation ability of the microbats which guides them on their foraging behavior. The BAT uses a combination of the major strengths of the PSO and the Harmony Search algorithm.

The succeeding subsection reviews the basics of two of the most popular swarm intelligence algorithms, i.e., PSO and the BAT algorithm.

PSO Algorithm

PSO is one of the most popular swarm based optimization algorithm. It was coined in the year 1995 by Kennedy and Eberhart (Kennedy and Eberhart, 1995). In PSO particles evolve in d-dimensional search space by the modulation of their movement according to their own flying experience and the flying experience of the neighboring particles.

The position and velocity associated with each particle is represented as a d dimensional vector i.e., $x_i = (x_{i1}, x_{i2}..........x_{id})$ and $V_i = (v_{i1}, v_{i2}..........v_{id})$ respectively. The best position each particle has attained so far is referred to as local best value (pbest) and is represented by $P_i = (p_{i1}, p_{i2}..........p_{id})$. The best position reached by any particle in the neighborhood is represented as $P_g = (p_{g1}, p_{g2}..........p_{gd})$ and is denoted as gbest. At every iteration, the position and velocities are updated using the following equations (Kennedy and Eberhart, 1995)

$$V_{ij}(t+1) = V_{ij}(t) + c_1 r_1 (p_{ij}(t) - x_{ij}(t)) + c_2 r_2 (p_{gj}(t) - x_{ij}(t)) \tag{1}$$

$$x_{ij}(t+1) = x_{ij}(t) + V_{ij}(t+1) \tag{2}$$

$j = 1, 2.........n$ where $n =$ dimensions, $i = 1, 2...N$ where N defines the number of particles, t denotes the iteration counter; r_1 and r_2 are random numbers uniformly distributed within the range of [0, 1], c_1, c_2 are called the cognitive and social learning parameters respectively. To increase the exploration capabilities and to avoid the premature convergence problem, inertia weight w was added to the previous velocity term which was suggested by Shi and Eberhart (Shi and Eberhart, 1998).

BAT Algorithm

BAT algorithm inspired from echolocation behavior of microbats follows certain procedures for position and velocity updating in accordance with the pulse frequency Q_i (Lu et al., 2017). The velocity v_i and position x_i corresponding the ith bat are defined in a d-dimensional search space. The new solutions are attained by updating x_i and v_i at each time step, t, and are mathematically given as (Yang, 2010)(Singh, Verma and Sharma, 2017):

$$Q_i = Q_{min} + (Q_{max} - Q_{min})\beta \tag{3}$$

$$v_i^t = v_i^{t-1} + (x_i^{t-1} - x^*)f_i \tag{4}$$

$$x_i^t = x_i^{t-1} + v_i^t \tag{5}$$

In eq. (3), β is a random number drawn from a uniform distribution in the range from {0 1}, Q_i is the frequency value related to the ith bat, Q_{max} and Q_{min} are the maximum and minimum frequency values. The v_i and x_i of the ith bat at the tth time step are denoted as v_i^t and x_i^t. x^* is the global best solution obtained by comparing and sorting the fitness value corresponding to all bat positions in accordance with the given objective function. For favoring exploitation around x^* a modification was proposed by Yang (Yang, 2010) and is mathematically denoted as:

$$x_{new} = x^* + \varepsilon A^t \tag{6}$$

Here, ε signify random value generated in the interval [-1, 1] and A^t is the mean loudness value at the tth time step for all the bats.

Furthermore, the rate of pulse emission, r_i and mean loudness, A_i are updated with iterations as given below:

$$A_i^{t+1} = \alpha A_i^t \tag{7}$$

$$r_i^{t+1} = r_i^0(1 - \exp(-\gamma t)) \tag{8}$$

In the above expression γ and α are constants and r_i^0 is the initial value of pulse emission rate of the ith bat.

EMPLOYED FITNESS CRITERIA AND ITS APPLICATION TO IMAGE SEGMENTATION PROCESS

MR image segmentation in the present work has been done using the concept of multilevel thresholding. Multilevel thresholding uses more than one threshold value to partition a given MR image (I) into multiple groups (M0, M1,…,Mk)via the following eq. (9)

$$M_0 = \{f(x,y) \in I \mid 0 \leq f(x,y) \leq t_1 - 1\}$$
$$M_1 = \{f(x,y) \in I \mid t_1 \leq f(x,y) \leq t_2 - 1\}$$
$$M_i = \{f(x,y) \in I \mid t_i \leq f(x,y) \leq t_{i+1} - 1\}$$
$$M_k = \{f(x,y) \in I \mid t_k \leq f(x,y) \leq L - 1\}$$

(9)

where $f(x,y)$ denote the intensity value at any spatial location (x, y), t_i (i=1,…, k) is the ith threshold value and k is the number of thresholds. Non parametric approaches are widely used for the computation of the multiple thresholds. In these approaches, thresholds are assigned to ensure that the histogram of thresholded image fulfills the desired criteria such as maximization of posterior entropy (Kapur, Sahoo and Wong, 1985; Tsallis, 1988; Cheng, Chen and Li, 1998), maximization of some measure of separability (Otsu, 1979), some index of fuzziness and fuzzy similarity measures (Li, Zhao and Cheng, 1995; Cheng and Lui, 1997) or minimizing Bayesian error measure (Kittler and Illingworth, 1986).

Various criteria for multilevel thresholding, computationally aided with evolutionary or swarm based optimization algorithms also exist in literature and significant among them are Kapur's Entropy (Manikandan et al., 2014), Tsallis Entropy (Agrawal et al., 2013), Cross Entropy (Yin, 2007; Horng, 2010; Horng and Liou, 2011; Tang et al., 2011), Renyi Entropy. (Sarkar et al., 2012)., Fuzzy Entropy (Yin et al., 2014) and the entropies calculated from the co-occurrence matrices (Mokji and Abu Bakar, 2007; Panda, Agrawal and Bhuyan, 2013).

In the current work, the efficacy of the Kapur's (Manikandan et al., 2014) and Tsallis entropy (Agrawal et al., 2013) was investigated for MR image segmentation. These criteria serve as a fitness function to be optimized using PSO and BAT algorithm resulting in the generation of the multiple thresholds. The optimal thresholds were then used to partition the given MR image into the CSF, WM, and the GM regions.

Before describing the step by step procedure involved in the computation of optimal thresholds, it is necessary to outline the mathematical formulation behind the construction of the fitness/objective function that is based on Kapur's and Tsallis entropy-based criterion. The succeeding subsection illustrates the mechanism for fitness function generation.

Kapur's Entropy

The procedure involved using Kapur's entropy is as follows:
Compute the normalized histogram(P_n) of gray level image, I which is denoted by $h(n)$

$$P_n = h(n) = \frac{f_n}{N}, \quad n = 0,1,2\ldots\ldots\ldots 255$$

(10)

where f_n is the observed frequency, i.e. number of pixels having gray level n and N is the total number of pixels in the picture. The mechanism of optimal multilevel thresholding is the process of dividing an image into multiple thresholds $\left(t_1,\ t_2, ...t_k\right)$ that maximizes the entropy (H) that is given as

$$H = -\sum_{n=0}^{t_1} P_{1n} ln P_{1n} - \sum_{n=t_1+1}^{t_2} P_{2n} ln P_{2n} \cdot \cdot \cdot - \sum_{n=t_k+1}^{255} P_{kn} ln P_{kn} \tag{11}$$

Alternatively, it is rewritten as

$$H = H_0 + H_1 + \ . \ . \ . \ + H_m \tag{12}$$

where

$$P_{1n} = \frac{P_n}{\sum_{n=0}^{t_1} P_n} \ ; \text{for } 0 \ \leq \ n \ < \ t_1 \tag{13}$$

$$P_{2n} = \frac{P_n}{\sum_{n=t_1+1}^{t_2} P_n} \ ; \text{for } t_1 \leq \ n \ < \ t_2 \tag{14}$$

$$P_{kn} = \frac{P_n}{\sum_{n=t_k+1}^{255} P_n} \ ; \text{for } t_k \leq \ n \ \leq \ 255 \tag{15}$$

$$[T_1,T_2,...,T_k] = \text{arg max} \left(\sum_{j=0}^{k} H_j\right) \tag{16}$$

As, the MR brain image primarily comprises of the WM, GM, CSF, and the background region so the goal of the segmentation algorithm would be the efficient delineation of these constituents through maximization of H as given in eq. (16). For partitioning the brain image into these constituents, three optimal thresholds would be needed.

Tsallis Entropy

The Tsallis Entropy for a non-extensive system is given by general formula as follows (Zhang and Wu, 2011; Agrawal et al., 2013)

$$S_q = \frac{1 - \sum_{i=1}^{q}(p_i)^q}{q-1} \tag{17}$$

where q denotes the entropic index specifying the degree of nonextensivity. The value of q was taken as four it yielded best segmentation results for most of the images. p_i denotes the probabilities of the pixel at gray level i. The cumulative probabilities for foreground class (A) and background class (B) can be defined as

$$w_A = \sum_{i=1}^{t} p_i \tag{18}$$

$$w_B = \sum_{i=t+1}^{L} p_i \tag{19}$$

The expression below gives normalization of probabilities

$$p^A = \frac{\{p_1, p_2, \dots \dots \dots p_t\}}{w_A} \tag{20}$$

$$p^B = \frac{\{p_{t+1}, p_{t+2}, \dots \dots \dots p_L\}}{w_B} \tag{21}$$

In the above expression, L signifies the total number of intensity levels in an image. The Tsallis entropy for each class is given as

$$S_q^A(t) = \frac{1 - \sum_{i=1}^{t}\left(p_i^A\right)^q}{q-1} \tag{22}$$

$$S_q^B\left(t\right) = \frac{1 - \sum_{i=t+1}^{L}\left(p_i^B\right)^q}{q-1} \qquad (23)$$

Total Tsallis entropy of image S_q (t) of an image is written as (Zhang and Wu, 2011; Agrawal et al., 2013)

$$S_q\left(\mathrm{t}\right) = S_q^A\left(t\right) + S_q^B\left(t\right) + \left(1-q\right) \times S_q^A\left(t\right) \times S_q^B\left(t\right) \qquad (24)$$

The optimum threshold value is obtained by maximization of Tsallis entropy given as

$$t^* = \arg(\max(S_q\left(\mathrm{t}\right)) \qquad (25)$$

Extending the above equation for multilevel thresholding gives eq. (26).

$$[T_1, T_2, ..., T_k] = \arg\max[S_q^1(t) + S_q^2(t) + ... + S_q^M(t) + (1-q)S_q^1(t)S_q^2(t)...........S_q^M(t)] \qquad (26)$$

where M =k+1 and

$$S_q^1\left(t\right) = \frac{1 - \sum_{i=1}^{t_1}\left(p_i^1\right)^q}{q-1} \qquad (27)$$

$$S_q^2\left(t\right) = \frac{1 - \sum_{i=t_1+1}^{t_2}\left(p_i^2\right)^q}{q-1} \qquad (28)$$

$$S_q^M\left(t\right) = \frac{1 - \sum_{i=t_k+1}^{L}\left(p_i^M\right)^q}{q-1} \qquad (29)$$

Here, M=k+1 and $p^1, p^2, ..., p^M$ corresponding to $S^1, S^2, ..., S^M$ can be obtained using $T_1, T_2, ..., T_k$ respectively.

Table 1. Step by step procedure to compute the optimal thresholds by incorporating the designed fitness criteria into the optimization framework

Sr. No.	Steps for the PSO Algorithm	Steps for the BAT Algorithm
1	The size of the swarm was taken to be forty, the number of dimensions was taken as three, i.e., equivalent to the number of thresholds, and the number of iterations were taken as 100	
2	Initialize the position of every particle in the range defined by the upper and lower bounds of the normal MRI zone	Initialize the position of every Bat in the range defined by the upper and lower bounds of the normal MRI zone
3	Initialize the velocities for each particle	Initialize the bats pulse frequency Q_i, loudness A_i and the pulse rate r_i
4	Evaluate the fitness function value $\left(\sum_{j=0}^{k} H_j\right)$ and $$[S_q^1(t) + S_q^2(t) + \ldots\ldots\ldots + S_q^M(t) + (1-q)S_q^1(t)S_q^2(t)\ldots\ldots\ldots S_q^M(t)]$$ for each particle/Bat position	
5	Selection of *pbest* and *gbest*: For the first iteration, the local best value i.e. *pbest* is equal to the current particle position, and *gbest* is the position value of particle at which objective function is maximum	Choose the best solution x^* for which the value of the objective function is maximum
6	Update the velocity and position using eq. (1) and (2).	Update the pulse frequency, velocity, and position of every bat using eq. (3), (4), and (5)
7	Update the *pbest* and *gbest* values: Check the fitness value at the updated particle position value, if it is better, i.e., greater than that of the *pbest* retained in memory set the current particle position value as the new *pbest*. From the updated *pbest*, select *gbest* as the particle position vector possesing the maximum entropy value.	**If** (*rand* (0,1) > r_i) then generate a local solution around the best solution (given by eq. (6)) **If** (*rand*< A_i & $f(x_i) > f(x^*)$), then accept new solutions Increase r_i and reduce A_i Rank the bats and find the current best value x^* (given by eq. (7) & (8))
8	Check for the convergence criteria, if not satisfied repeat steps 4 to 7. For this maximization, problem number of iterations was used as the convergence criteria.	

For Kapur's entropy the expression given by eq. (16) was employed as fitness criteria and for Tsallis entropy the expression given by eq. (26) was used as a fitness function. Higher value of these fitness functions indicates better homogeneity of the segmented regions.

The next stages briefly describe the steps for the incorporation of the designed fitness criteria (eq. (16) and eq. (26)) into an optimization framework to compute the appropriate thresholds for the segmentation. Steps are given separately for PSO and BAT optimization algorithm and they are tabulated below (Table 1):

RESULTS AND DISCUSSIONS

To validate the efficacy of the different objective functions computationally aided with the evolutionary algorithm for the image segmentation, simulated MR brain images from the Brain web database (http://brainweb.bic.mni.mcgill.ca/brainweb) were taken. The simulations were based on an anatomical model of the normal brain which can serve as ground truth for the validation of any algorithm. The details of the images taken from this database are as follows: Phantom_name=normal, protocol=ICBM, modality=T1, Slice_thickness=1mm, Noise=0% and intensity non-uniformity (INU) =0%. The algorithm was implemented on 20 coronal slices of T1_ ICBM_ normal_ 1mm_ pn0_ rf0 simulated brain phantom. The phantom dimensions were $181 \times 217 \times 181$ voxels, with a step size equal to 1mm.

The segmentation process was preceded by skull stripping procedure, as the pixels present in the brain tissues have the intensities similar to the skull region. The skull region was extracted by first converting the MR image to binary image using Otsu's method (Otsu, 1979). After that, a search was made for the largest connected component. Finally, only the pixels present in that largest component were retained corresponding to the brain region. The segmentation results were evaluated using Dice as a similarity measure. The Dice measure computes the similarity between two regions and is defined as (Agrawal, Panda and Dora, 2014; Singh and Garg, 2014)

$$Dice = 2 \times \frac{I_{gt} \cap I_{seg}}{I_{gt} + I_{seg}} \tag{30}$$

where I_{gt} refers to the ground truth image and I_{seg} represents segmented image. A higher value of Dice corresponds to more exact segmentation. Table I. shows the values of the Dice corresponding to WM, GM and CSF regions. It is observed that the segmentation results obtained with the BAT algorithm are closer to the ground truth region. The results for the 90th coronal slice were also compared with those obtained using fuzzy clustering approach proposed by Agarwal et al. (Agrawal, Panda and Dora, 2014) and (Kaur, Saini and Gupta, 2018). From the tabulated results in Table 2 and Table 3, it is concluded that Tsallis entropy outperforms Kapur's entropy and the fuzzy clustering approach for both the CSF and WM regions. Moreover, segmentation results obtained using the BAT algorithm are better than the works reported by (Kaur, Saini and Gupta, 2018) where PSO algorithm has been used for obtaining the optimal set of thresholds. The average value of Dice obtained using the BAT algorithm for Tsallis entropy were 0.972238, 0.837515, and 0.887657 which are better than that obtained using the PSO algorithm that resulted in an average value equal to 0.967279, 0.828330, and 0.878031 for the WM, GM, and the CSF. Qualitatively, the segmentations obtained using the BAT algorithm for slice 90 are given in figure 1.

Better performance of the Tsallis entropy can be attributed to the fact that it is able to capture the difference in the texture information present in the various tissue constituents more effectively in contrast to the Kapur's entropy. It has also proved to be proficient in seizing the short and the long range correlation among the pixels belonging to the same object in an image. Superior performance of the tsallis entropy for natural image segmentation was also ascertained in the works by (Zhang and Wu, 2011) where optimal thresholds were obtained using the Tsallis entropy in contrast to the Kapur's entropy criteria. Another reason for the improvement in the thresholding results is that the tsallis entropy criteria make

Figure 1 (a) Simulated T1 MR image slice 90; (b),(c),(d) represent the ground truth CSF, WM and GM regions for slice 90; (e) and (i) segmented slice 90 using Tsallis and Kapur's entropy optimized by BAT algorithm; (f),(g),(h) and (j),(k),(l) represent the delineated CSF, WM and GM regions for slice 90 using Tsallis and Kapur's entropy when maximized using BAT algorithm

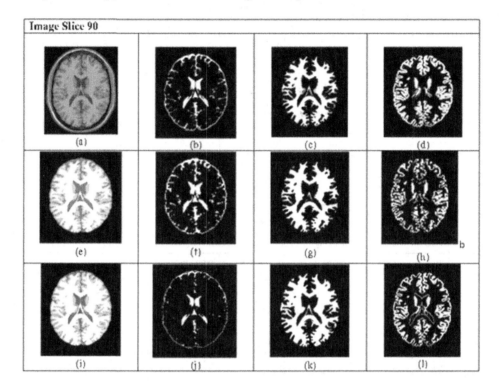

use of the global and the objective property of the image histogram to compute the optimum threshold for segmentation. Moreover, BAT algorithm exhibits better results in contrast to the PSO algorithm for both the entropies as it circumvents the drawback of local trapping or limited exploration and the exploitation capabilities existing in PSO.

ADVANTAGES AND LIMITATIONS OF THE PROPOSED WORK

The advantage of the presented work is that it is a fully automatic multilevel thresholding algorithm for MR image segmentation. This approach successfully extracts the region of interest by capturing the gradual and sharp intensity variations existing in MR tumor images having vague boundaries. The proposed method employs one of the recent optimization algorithm, i.e., BAT, for the generation of the optimal thresholds which has low computational complexity than exhaustive search methods and better exploration capability as compared to PSO. Moreover, the method does not require any initialization by the clinician, the algorithm does not need any training or learning phase which generalizes its applicability to the diversified set of images with fuzzy boundaries, poor contrast and those acquired from the multiple centres. Clinically, the automated approach is expected to relieve the radiologist from the

Table 2. Comparison of the Dice coefficient for the different brain tissue constituents obtained by maximizing the objective function through the PSO and the BAT optimization algorithm

Subject (Slice No.)	Employed Optimization Criteria	Dice for WM (Kapur Entropy)	Dice for WM (Tsallis Entropy)	Dice for GM (Kapurs Entropy)	Dice for GM (Tsallis Entropy)	Dice for CSF (Kapurs Entropy)	Dice for CSF (Tsallis Entropy)
90	PSO	0.948975	0.991115	0.853233	0.845863	0.562622	0.885730
	BAT	0.950611	0.992318	0.858213	0.847154	0.613981	0.890503
91	PSO	0.956445	0.975805	0.853591	0.820053	0.541796	0.920855
	BAT	0.970001	0.978132	0.859318	0.832590	0.562143	0.928110
92	PSO	0.962848	0.967729	0.864248	0.820595	0.607280	0.899172
	BAT	0.971421	0.980007	0.873291	0.849171	0.625543	0.901563
93	PSO	0.969091	0.978254	0.876662	0.826524	0.614796	0.892097
	BAT	0.981130	0.984156	0.883520	0.831025	0.635210	0.911725
94	PSO	0.956030	0.972219	0.855376	0.815040	0.653992	0.923099
	BAT	0.961173	0.978113	0.861053	0.826142	0.665231	0.931125
95	PSO	0.946377	0.987615	0.864584	0.863855	0.583642	0.910384
	BAT	0.957703	0.989315	0.874472	0.871583	0.616921	0.923179
96	PSO	0.943621	0.970802	0.840561	0.822186	0.574307	0.901584
	BAT	0.953121	0.973211	0.853649	0.825610	0.588317	0.911453
97	PSO	0.939694	0.949904	0.847860	0.763720	0.501460	0.850677
	BAT	0.940012	0.952683	0.852130	0.772139	0.520021	0.863110
98	PSO	0.946455	0.973008	0.862461	0.795258	0.527177	0.897427
	BAT	0.953180	0.987665	0.871123	0.801538	0.530071	0.901129
99	PSO	0.941782	0.973895	0.859087	0.874090	0.496421	0.909383
	BAT	0.950091	0.987521	0.861157	0.881482	0.504419	0.918371
100	PSO	0.946350	0.994791	0.854937	0.821111	0.446252	0.907799
	BAT	0.951559	0.995100	0.862150	0.830012	0.465211	0.913720
101	PSO	0.945977	0.978959	0.864723	0.860672	0.357519	0.901358
	BAT	0.951103	0.981213	0.871140	0.871871	0.381190	0.921130
102	PSO	0.941821	0.983371	0.863633	0.870157	0.782760	0.896819
	BAT	0.952140	0.984325	0.876351	0.884710	0.796015	0.911063
103	PSO	0.919264	0.951415	0.831798	0.811852	0.763524	0.866623
	BAT	0.925001	0.964150	0.842190	0.822531	0.772401	0.872250
104	PSO	0.920248	0.945363	0.825959	0.829434	0.777299	0.851541
	BAT	0.931401	0.9510032	0.831095	0.837925	0.785120	0.861132
105	PSO	0.942690	0.970668	0.877872	0.720241	0.716343	0.867234
	BAT	0.951126	0.972251	0.883915	0.731520	0.726901	0.874452
106	PSO	0.920248	0.938944	0.825762	0.851660	0.768102	0.827491
	BAT	0.931541	0.941003	0.841172	0.861701	0.778143	0.834725

continued on following page

Table 2. Continued

Subject (Slice No.)	Employed Optimization Criteria	Dice for WM (Kapur Entropy)	Dice for WM (Tsallis Entropy)	Dice for GM (Kapurs Entropy)	Dice for GM (Tsallis Entropy)	Dice for CSF (Kapurs Entropy)	Dice for CSF (Tsallis Entropy)
107	*PSO*	0.931178	0.949793	0.864266	0.856391	0.738170	0.831475
	BAT	0.944101	0.953421	0.871325	0.866542	0.742180	0.844250
108	*PSO*	0.913493	0.969766	0.833108	0.827920	0.746338	0.850103
	BAT	0.925673	0.970003	0.838912	0.831529	0.751338	0.860051
109	*PSO*	0.893989	0.922175	0.800784	0.869972	0.716183	0.769765
	BAT	0.900131	0.929174	0.811521	0.873530	0.721850	0.780101
Mean Value	*PSO*	0.939329	0.967279	0.851025	0.828330	0.623799	0.878031
	BAT	0.947611	0.972238	0.858885	0.837515	0.63911	0.887657

Table 3. Segmentation evaluation in terms of dice measure in contrast to the existing works on Brain tissue segmentation

Slice no.	Brain Tissues	(Agrawal, Panda and Dora, 2014)	Kapurs Entropy (PSO Algorithm) (Kaur, Saini and Gupta, 2018)	Tsallis Entropy (PSO Algorithm) (Kaur, Saini and Gupta, 2018)	Kapurs Entropy (BAT Algorithm)	Tsallis Entropy (BAT Algorithm)
Slice 90	CSF	0.6623	0.562622	0.885730	0.613981	**0.890503**
	GM	0.8941	0.853233	0.845863	0.858213	0.847154
	WM	0.9684	0.948975	0.991115	0.950611	**0.992318**

tedious task of manually labelling the tissue constituents from the slices. Additionally, such an approach is expected to reduce the interobserver variability.

Both the Kapur's and the Tsallis entropy are intensity based multilevel thresholding techniques. They suffer from the limitation that the spatial correlation of the pixels has been ignored while computing the thresholds. For the images having the similar type of histogram but different texture information, the intensity based thresholding yields the same value of thresholds which is inappropriate.

The recent segmentation methods like those based on texture features and random forest classifier as proposed in the works by (Reza and Iftekharuddin, 2013) and Graph-based concurrent brain tumor segmentation given in (Parisot et al., 2014) suffer from the drawback that they need the pre-processing stages like registration, bias field correction, tumor localization, and a training phase.

The proposed approach is advantageous in context to these methods in the manner that it needs, i) no preprocessing stages like denoising, registration, and bias field correction, ii) no tumor localization, and iii) no training phase.

One of the possible open areas of research related to present work is exploring other entropies that incorporate spatial distribution of pixels entrenched in the GLCM sub-blocks along with the intensity information for multilevel image segmentation through which an increased value of Dice can be obtained for all the three regions. Future works will also be focused on extending the approach for the segmentation of diseased MRI image volumes.

CONCLUSION

In this paper PSO and BAT based multilevel thresholding using Kapur's and Tsallis entropy were explored for the segmentation of the brain image into its various tissue constituents. The method works well for normal brain MR images which have a multimodal histogram by selecting the optimal thresholds via the entropy maximization procedure. The performance of Kapur's and the Tsallis entropy is validated both quantitatively and qualitatively on the benchmark T1 axial brain MR images from the brain web database. Quantitatively the performance is assessed using the Dice measure. From the experimental results, it was seen that Tsallis entropy when optimized using the BAT works efficiently for the segmentation of CSF and WM regions in contrast to Kapur's entropy, fuzzy clustering approach, and the PSO based method as indicative by the Dice value that was equal to 0.890503 and 0.992318 for the typical 90th slice from the database. Better results were achieved because both the short range and the long range correlations existing in the pixels belonging to the same object were effectively seized via the tsallis entropy when optimized via the BAT algorithm. The parameter of the Tsallis entropy can be fine-tuned to further improvise the image thresholding results. One of the main advantages of the tsallis entropy based multilevel thresholding scheme is that it is computationally simple, independent of the prior anatomical knowledge, or the bias field correction that confines the application of many existing state of art approaches related to the medical image segmentation. Moreover, optimization using the BAT algorithm further improvise the segmentation results as it results in increase in the diversity of the search space resulting in optimal threshold values. The exploration of other entropies can be looked in future through which a higher value of Dice can be achieved for all the brain tissue constituents and analyzing the computational complexity of different evolutionary algorithms.

REFERENCES

Agrawal, S., Panda, R., Bhuyan, S., & Panigrahi, B. K. (2013). Tsallis entropy based optimal multilevel thresholding using cuckoo search algorithm. *Swarm and Evolutionary Computation. Elsevier, 11*(1), 16–30. doi:10.1016/j.swevo.2013.02.001

Agrawal, S., Panda, R., & Dora, L. (2014). A study on fuzzy clustering for magnetic resonance brain image segmentation using soft computing approaches. *Applied Soft Computing, 24*, 522–533. doi:10.1016/j. asoc.2014.08.011

Cheng, H. D., Chen, J.-R., & Li, J. (1998). Threshold selection based on fuzzy c-partition entropy approach. *Pattern Recognition, 31*(7), 857–870. doi:10.1016/S0031-3203(97)00113-1

Cheng, H. D., & Lui, Y. M. (1997). Automatic bandwidth selection of fuzzy membership functions. *Information Sciences*, *103*(1–4), 1–21. doi:10.1016/S0020-0255(97)00057-1

Corso, J. J., Sharon, E., Dube, S., El-Saden, S., Sinha, U., & Yuille, A. (2008). Efficient multilevel brain tumor segmentation with integrated bayesian model classification. *IEEE Transactions on Medical Imaging*, *27*(5), 629–640. doi:10.1109/TMI.2007.912817 PMID:18450536

De, A., Sharma, D., Mata, S., & Devi, V. (2010). Masking based Segmentation of Diseased MRI Images. *International Conference on Information Science and Applications (ICISA)*, 1–7. 10.1109/ICISA.2010.5480274

Djerou, L., Khelil, N., Dehimi, H. E., & Batouche, M. (2009). Automatic Multilevel Thresholding Using Binary Particle Swarm Optimization for Image Segmentation. In *International Conference of Soft Computing and Pattern Recognition, 2009. SOCPAR '09*. Malacca: IEEE. 10.1109/SoCPaR.2009.25

Dou, W., Ruan, S., Chen, Y., Bloyet, D., & Constans, J.-M. (2007). A framework of fuzzy information fusion for the segmentation of brain tumor tissues on MR images. *Image and Vision Computing*, *25*(2), 164–171. doi:10.1016/j.imavis.2006.01.025

El Aziz, M. A., & Hassanien, A. E. (2016). Modified cuckoo search algorithm with rough sets for feature selection. *Neural Computing and Applications. Springer*, *29*(4), 925–934. doi:10.100700521-016-2473-7

Gao, H., Xu, W., Sun, J., & Tang, Y. (2010). Multilevel Thresholding for Image Segmentation Through an Improved Quantum-Behaved Particle Swarm Algorithm. *IEEE Transactions on Instrumentation and Measurement*, *59*(4), 934–946. doi:10.1109/TIM.2009.2030931

Georgiadis, P., Cavouras, D., Kalatzis, I., & Daskalakis, A. (2007). Non-linear Least Squares Features Transformation for Improving the Performance of Probabilistic Neural Networks in Classifying Human Brain Tumors on MRI. Computational Science and Its Applications – ICCSA 2007, 239–247. doi:10.1007/978-3-540-74484-9_21

Georgiadis, P., Cavouras, D., Kalatzis, I., Daskalakis, A., Kagadis, G. C., Sifaki, K., ... Solomou, E. (2008). Improving brain tumor characterization on MRI by probabilistic neural networks and non-linear transformation of textural features. *Computer Methods and Programs in Biomedicine*, *89*(1), 24–32. doi:10.1016/j.cmpb.2007.10.007 PMID:18053610

Gondal, A. H., & Khan, M. N. A. (2013). A review of fully automated techniques for brain tumor detection from MR images. *International Journal of Modern Education and Computer Science. Modern Education and Computer Science Press*, *5*(2), 55–61.

Hemanth, D. J., Vijila, C. K. S., Selvakumar, A. I., & Anitha, J. (2013). Distance metric-based time-efficient fuzzy algorithm for abnormal magnetic resonance brain image segmentation. *Neural Computing & Applications*, *22*(5), 1013–1022. doi:10.100700521-011-0792-2

Hongmei, T., Cuixia, W., Liying, H., & Xia, W. (2010). Image Segmentation Based on Improved PSO. In *International Conference on Computer and Communication Technologies in Agriculture Engineering Image*. Chengdue: IEEE.

Horng, M. H. (2010). Multilevel minimum cross entropy threshold selection based on the honey bee mating optimization. *Expert Systems with Applications*, *37*(6), 4580–4592. doi:10.1016/j.eswa.2009.12.050

Horng, M.-H., & Liou, R.-J. (2011). Multilevel minimum cross entropy threshold selection based on the firefly algorithm. *Expert Systems with Applications*, *38*(12), 14805–14811. doi:10.1016/j.eswa.2011.05.069

Kapur, J. N., Sahoo, P. K., & Wong, A. K. C. (1985). A new method for gray-level picture thresholding using the entropy of the histogram. *Computer Vision Graphics and Image Processing*, *29*(3), 273–285. doi:10.1016/0734-189X(85)90125-2

Kaur, T., Saini, B. S., & Gupta, S. (2016). Optimized Multi Threshold Brain Tumor Image Segmentation Using Two Dimensional Minimum Cross Entropy Based on Co-occurrence Matrix. In *Medical Imaging in Clinical Applications* (pp. 461–486). Springer International Publishing. doi:10.1007/978-3-319-33793-7_20

Kaur, T., Saini, B. S., & Gupta, S. (2018). A comparative study on Kapur's and Tsallis entropy for multilevel thresholding of MR images via particle swarm optimisation technique. *Int. J. Computing Systems in Engineering*, *4*(2/3), 156–164. doi:10.1504/IJCSYSE.2018.091395

Kennedy, J., & Eberhart, R. (1995). Particle swarm optimization. In *Proceedings of ICNN'95 - International Conference on Neural Networks*. Perth, Australia: IEEE. 10.1109/ICNN.1995.488968

Kittler, J., & Illingworth, J. (1986). Minimum error thresholding. *Pattern Recognition*, *19*(1), 41–47. doi:10.1016/0031-3203(86)90030-0

Li, X., Zhao, Z., & Cheng, H. D. (1995). Fuzzy entropy threshold approach to breast cancer detection. *Information Sciences - Applications*, *4*, 49–56.

Lin, M., & Hua, Z. (2009). Improved PSO Algorithm with Adaptive Inertia Weight and Mutation. *World Congress on Computer Science and Information Engineering*, 622–625. 10.1109/CSIE.2009.428

Lu, S., Qiu, X., Shi, J., Li, N., Lu, Z.-H., Chen, P., … Zhang, Y. (2017). A pathological brain detection system based on extreme learning machine optimized by bat algorithm. *CNS & Neurological Disorders-Drug Targets (Formerly Current Drug Targets-CNS & Neurological Disorders)*, *16*(1), 23–29.

Mahdavi, M., Fesanghary, M., & Damangir, E. (2007). An improved harmony search algorithm for solving optimization problems. *Applied Mathematics and Computation*, *188*(2), 1567–1579. doi:10.1016/j.amc.2006.11.033

Manikandan, S., Ramar, K., Iruthayarajan, M. W., Srinivasagan, K. G. G., Willjuice Iruthayarajan, M., & Srinivasagan, K. G. G. (2014). Multilevel thresholding for segmentation of medical brain images using Real coded Genetic Algorithm. *Measurement*, *47*(1), 558–568. doi:10.1016/j.measurement.2013.09.031

Mokji, M. M., & Abu Bakar, S. A. R. (2007). Adaptive thresholding based on co-occurrence matrix edge information. *Journal of Computers*, *2*(8), 44–52. doi:10.4304/jcp.2.8.44-52

Nakib, A., Roman, S., Oulhadj, H., & Siarry, P. (2007). Fast brain MRI segmentation based on two-dimensional survival exponential entropy and particle swarm optimization. *Proceedings of the 29th Annual International Conference of the IEEE EMBS*, 5563–6. 10.1109/IEMBS.2007.4353607

Otsu, N. (1979). A threshold selection method from gray-level histograms. *IEEE Transactions on Systems, Man, and Cybernetics*, *SMC-9*(1), 62–66. doi:10.1109/TSMC.1979.4310076

Panda, R., Agrawal, S., & Bhuyan, S. (2013). Edge magnitude based multilevel thresholding using Cuckoo search technique. *Expert Systems with Applications*, *40*(18), 7617–7628. doi:10.1016/j.eswa.2013.07.060

Parisot, S., Wells, W., Chemouny, S., Duffau, H., & Paragios, N. (2014). 'Concurrent tumor segmentation and registration with uncertainty-based sparse non-uniform graphs', *Medical Image Analysis. Elsevier B.*, *18*(4), 647–659. PMID:24717540

Reza, S., & Iftekharuddin, K. M. (2013). Multi-class Abnormal Brain Tissue Segmentation Using Texture Features. In *MICCAI Challenge on Multimodal Brain Tumor Segmentation* (pp. 38–42). Nagoya, Japan: IEEE.

Sarkar, S., Sen, N., Kundu, A., Das, S., & Chaudhuri, S. S. (2012). A differential evolutionary multilevel segmentation of near infra-red images using renyi's entropy. *International Conference on Frontiers of Intelligent Computing: Theory and Applications*, 699–706.

Sathya, P. D., & Kayalvizhi, R. (2010). Optimum multilevel image thresholding based on tsallis entropy method with bacterial foraging algorithm. *International Journal of Computer Science Issues*, *7*(5), 336–343.

Shi, Y., & Eberhart, R. (1998). A modified particle swarm optimizer. In *IEEE World Congress on Computational Intelligence*. Anchorage, AK: IEEE.

Singh, M., Verma, A., & Sharma, N. (2017). Bat optimization based neuron model of stochastic resonance for the enhancement of MR images. *Biocybernetics and Biomedical Engineering*, *37*(1), 124–134. doi:10.1016/j.bbe.2016.10.006

Singh, P. P., & Garg, R. D. (2014). Classification of high resolution satellite images using spatial constraints-based fuzzy clustering. *Journal of Applied Remote Sensing*, *8*(1).

Staal, F. J. T., Van Der Luijt, R. B., Baert, M. R. M., Van Drunen, J., Van Bakel, H., Peters, E., & ... . (2002). A novel germline mutation of PTEN associated with brain tumours of multiple lineages. *British Journal of Cancer*, *86*(10), 1586–1591. PMID:12085208

Tang, K., Yuan, X., Sun, T., Yang, J., & Gao, S. (2011). An improved scheme for minimum cross entropy threshold selection based on genetic algorithm. *Knowledge-Based Systems. Elsevier B*, *24*(8), 1131–1138.

Tsallis, C. (1988). Possible generalization of boltzmann- gibbs statistics. *Journal of Statistical Physics*, *52*(1), 479–487. doi:10.1007/BF01016429

Yang, X.-S. (2010). A new metaheuristic bat-inspired algorithm. In *Nature inspired cooperative strategies for optimization (NICSO 2010)* (pp. 65–74). Springer. doi:10.1007/978-3-642-12538-6_6

Yin, P.-Y. (2007). Multilevel minimum cross entropy threshold selection based on particle swarm optimization. *Applied Mathematics and Computation*, *184*(2), 503–513. doi:10.1016/j.amc.2006.06.057

Yin, S., Zhao, X., Wang, W., & Gong, M. (2014). Efficient multilevel image segmentation through fuzzy entropy maximization and graph cut optimization. *Pattern Recognition*, *47*(9), 2894–2907. doi:10.1016/j.patcog.2014.03.009

Zacharaki, E. I., Wang, S., Chawla, S., & Soo, D. (2009). Classification of brain tumor type and grade using MRI texture and shape in a machine learning scheme. *Magnetic Resonance in Medicine*, *62*(6), 1609–1618. doi:10.1002/mrm.22147 PMID:19859947

Zhang, Y., & Wu, L. (2011). Optimal Multi-Level Thresholding Based on Maximum Tsallis Entropy via an Artificial Bee Colony Approach. *Entropy (Basel, Switzerland)*, *13*(4), 841–859. doi:10.3390/e13040841

Chapter 10
Advancements in Data Security and Privacy Techniques Used in IoT–Based Hospital Applications

Ankita Tiwari
Amity University, India

Raghuvendra Pratap Tripathi
Amity University, India

Dinesh Bhatia
North Eastern Hill University, India

ABSTRACT

The risk of encountering new diseases is on the rise in medical centers globally. By employing advancements in medical sensors technology, new health monitoring programs are being developed for continuous monitoring of physiological parameters in patients. Since the stored medical data is personal health record of an individual, it requires delicate and secure handling. In wireless transmission networks, medical data is disposed of to avoid loss due to alteration, eavesdropping, etc. Hence, privacy and security of the medical data are the major considerations during wireless transfer through Medical Sensor Network of MSNs. This chapter delves upon understanding the working of a secure monitoring system wherein the data could be continuously observed with the support of MSNs. Process of sanctioning secure data to authorized users such as physician, clinician, or patient through the key provided to access the file are also explained. Comparative analysis of the encryption techniques such as paillier, RSA, and ELGamal has been included to make the reader aware in selecting a useful technique for a particular hospital application.

DOI: 10.4018/978-1-5225-7952-6.ch010

INTRODUCTION

A medical application necessitates treating patient care beyond the healthcare continuum. The healthcare continuum includes homecare, hospital, and long-term care facility. The medical devices which are connected through the Internet are referred as Internet of Things (IoT) applications. IoT applications have been widely investigated, forecasted for widespread future use even located on small scale. Any hospital that starts "smart beds" programme, can detect whether the hospital bed is occupied or not, analyses when the patient requires assistance to use the lavatory or move around and send desired information to the available nurse or nearest hospital staff for patient support (R. Babu, 2015). This smart bed has self-adjustable features, according to the appropriate patient load and nature of support required which can be provided without manual assistance. Some other areas where smart management is being used are home medication dispensers to automatically upload patient data to a cloud server when medication should be avoided or any other health symptoms which require immediate attention of the nursing staff or at home medical care personnel (Chouffani, 2016).

The definition of IoT given by IEEE is: "…a self-configured and adaptive system consisting of networks of sensors and smart objects whose purpose is to interconnect "all" things, including every day and industrial objects, in such a way as to make them intelligent, programmable and more capable of interacting with humans" (Internet of Things, 2018). The information provided by Gartner (Garthner, 2018) is that excluding cell phones, tablets, and computers, there are more than 8.5 billion devices connected through internet frequently which is a large number of devices connected online.

Nowadays, advancement in the proliferation and bioengineering of body sensor platforms has authorized the recognition of mobile health and pervasive systems. In this system, sensors are placed on the patient's body. These sensors record the data and send it to end user. Data transfer and collection must be private and secured because of using open network environment and mobile system considering patient safety aspects (Halperin, Heydt-Benjamin, Fu, Kohno, & Maisel, 2008) (Kumar & Lee., 2013). Some medical devices in present market are unguarded to attacks (Halperin, Heydt-Benjamin, Fu, Kohno, & Maisel, 2008) (Radclliffe., 2011). We contemplate a comprehensive system architecture where some

Figure 1. IoT healthcare network (IoThNet) issues

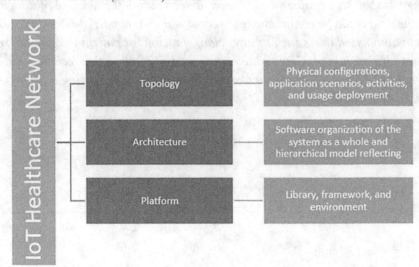

specified technologies are combined to support the crucial patient's data security aspects in MSN based mobile health system.

This security approach depends on standardized protocol i.e. Host Identity Protocol (HIP) (Gurtov, Komu, & Moskowitz., 2009). Till now, HIP has succeeded some promising security algorithms for IoT devices and mobile networks (Heer, 2007) (Moskowitz., 2012) (Olivereau., 2012) (Urien., 2013). In this chapter, review of advancement in data security and privacy technologies by employing IoT in the medical world has been mentioned.

RELATED WORK

Medical Sensing

There is a long history of utilizing sensors in prescription and general wellbeing (Aberg, Togawa, & Spelman, 2002) (Wilson, 1999). Installed in an assortment of restorative instruments for use at doctor's facilities, center, and homes, sensors give patients and their human services suppliers understanding into physiological and physical wellbeing states that are basic to the location, determination, treatment, and administration of infirmities. A lot of present day solution would basically not be conceivable nor be practical without sensors, for example, thermometers, pulse screens, glucose screens, EKG, PPG, EEG, and different types of imaging sensors. The capacity to quantify physiological state is likewise basic for interventional gadgets, for example, pacemakers and insulin pumps.

Restorative sensors consolidate transducers for recognizing electrical, warm, optical, compound, hereditary, and different signs with physiological starting point with flag handling calculations to appraise highlights demonstrative of a man's wellbeing status. Sensors past those that specifically measure wellbeing state have additionally discovered use in the act of prescription. For instance, area and closeness detecting advancements (Khan & Skinner, 2002) are being utilized for enhancing the conveyance of patient consideration and work process productivity in doctor's facilities (Emory & Lenert, 2005), following the spread of maladies by general wellbeing organizations (Hanjagi, Srihari, & Rayamane, 2007), and observing individuals' wellbeing related practices (e.g., movement levels) and introduction to negative natural components, for example, contamination (Patrick, 2007). There are three particular measurements along which progresses in therapeutic detecting advancements are occurring. We expound on every one of the three in the following passages that pursue.

Sensing Modality

Growth and advancement in modern day technologies, for example, MEMS, imaging, and microfluidic and nano-fluidic lab-on-chip are prompting new types of synthetic, organic, and genomic detecting and investigations accessible outside the bounds of a research center at the purpose of-care. By empowering new modest indicative abilities, these detecting advances guarantee to upset human services both regarding settling general wellbeing emergency because of irresistible illnesses (Yager, et al., 2006) and furthermore empowering early location and customized medicines.

Size and Cost

Most therapeutic sensors have customarily been too expensive and complex to be utilized outside of clinical situations. Be that as it may, ongoing advancements in microelectronics and registering have made numerous types of restorative detecting all the more easily available to people at their homes, work places, and other living spaces.

The first to rise (Aberg, Togawa, & Spelman, 2002) were convenient therapeutic sensors for home utilization (e.g., circulatory strain and blood glucose screens). By empowering, continuous estimations of basic physiological information without expecting visits to the specialist, these instruments upset the administration of illnesses, for example, hypertension and diabetes.

Next, walking medicinal sensors, whose little frame factor enabled them to be worn or conveyed by a man, came into existence (Aberg, Togawa, & Spelman, 2002). Such sensors empower people to constantly gauge physiological parameters while connected with routine life exercises. Models incorporate wearable pulse and physical movement screens and Holter screens. These gadgets target wellness lovers, wellbeing cognizant people and watch heart or neural occasions that may not show amid a short visit to the specialist.

All the more as of late implanted medicinal sensors incorporated with assistive and prosthetic gadgets for geriatrics (Wu, et al., 2008) and orthotics (Dunkels, Gr¨onvall, & Voigt, 2004) have been developed in recent past.

At last, we are seeing the development of implantable restorative sensors for persistently estimating inner wellbeing status and physiological signs. At times the reason for existing is to consistently screen wellbeing parameters that are not remotely accessible, for example, intraocular weight in glaucoma patients (Dresher & Irazoqui, 2007). The objective in different cases is to utilize the estimations as triggers for physiological intercessions that avoid approaching unfavorable occasions (e.g., epileptic seizures (Raghunathan, Ward, Roy, & Irazoqui, 2009)) and for physical help (e.g., mind controlled engine prosthetics (Linderman, et al., 2008)). Given their implantable nature, these gadgets confront serious size requirements and need to impart and get control remotely.

Connectivity

Driven by advances in data innovation, medicinal sensors have turned out to be progressively interconnected with different gadgets. Early therapeutic sensors were to a great extent confined with incorporated user interfaces (UIs) for showing their estimations.

In this way, sensors wound up fit for interfacing to outer gadgets by means of wired interfaces, for example, RS 232, USB, and Ethernet. All the more as of late, restorative sensors have joined remote associations, both short-run, for example, Bluetooth, Zigbee, and close field radios to convey remotely to close-by PCs, PDAs, or cell phones, and long-extend, for example, WiFi or cell correspondences, to discuss specifically with distributed computing administrations. Other than the accommodation of tether less activity, such remote associations allow sensor estimations to be sent to parental figures while patients experience their day by day work life far from home, hence proclaiming a time of universal on-going therapeutic detecting. We take note of that with compact and mobile sensors, the wired or remote availability to distributed computing assets is irregular (e.g., network might be accessible just when the sensor is in cell inclusion territory or docked to the client's home PC).

Accordingly such sensors can likewise record estimations in non-volatile memory for transferring at a later time when they can be imparted to medicinal services staff and further investigated.

Wireless Sensor Platforms

Late years have seen the development of different implanted figuring stages that incorporate preparing, stockpiling, remote systems administration, and sensors. These inserted figuring stages offer the capacity to detect physical wonders at fleeting and spatial constancies that were already unfeasible. Installed processing stages utilized for medicinal services applications extend from cell phones to specific remote detecting stages, known as bits, that have considerably more stringent asset limitations as far as accessible figuring power, memory, organize data transfer capacity, and accessible vitality.

Existing bits regularly utilize 8 or 16-bit microcontrollers with several KBs of RAM, many KBs of ROM for program stockpiling and outer stockpiling as Flash memory. These gadgets work at a couple of milliwatts while running at around 10 MHz (Polastre, Szewczyk, & Culler, 2005). A large portion of the circuits can be controlled off, so the backup power can be around one microwatt. In the event that such a gadget is dynamic for 1% of the time, its normal power utilization is only a couple of microwatts empowering long haul activity with two AA batteries. Bits are normally furnished with low-control radios, for example, those agreeable with the IEEE 802.15.4 standard for remote sensor systems. Such radios as a rule transmit at rates between 10-250 Kbps, expend around 20-60 milliwatts, and their correspondence extend is normally estimated in several meters. At last, bits incorporate various simple and computerized interfaces that empower them to associate with a wide assortment of ware sensors.

These equipment developments are paralleled by advances in installed working frameworks (Dunkels, Grönvall, & Voigt, 2004) (Hil, Szewczyk, Woo, Hollar, Culler, & Pister, 2000), segment based programming dialects (Gay, Levis, Von Behren, Welsh, Brewer, & Culler, 2014), and organizing conventions (Gnawali, Fonseca, Jamieson, Moss, & Levis, 2009) (Buettner, Yee, Anderson, & Han, 2006). Rather than asset compelled bits, cell phones give all the more great microchips, bigger information stockpiling, and higher system data transfer capacity through cell and IEEE 802.11 remote interfaces to the detriment of higher vitality utilization. Their corresponding attributes make cell phones and bits integral stages appropriate for various classifications of medicinal services applications, which is discussed in following sections of this chapter.

MEDICAL SENSOR NETWORK

When sensors are implanted within patient body or wearable, these sensors web to form a network. This network is called as medical sensor network (MSN). These sensor webs receive the information from its surrounding and save in its personal information space. The saved data is sent to remote monitoring systems or prescription systems with information sent to the physician. Figure 3 shows the basic architecture of MSN. The MSN refers to the positioning of different sensors of an IoT medical network and designate representable outline of seamless medical environments. In figure 2, it is shown that a heterogeneous computing network receives and collects a huge amount of sensor data and vital signs such as body temperature, blood pressure (BP), oxygen saturation, and electrocardiograms (ECG) and generates a general IoT medical topology.

Figure 2. Sensor web on human body or patient's body

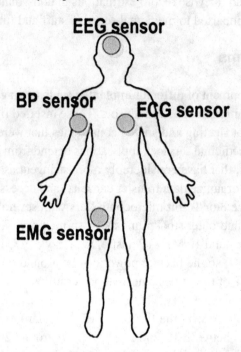

Figure 3. Medical sensor network or body sensor network and its backend services

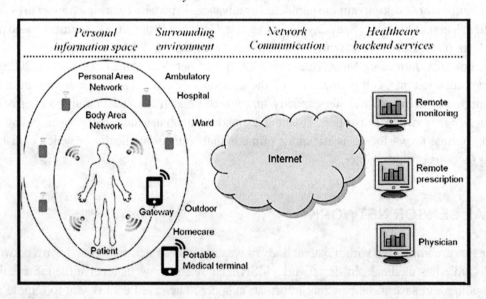

At the time of data transmission through wired or wireless medium, there may be a probability of data or information loss. Wireless data transmission is used for sending data from sensors to other place. At the time of wireless data transmission, there are some encryption methods available, which are used to secure data to maintain patient confidentiality. When the sensor web connects with network, it forms a body sensor network (BSN).

Architecture of MSN

The MSN architecture alludes to a frame for the description of MSN physical elements, its working principles, techniques, and their functional organization. In figure 3, the basic architecture of ambient assisted bio device and telehealth endorsed by Continua Health Alliance has been explained. The main key issues that have been recognized for MSN architecture (Shahamabadi, Ali, Varahram, & Jara, 2013) include multimedia streaming, reliable interaction between caregivers and IoT gateways, and the inter-functionality of IoT gateway and wireless personal area network (WPAN)/ wireless local area network (WLAN).

6LoWPAN is based on IPv6, and used for designing MSN architecture (Imadali, Karanasiou, Petrescu, Sifniadis, Veque, & Angelidis, 2012) (Jara, Zamora, & Skarmeta, Jun. 2012) (Maglogiannis, 2012). In (Bormann, 2009), the layer structure of 6LoWPAN is defined which is shown in figure 4. According to the MSN concept, body sensor applications of IPv6 and 6LoWPAN, and the sensor devices for data sending over 802.15.4 protocol. With the help of transmission line protocol (UDP: user datagram protocol), data is received at sensor nodes.

Medical systems have been surveyed for vehicular networks. The medical data, which is captured, have been evaluated with IPv6 application protocol (Imadali, Karanasiou, Petrescu, Sifniadis, Veque, & Angelidis, 2012). Moreover, mobile IPv6 (MIPv6) is not supported by 6LoWPAN, it is a subset of IPv6 protocol versatility. For introducing mobility to 6LoWPAN, there is a protocol proposed in (Shahamabadi, Ali, Varahram, & Jara, Jul. 2013), and data is transferred among base networks, mobile patient nodes and visited networks.

Healthcare Applications

Remotely organized sensors empower thick spatiotemporal testing of physical, physiological, mental, subjective, and social procedures in spaces running from individual to structures to significantly bigger scale ones. Such thick inspecting crosswise over spaces of various scales is bringing about tangible data based social insurance applications which, dissimilar to those portrayed in Section-Medical Sensing, circuit and total data gathered from numerous dispersed sensors. Also, the modernity of detecting has expanded immensely with the advances in shabby and small scale, yet excellent sensors for home that individuals can utilize, the improvement of refined machine learning calculations that empower complex conditions, for example, stress, sadness, and dependence on gathered information from tactile data, lastly the rise of unavoidable Internet availability encouraging convenient spread of sensor data to guardians.

In what pursues, we present a rundown of medicinal services applications empowered by these advancements. Observing in Mass-Casualty Disasters, while triage conventions for crisis therapeutic administrations as of now exist (Hodgetts & Mackaway-Jones, 1995). Their adequacy can rapidly corrupt with expanding number of exploited people. In addition, there is a need to enhance the evaluation of the people on call's wellbeing status amid such mass-loss catastrophes. The expanded compactness, adaptability, and quickly deployable nature of remote detecting frameworks can be utilized to naturally report the triage levels of various unfortunate casualties and ceaselessly track the wellbeing status of people on call at the fiasco scene all the more viably.

Vital Sign Monitoring in Hospitals

Remote detecting innovation helps to address different disadvantages related with wired sensors that are regularly utilized in healing centers and crisis rooms to screen patients (Ko, 2010). The natural scatter of wires appended to a patient isn't awkward for patients prompting confined portability and more uneasiness, but on the other hand is difficult to oversee for the staff. Very normal are consider separations of sensors by tired patients and disappointments to reattach sensors legitimately as patients are moved around in a doctor's facility and gave off crosswise over various units. Remote detecting equipment, those are less recognizable and have diligent system availability to backend restorative record frameworks help lessen the tangles of wires and patient tension, while additionally diminishing the event of mistakes.

At-Home and Mobile Aging

As individuals age, they encounter an assortment of subjective, physical, and social changes that test their wellbeing, autonomy and personal satisfaction (Wood, Fang, Stankovic, & He, 2006). Illnesses, for example, diabetes, asthma, perpetual obstructive pneumonic sickness, congestive heart disappointment, and memory decay are trying to screen and treat. These sicknesses can profit by patients playing a functioning job in the observing procedure. Remotely arranged sensors implanted in individuals' living spaces or carried on the individual can gather data about close to home physical, physiological, and social states with examples progressively and all over. Such information can likewise be associated with social and natural setting. From such "living records", valuable deductions about wellbeing and prosperity can be drawn. This can be utilized for mindfulness and individual examination to help with rolling out conduct improvements, and to impart to parental figures for early location and mediation. In the meantime such techniques are successful and financial methods for checking age-related diseases.

Assistance With Motor and Sensory Decline

Another utilization of remote arranged detecting is to give dynamic help and direction to patients adapting to declining tactile and engine capacities. We are seeing the development of new sorts of shrewd assistive gadgets that make utilization of data about the patient's physiological and physical state from sensors worked in the gadget, worn or even embedded on the client's individual, and installed in the environment. These clever assistive gadgets cannot just tailor their reaction to singular clients and their present setting, yet in addition give the client and their guardian's essential criticism for longer-term preparing. Conventional assistive gadgets, for example, sticks, props, walkers, and wheel seats can combine data from implicit and outer sensors to furnish the clients with nonstop customized input and direction towards the right use of the gadgets. Such gadgets can likewise adjust the physical qualities of the gadget regarding the unique situation and an endorsed preparing or recovery regimen (Wu, et al., 2008). Moreover, remote arranged detecting empowers new sorts of assistive gadgets, for example, way-discovering (Coughlan, 2007) and strolling route (Bohonos, 2007) for the outwardly debilitated.

Large-Scale In-Field Medical and Behavioral Studies

Wearable sensors together with sensor-prepared Internet-associated cell phones have started to change restorative and general wellbeing research thinking by empowering conduct and physiological information

Figure 4. Protocol stack of different layers in 6LoWPAN
Source: Bormann, 2009

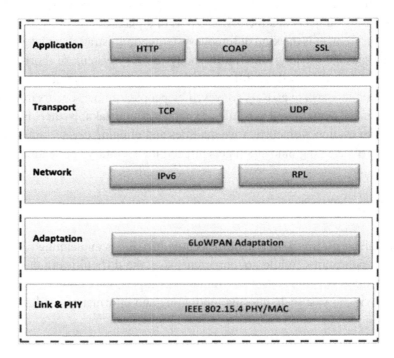

to be persistently gathered from an extensive number of dispersed subjects as they lead their everyday lives. With their capacity to give understanding into subject expresses that can't be repeated in controlled clinical and lab settings and that can't be estimated from PC helped review self-report techniques, such detecting frameworks are getting to be basic to restorative, mental, and social research. In reality, a noteworthy objective of the Exposure Biology program under NIH's Genes and Environment Initiative (GEI) is to grow such field deployable detecting instruments to evaluate exposures to condition (e.g., psychosocial push, habit, toxicants, consume less calories, physical action) unbiased, consequently, and for quite a long time at any given moment in the members' indigenous habitats. Specialists, both inside the GEI program and somewhere else, have additionally perceived the utility of such detecting in making estimations for longitudinal investigations going from the size of people to substantial populaces (Krumm, 2007).

As the four precedents above show, the applications empowered by remote organized detecting innovations are disseminated over different measurements. One measurement is the spatial and fleeting extent of circulated detecting. The spatial extension can extend from tangible perceptions of wellbeing status made when an individual is kept to a building (e.g., home, doctor's facility) or an all-around characterized locale (e.g., fiasco site) to perceptions made as an individual moves around throughout day by day life. The worldly extension can go from perceptions made for the span of a sickness or an occasion to long haul perceptions made for dealing with a long haul malady or for general wellbeing purposes. Diverse spatial and transient degrees put distinctive limitations on the accessibility of vitality and correspondences framework, and distinctive necessities on ergonomics.

A second measurement is that of the gathering size, which can go from an individual patient at home, to gatherings of patients at a healing center and exploited people at debacle locales, and the distance to vast scattered populace of subjects in a medicinal report or a plague.

The last basic measurement is the kind of remote systems administration and detecting advances that are utilized: on-body sensors with long range radios, body-territory systems of short-run on-body sensors with a long-go portal, sensors embedded in-body with remote correspondence and power conveyance, remote sensors inserted in assistive gadgets conveyed by people, remote sensors implanted in the earth, and sensors installed in the omnipresent versatile cell phones. Unmistakably, there is a rich decent variety of remote detecting innovation with correlative qualities and obliging diverse applications. Ordinarily, in excess of one kind of detecting innovation gets utilized for a solitary application.

TECHNICAL CHALLENGES

In the sections that tail we portray a portion of the center difficulties in planning remote sensor systems for social insurance applications. While not comprehensive, the difficulties in this rundown length an extensive variety of subjects, from center PC frameworks topics, for example, versatility, unwavering quality, and productivity, to vast scale information mining and information affiliation issues, and even lawful issues.

Trustworthiness

Medicinal services applications force strict necessities on end-to-end framework dependability and information conveyance. For instance, beat oximetry applications, which measure the levels of oxygen in a man's blood, must convey no less than one, estimation at regular intervals (Intille, 2006). Besides, end-clients require estimations that are sufficiently exact to be utilized in restorative research. Utilizing a similar heartbeat oximetry model, estimations must go astray at most 4% from the real oxygen fixations in the blood (Intille, 2006). At long last, applications that consolidate estimations with activation, for example, control of mixture pumps and patient controlled absence of pain (PCA) gadgets, force imperatives on the conclusion to-end conveyance inertness. We term the blend of information conveyance and quality properties the dependability of the framework and guarantee that therapeutic detecting applications require elevated amounts of reliability.

Various components confuse the frameworks' capacity to give the dependability that applications require. To begin with, restorative offices, where a portion of these frameworks will be conveyed, can be exceptionally unforgiving conditions for radio recurrence (RF) correspondences. This brutality is the consequence of auxiliary factors, for example, the nearness of metal entryways and dividers and also consider exertion to give radiation protecting, for instance in working rooms that utilization fluoroscopy for orthopedic techniques. Truth be told, Ko et al. as of late found that parcel misfortunes for radios following the IEEE 802.15.4 standard is higher in healing facilities than other indoor conditions (Liao, Fox, & Kautz, 2005). Also, gadgets that utilization 802.15.4 radios are powerless to impedance from WiFi systems, Bluetooth gadgets, and cordless telephones which are all intensely utilized in numerous healing centers.

The effect of hindrances and impedance is exacerbated by the way that most remote sensor organize frameworks utilize low power radios to accomplish long framework lifetimes (i.e., expanding the battery re-charging cycle). The other ramifications of utilizing low-control radios are that the system throughput of these gadgets is restricted. For instance, the hypothetical most extreme throughput of IEEE 802.15.4 radios is 250 Kbps and much lower by and by because of imperatives presented by MAC conventions also, multi-bounce interchanges. Considering that applications, for example, movement and action observing catch many examples every second, these throughput limits imply that a system can bolster few gadgets or that just a subset of the estimations can be conveyed progressively.

Sometimes the nature of the information gathered from remote detecting frameworks can be endangered not by sensor blames and breakdowns, but rather by client activities. This is genuine notwithstanding for cell phone based detecting frameworks for which huge numbers of the previously mentioned RF challenges are less serious. Considering that remote detecting frameworks for social insurance will be utilized by the elderly and medicinal staff with small preparing, misfortune in quality because of administrator abuse is a major concern. In addition, since remote detecting empowers persistent accumulation of physiological information under conditions not initially imagined by the sensors' engineers, the gathered estimations might be dirtied by an assortment of antiquities. For instance, movement antiques can affect the nature of pulse and breath estimations. In this manner, assessing the nature of estimations gathered under questionable conditions is a noteworthy test that WSNs for human services must address. Thus, this test implies that WSNs need to utilize methods for mechanized information approval and purifying and interfaces to encourage and check their right establishment. To wrap things up, WSNs in social insurance ought to give metadata that illuminate information shoppers of the nature of the information conveyed.

Privacy and Security

Remote sensor arrangements in human services are utilized to decide the exercises of every day living (ADL) and give information to longitudinal examinations. It is then simple to see that such WSNs additionally present chances to disregard protection. Besides, the significance of anchoring such frameworks will keep on ascending as their appropriation rate increments.

The main protection challenge experienced is the ambiguous determination of security. The Heath Insurance Portability and Accountability Act (HIPPA) by the U.S. government is one endeavor to characterize this term. One issue is that HIPPA and in addition different laws characterize protection utilizing human dialect (e.g., English), consequently, making a semantic bad dream. The protection detail dialects have been produced to determine security arrangements for a framework formally. Once the protection details are determined, medicinal services frameworks must authorize this security and furthermore have the capacity to express clients' solicitations for information get to and the framework's arrangements. These solicitations ought to be assessed against the predefined approaches with the end goal to choose on the off chance that they ought to be conceded or denied. This structure offers ascend to numerous new research moves, some extraordinary to WSNs, as we depict in the passages that pursue.

1. Since setting can influence security, approach dialects must have the capacity to express extraordinary kinds of setting from nature, for example, time, space, physiological parameter detecting, ecological detecting, and stream based loud information. Also, the greater part of the setting must be gathered and assessed continuously. Since setting is so focal it should likewise be available in a protected and precise way.

2. There is a need to speak to various kinds of information proprietors and demand subjects in the framework and in addition outside clients and their rights when diverse areas, for example, helped living offices, doctor's facilities, and drug stores cooperate. One of the more troublesome protection issues happens while collaborating frameworks have their own security strategies. Therefore, irregularities in such strategies may emerge crosswise over various frameworks. Hence, on-line consistency checking and notice alongside goals plans are required.

3. There is a need to present to abnormal state collecting solicitations, for example, questioning the normal, greatest, or least perusing of determined detecting information. This security capacity must be bolstered by anonym zing accumulation capacities. This need emerges for applications identified with longitudinal examinations and person to person communication.

4. There is a need to help not just adherence to protection for information inquiries (e.g., information pull demands), yet additionally the security for push setup solicitations to set framework parameters (e.g., for private utilize or arranging particular restorative actuators).

5. Because WSNs screen and control a huge assortment of physical parameters in various settings, it is important to endure a high level of elements and conceivably even permit impermanent security infringement with the end goal to meet practical, wellbeing or execution prerequisites. For instance, an individual wearing an EKG may encounter heart arrhythmia and the continuous announcing of this issue outweighs some current protection prerequisites. At the end of the day to send a crisis caution rapidly it might be important to avoid different security assurances. At whatever point such infringement happen, center medicinal services staff individuals must be advised of such occurrences.

Notwithstanding strategy and database question protection infringement, WSNs are helpless to new side channel security assaults that gain data by watching the radio transmissions of sensors to find private exercises, notwithstanding when the transmissions are encoded. This physical layer assault needs just the season of transmission and the unique finger impression of each message, where a unique mark is an arrangement of highlights of a RF waveform that are exceptional to a specific transmitter. Along these lines, this is known as the Fingerprint and Timing-based Snooping (FATS) assault (Srinivasan, Stankovic, & Whitehouse, 2008).

To execute a FATS assault, a foe records stealthily on the sensors' radio to gather the timestamps and fingerprints of every radio transmission. The enemy at that point utilizes the fingerprints to connect each message with an extraordinary transmitter, and utilizations various periods of induction to derive the area and sort of every sensor. When this is known, different private client exercises and wellbeing conditions can be deduced.

For instance, Srinivasan et al. present this exceptional physical layer security assault and propose arrangements regarding a savvy home situation (Srinivasan, Stankovic, & Whitehouse, 2008). Three layers of surmising are utilized in their work. To begin with, sensors in a similar room are grouped dependent on the closeness of their transmission designs. At that point the general transmission example of each room is passed to a classifier, which consequently distinguishes the sort of room (e.g., washroom or kitchen). Once the kind of room is recognized, the transmission example of every sensor is passed to another classifier, which consequently distinguishes the sort of sensor (e.g., a movement sensor or a cooler entryway). From this data, the foe effortlessly recognizes a few exercises of the home's inhabitants, for example, cooking, showering, and toileting, all with reliably high exactness. From such data it is then conceivable to derive the occupants' wellbeing conditions. Luckily, numerous arrangements with various tradeoffs are feasible for this kind of physical layer assault. Such arrangements incorporate (i) weakening the flag outside of the home to build the bundle misfortune proportion of the spy, (ii) occasionally transmitting radio messages regardless of whether the gadget has information to be sent, (iii) haphazardly postponing radio messages to shroud the time that the relating occasions happened, (iv) concealing the unique mark of the transmitter, and (v) transmitting counterfeit information to copy a genuine occasion.

Sadly, a foe can join data accessible from many (outside) sources with physical layer data to make deductions considerably more precise and intrusive. New arrangements that are practical, address physical layer information, secure against derivations dependent on accumulations of related information, and still allow the first usefulness of the framework to work successfully are required.

A related essential issue, yet unsolved in WSNs is managing security assaults. Security assaults are particularly dangerous to low-control WSN stages in view of a few reasons including the strict asset requirements of the gadgets, negligible openness to the sensors and actuators, and the inconsistent idea of low-control remote correspondences. The security issue is additionally exacerbated by the perception that transient and changeless arbitrary disappointments are regular in WSNs and such disappointments are vulnerabilities that can be misused by assailants. For instance, with these vulnerabilities it is workable for an aggressor to misrepresent setting, adjust get to rights, make disavowal of administration, and, as a rule disturb the task of the framework. This could result in a patient being denied treatment, or more regrettable, accepting the wrong treatment.

Having as a primary concern with one such kind of difficulties, new lightweight security arrangements that can work in these open and asset constrained frameworks are required. Arrangements that adventure the extensive measure of excess found in numerous WSN frameworks are being sought after. This excess makes awesome potential for outlining WSN frameworks that constantly give their objective administrations regardless of the presence of disappointments or assaults. At the end of the day, to meet reasonable framework prerequisites that get from extensive and unattended activity, WSNs must have the capacity to keep on working tastefully and adequately recoup from security assaults. WSNs should likewise be sufficiently adaptable to adjust to assaults not foreseen amid outline or organization time. Work, for example, the one proposed by Wood et al. gives a case of how such issues are tended to, by proposing to plan a self-recuperating framework with the nearness and discovery of assaults, as opposed to attempting to fabricate a totally secure framework (Wood, Fang, Stankovic, & He, 2006).

Data Security

Now a day's data security is one of the basic needs in every sector which include medical, bank, education, defense etc. In almost every field data is transmitted and received through various mediums. There are several encryption algorithms available which provides security to this transmitted data or information. In medical data, the confidential information is in the form of patients name, age, blood group, weight, height etc. which needs to be made secure to prevent its misuse or theft. This is the time to store the data with Internet of Things (IoT), because it is one of the secure place to store patient data for long time duration.

When we talk about data security the first question arises that, "what is the need of data security in medical information?" As it is well know that the identity and privacy breach thefts including medical information are on growth. Ponemon Institute reported (Ponemon Organization, 2015) that since 2010, there is 125 percent increase in criminal attack on medical data which is the main leading cause of information breaches. In the research (Ponemon Organization, 2015), it is also observed that 91 percent of medical organizations have suffered from minimum one data breach, which leads to the loss of more than $2 million.

According to American action forum (Hayes, 2015), it is found that since 2009, medical data breaches have cost the health care system more than $50 billion which is a huge cost. Moreover, medical data cannot be wracked easily, whereas other records such as bank cards can be cancelled quickly. Medical breaches are not only caused by theft, this may also cause by an inadvertent error. Therefore, preventing the data from theft and breaches there is a need to apply specialized data encryption algorithms which have been explained in the section "Data Encryption Techniques".

Figure 5. Cost of data breach per record compromised
Source: Ponemon Organizaztion, 2015

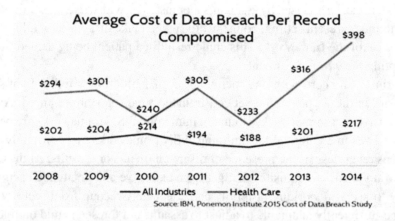

Figure 6. Number of record breaches per year
Source: Hayes, 2015

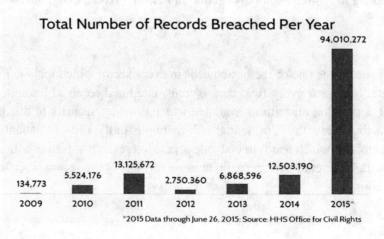

Resource Scarcity

With the end goal to empower little gadget sizes with sensible battery lifetimes, normal remote sensor hubs make utilization of low-control segments with unobtrusive assets. Figure 1 demonstrates a run of the mill wearable sensor hub for therapeutic applications, the SHIMMER stage (Ngoc, 2008). The SHIMMER contains an implanted microcontroller (TI MSP430; 8 MHz clock speed; 10 KB RAM; 48 KB ROM) and a low-control radio (Chipcon CC2420; IEEE 802.15.4; 2.4 GHz; 250 Kbps PHY information rate). The aggregate gadget control spending plan is roughly 60 milliwatts when dynamic, with a rest control deplete of a couple of microwatts. This outline allows little, re-chargeable batteries to keep up gadget lifetimes of hours or days, contingent upon the application's obligation cycles.

There is a great degree constrained calculation, correspondence, and vitality assets of remote sensor hubs prompt various difficulties for framework plan. Programming must be outlined precisely in view of these asset requirements. The insufficient memory requires the utilization of lean, occasion driven simultaneousness models, and blocks customary OS plans. Computational strength and radio transfer speed are both restricted, necessitating that sensor hubs exchange off calculation and correspondence overheads, for instance, by playing out an unassuming measure of on-board preparing to diminish information transmission prerequisites. At last, application code must be to a great degree cautious with the hub's constrained vitality spending plan, restricting radio correspondence and information handling to broaden the battery lifetime.

While cell phone based frameworks regularly appreciate all the more handling force and remote transmission capacity, the way that they are less adaptable contrasted with adjustable bit stages, confines their ability to forcefully preserve vitality. This prompts shorter re-charge cycles and can restrict the kinds of utilizations that cell phones can bolster.

Figure 7. SHIMMER wearable sensor platform

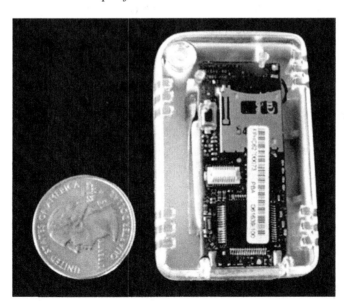

Another thought for low-control detecting stages is the variance in the asset stack experienced by sensor hubs. Contingent upon the patient's condition, the sensor information being gathered, and the nature of the radio connection, sensor hubs may encounter a wide variety in correspondence and handling load after some time. For instance, if sensor hubs perform multihop directing, a given hub might be required to forward bundles for at least one different hubs alongside transmitting its very own information. The system topology can change after some time, because of hub portability and natural variances in the RF medium, actuating erratic examples of vitality utilization for which the application must be readied.

DATA ENCRYPTION TECHNIQUES

Encryption is a process of encoding an information or data in order to allow only a sanctioned person to access it. The encryption doesn't avert interference, but contradict the comprehensible content to a future interceptor.

Paillier Cryptosystem

This cryptosystem was invented by Pascal Paillier. It was invented in 1999. It is the probabilistic asymmetric cryptographic algorithm for the public key cryptography (Paillier, 1999). The nth residue classes' computation is accepted to be computationally complex. Paillier cryptosystem is an intractability assumption based on decisional composite residuosity assumption (DCRA) (Paillier, 1999). This cryptography scheme is an additive homomorphic encryption method. The homomorphic cryptosystem means that, the encryption of m_1 and m_2 is $m_1 + m_2$.

There are so many encryption algorithm based on additive homomorphic methods. It is most efficient among all of them. Paillier encryption method is an augmentation of Okamoto-Uchiyama scheme (Okamoto & Uchiyama, 1998). As the security parameter is n. Two n bit prime values a and b are selected randomly $N = ab$. It $x \in B$ is an unsystematic base. To cipher any information $m < N$, one selected a random number $y \in \mathbb{Z}_N^*$ calculates the encrypted text as:

$$c = x^m y^N \bmod N^2 \tag{1}$$

When receiving an encrypted text c, it is examined that $c < N^2$. If the condition is true then the message m is decrypted as:

$$m = L\left(c^{\lambda(N)} \bmod N^2\right) / L\left(x^{\lambda(N)} \bmod e N^2\right) \bmod N \tag{2}$$

Paillier cryptosystem has useful properties like product of coded information results in the summation of the real information mod n:

$$D\left[E\left(m_1\right) * E\left(m_2\right) \bmod n^2\right] = m_1 + m_2 \bmod n \tag{3}$$

It is also raising an encrypted text to constant power output in multiple of original message text:

$$D\left[E\left(m\right)^{k}\,modn^{2}\right] = k*mmodn \tag{4}$$

RSA (Rivest-Shamir-Adleman) Cryptosystem

In 1977, the concept of RSA encryption method was first introduced by Ron Rivest and his team (Rivest, Shamir, & Adleman, 1978). In 1983, RSA cryptosystem founded RSA Data Security which was publically released in 2000. This algorithm is widely used for encrypting messages. The key size of private key is around $1024\,to\,4096$ bit. The basic principle of RSA cryptosystem is to find three large non-negative integers e, d and n i.e. modular exponentiation of all integers m (with $0 \leq m < n$):

$$\left(m^{e}\right)^{d} \equiv m\left(modn\right) \tag{5}$$

As we have the knowledge of e, n and m, it is very difficult to find the value of d from above given expression. Moreover, in some operations the above equation can be written as:

$$\left(m^{d}\right)^{e} \equiv m\left(modn\right) \tag{6}$$

This cryptosystem includes the private and public key, where public key is universal and used for encryption. The private key is used for decrypting as well as encrypting the information in a reasonable time frame. That is the reason; this algorithm has become universally applied asymmetric cryptosystem (Diffie & Hellman, 1976). This algorithm provides a system of assuring the integrity, confidentiality, non-reputability and authenticity of electronic information transmission and data storage. RSA algorithm works on different protocols such as OpenPGP (Open and free version of Pretty Good Privacy), SSH (Secure Shell), SSL/TLS (Secure Socket Layer/ Transport Layer Security), and S/MIME (Secure/ Multipurpose Internet Mail Extensions) for digital signature and encrypting the information. Signature verification is one of the most common operations performed by RSA cryptosystem in IT applications (Cormen, Leiserson, Rivest, & Stein, 2001).

ELGamal Cryptosystem

This is an asymmetric key encryption system algorithm, generally used for public key encryption. This encryption system is designed on the basis of Diffie-Hellman key exchange model. In 1985, Taher Elgamal explained that, the system creates another layer of security by using an asymmetrically encryption keys, which were previously used only for symmetric information encryption (ElGamal, 1985). This encryption system is used in recent version of PGP (Zimmermann, 2010), GNU Privacy Guard software (Hansen, 2012) and other encryption methods. ELGamal signature scheme (Nyberg & Rueppel, 1996) is different from ELGamal encryption and it is the root for Digital Signature Algorithm (Digital Signature Standard (DSS), 1994)

ELGamal cryptography can be explained as a cyclic group G (Hazewinkel & Michiel, 1994). Its security is influenced by a particular problem in G, this problem is related to computing discrete logarithms. This cryptosystem consists of three steps: key generation, encryption and decryption algorithm.

Key Generation

"The key generation algorithm includes following steps:

- Alice initiates an efficient explanation of the cyclic group G with generator g and order n.
- Alice selected a p randomly from $\{1,...,q-1\}$.
- Alice computes $h := g^p$
- Alice issues h, associated with the explanation of G, g, q as the public key. Alice kept p as the private key, which need to be secure" (ElGamal, 1985).

Encryption

"The algorithm includes following steps to encryption the original information m in form of Alice public key G, g, q

- Bob selected r from $\{1,...,q-1\}$, and then compute $c_1 := g^r$
- Bob computed the split secret $s := h^r := g^{pr}$
- Bob plans to convert his message m into m' of G.
- Bob computes $c_2 := m' * s$.
- Bob transmits his cipher text to Alice $\left(c_1 c_2\right) = \left(g^r, m' * h\right) = \left(g^r, m' * g^{pr}\right)$

In this encryption method it is easy to calculate h^r, if new message m' is known. This is the reason to generate a new r for every other message. That is the reason to call r as an ephemeral key (Ephemeral Key, 2018)."

Decryption

The algorithm works in following steps to decode the cipher text $\left(c_1 c_2\right)$ with the Alice's private key p.

- Alice computes the shared encrypted message $s := c_1^p$
- After first step Alice calculates $m' := c_2 * s^{-1}$. Now Alice retrieves the plain text information m, where G group is having s.

This decryption algorithm forms the message which was send, since:

$$c_2 s^{-1} = m' * h^r * \left(g^{pr}\right)^{-1} = m' * g^{pr} * g^{-pr} = m' \tag{7}$$

This cryptosystem is generally used in hybrid encryption to encode the message with symmetric cryptosystem. The algorithm is used to encrypt the message using symmetric key encryption. This is the reason that ELGamal like asymmetric cryptosystems are generally slower that symmetric cryptosystems for a same level of security (ElGamal, 1985).

DISSCUSSION AND CONCLUSION

The IoT has demonstrated its presence in our lives, from dealing at an essential level to the social relationship. It has included a new prospective into internet by authorizing communications among objects, livings and non-livings, and building an intelligent and smart world. The IoT has conducted with a vision of "anywhere, anything, anytime, anyway" interactions in real sense. It is perceived that it should be contemplated as the fundamental part of the prevailing internet depending on IoTs future ways, and it is obvious to become different from the available levels of internet compared to what we use and see in our daily lives. Therefore, the conceptual frame comes in the limelight. The Architecture is a substructure of technology that authorizes things to connect each other and communicate with same or different objects by striking human being to be the layer on it. In reality, it is understandable that the present IoT paradigms, which encourages in the direction machine to machine (M2M) interactions, is now getting restricted by so many factors.

In this chapter, the essential components for the IoTs community were examined. The parameters of IoT devices, is requisite to offer established multimedia data transfer. The present module is able to offer the requisite bitrate of text data streaming and transmission were chosen. Furthermore, the bitrate interval dependency was examined for systems working on Bluetooth and Wi-Fi technologies. These analysis were held as a generalised form of the algorithms being advanced for instinctive connection of the IoT modules. The algorithms allow the encryption of the data file with the use of three different algorithms: Paillier cryptosystem, RSA cryptosystem and ELGamal cryptosystem. The performance is checked after the encryption and decryption of data files using these algorithms. The concluding results show that every algorithm has different ability and status to make the data safe. Hence, it is required to decide and finalise the algorithm based on the type of data. However, the results vary depending on the property and size of data file.

FUTURE SCOPE

Wireless Senor Network (WSN) is a conventional technology formed of small size battery operated "motes" with radio communication and limited calculation capabilities. This methodology has the ability to study of resuscitative care and impact the delivery by permitting the device to be fully automated and automatically collect the vital signs from the patient care unit. This collected data would be used for correlation with hospital records, long term observation of the patient and real-time triage. These automated networks would help to provide a better observation environment to the post-operative patient, provide continuous monitoring during neuro-rehabilitation period in ambulatory atmosphere, monitor elderly person at home and patient suffering from lung diseases such as chronic obstructive pulmonary disease (COPD). This work can be extended by including artificial intelligence to the WSN, which is helpful in exploring data robustness, distributed storage, parallel distribution computation and automatic sensor reading classification. The automatic sensor reading classification would assist the physicians in early detection of diseases.

This work can also be extended by designing architecture of remote patient monitoring system. In this system wireless sensor nodes would be able to detect various other environment factors and add to the security of the system. It can be used in home, hospitals, and ambulatory, where it would implement a real time patient monitoring, by which the doctor can watch the patients on remote location and provide the first aid advice to patients.

REFERENCES

Aberg, P. A., Togawa, T., & Spelman, F. A. (2002). Sensors in Medicine and Healthcare. *Wiley-VCH, 15*(3), 152-169.

Babu, A. K. (2015). A Survey on the Role of IoT and Cloud in Health Care. *International Journal of Scientific Engineering and Technology Research, 4*(12), 2217–2219.

Bohonos, S. L. (2007). Universal real-time navigational assistance (URNA): an urban bluetooth beacon for the blind. In *1st ACM SIGMOBILE international workshop on Systems and networking support for healthcare and assisted living environments* (pp. 83-88). New York: ACM.

Bormann, Z. S. (2009). *6LoWPAN: The Wireless Embedded Internet* (1st ed.). London: Wiley.

Buettner, M., Yee, G. V., Anderson, E., & Han, R. (2006). X-MAC: a short preamble MAC protocol for duty-cycled wireless sensor networks. In *4th international conference on Embedded networked sensor systems* (pp. 307-320). ACM.

Chouffani, R. (2016, November). *Can we expect the Internet of Things in healthcare?* Retrieved from http://internetofthingsagenda.techtarget.com/feature/Can-we-expect-the-Internet-of-Things-in-healthcare

Cormen, T. H., Leiserson, C. E., Rivest, R. L., & Stein, C. (2001). Introduction to Algorithms (2nd ed.). MIT Press and McGraw-Hill.

Coughlan, J. (2007). Color targets: Fiducials to help visually impaired people find their way by camera phone. *EURASIP Journal on Image and Video Processing, 12*(1), 96–111.

Diffie, W., & Hellman, M. (1976). New directions in cryptography. *IEEE Transactions on Information Theory, 22*(6), 644–654. doi:10.1109/TIT.1976.1055638

Digital Signature Standard (DSS). (1994, May 19). Retrieved from FIPS PUB 186: csrc.nist.gov

Dresher, R., & Irazoqui, P. (2007). A Compact Nanopower Low Output Impedance CMOS Operational Amplifier for Wireless Intraocular Pressure Recordings. In *29th Annual International Conference of the IEEE* (pp. 6055-6058). Engineering in Medicine and Biology Society. 10.1109/IEMBS.2007.4353729

Dunkels, A., Gr"onvall, B., & Voigt, T. (2004). Contiki - a lightweight and flexible operating system for tiny networked sensors. In *First IEEE Workshop on Embedded Networked Sensors (Emnets-I)* (pp. 15-26). IEEE. 10.1109/LCN.2004.38

ElGamal, T. (1985). A Public-Key Cryptosystem and a Signature Scheme Based on Discrete Logarithms. *IEEE Transactions on Information Theory*, *31*(4), 469–472. doi:10.1109/TIT.1985.1057074

Emory, F. A., & Lenert, L. A. (2005). MASCAL: RFID Tracking of Patients, Staff and Equipment to Enhance Hospital Response to Mass Casualty Events. In *The AMIA Annual Symposium* (pp. 261-265). AMIA.

Ephemeral Key. (2018, June 7). Retrieved from Wikipedia: https://en.wikipedia.org/wiki/Ephemeral_key

Garthner. (2018, May). *Gartner Technical Research*. Retrieved from Internet of Things: http://www.gartner.com/technology/research/internet-of-things/

Gay, D., Levis, P., Von Behren, R., Welsh, M., Brewer, E., & Culler, D. (2014). The nesC language: A holistic approach to networked embedded systems. *ACM SIGPLAN Notices*, *49*(4), 41–51. doi:10.1145/2641638.2641652

Gnawali, O., Fonseca, R., Jamieson, K., Moss, D., & Levis, P. (2009). Collection tree protocol. In *7th ACM conference on embedded networked sensor systems* (pp. 1-14). ACM.

Gurtov, A., Komu, M., & Moskowitz, R. (2009). Host Identity Protocol (HIP): Identifier/locator split for host mobility and multihoming. *Internet Protocol Journal*, *12*(1), 27–32.

Halperin, D., Heydt-Benjamin, T. S., Fu, K., Kohno, T., & Maisel, W. H. (2008). Security and privacy for implantable medical devices. *IEEE Pervasive Computing*, *7*(1), 30–39. doi:10.1109/MPRV.2008.16

Hanjagi, A., Srihari, P., & Rayamane, A. (2007). A public health care information system using GIS and GPS: A case study of Shiggaon. *Springer: GIS for Health and the Environment*, *5*(1), 243–255.

Hansen, R. (2012, Jan.). *Gnu Privacy Guard*. Retrieved from GnuPG: https://www.gnupg.org/faq/gnupg-faq.html#compatible

Hayes, T. O. (2015, August 6). *American Action Forum*. Retrieved from https://www.americanactionforum.org/research/are-electronic-medical-records-worth-the-costs-of-implementation/

Hazewinkel & Michiel. (1994). Cyclic group. In *Encyclopedia of Mathematics*. Springer Science+Business Media B.V. / Kluwer Academic Publishers.

Heer, T. (2007). LHIP lightweight authentication extension for HIP. *IETF*, *12*(3), 290–230.

Hil, J., Szewczyk, R., Woo, A., Hollar, S., Culler, D., & Pister, K. (2000). System architecture directions for network sensors. *Operating Systems Review*, *34*(5), 93–104. doi:10.1145/384264.379006

Hodgetts, T., & Mackaway-Jones, K. (1995). *Major Incident Medical Management and Support, the Practical Approach*. BMJ Publishing Group.

Imadali, S., Karanasiou, A., Petrescu, A., Sifniadis, I., Veque, V., & Angelidis, P. (2012). eHealth service support in IPv6 vehicular networks. In *IEEE Int. Conf. Wireless Mobile Comput., Netw. Commun. (WiMob)* (pp. 579-585). London: IEEE Digital eXplore. 10.1109/WiMOB.2012.6379134

Internet of Things. (2018, May). Retrieved from IEEE: http://iot.ieee.org/about.html

Intille, S. S. (2006). Using a live-in laboratory for ubiquitous computing research. In *International Conference on Pervasive Computing* (pp. 349-365). Berlin: Springer. 10.1007/11748625_22

Jara, A. J., Zamora, M. A., & Skarmeta, A. (2012). Knowledge acquisition and management architecture for mobile and personal health environments based on the Internet of Things. In *IEEE Int. Conf. Trust, Security Privacy Comput. Commun. (TrustCom)* (pp. 1811-1818). IEEE Digital eXplore. 10.1109/TrustCom.2012.194

Khan, O. A., & Skinner, R. (2002). *Geographic Information Systems and Health Applications.* IGI Globa.

Ko, J. L.-E., Dutton, R. P., Lim, J. H., Chen, Y., Musvaloiu-E, R., Terzis, A., ... Selavo, L. (2010). MEDiSN: Medical emergency detection in sensor networks. *ACM Transactions on Embedded Computing Systems, 10*(1), 89–101. doi:10.1145/1814539.1814550

Krumm, J. (2007). Inference attacks on location track. In *International Conference on Pervasive Computing* (pp. 127-143). Berlin: Springer. 10.1007/978-3-540-72037-9_8

Kumar, P., & Lee, H. (2013). Security issues in healthcare applications using wireless medical sensor networks: A survey. *Sensors (Basel), 12*(1), 55–91. doi:10.3390120100055 PMID:22368458

Liao, L., Fox, D., & Kautz, H. (2005). BLocation-based activity recognition using relational Markov networks. *19th Int. In Joint Conf. Artif. Intell.,* 773-778.

Linderman, M. D., Santhanam, G., Kemere, C. T., Gilja, V., O'Driscoll, S., Yu, B. M., ... Meng, T. (2008). Signal processing challenges for neural prostheses. *IEEE Signal Processing Magazine, 25*(1), 18–28. doi:10.1109/MSP.2008.4408439

Maglogiannis, C. D. (2012). Bringing IoT and cloud computing towards pervasive healthcare. In *Int. Conf. Innov. Mobile Internet Services Ubiquitous Comput. (IMIS),* (pp. 922-926). Academic Press.

Moskowitz, R. (2012). HIP Diet EXchange (DEX): Draft-moskowitz-hip-dex-00. *Standards Track, 19*(5), 120–135.

Ngoc, T. V. (2008). *Medical applications of wireless networks.* Washington, DC: Recent Advances in Wireless and Mobile Networking.

Nyberg, K., & Rueppel, R. A. (1996). Message recovery for signature schemes based on the discrete logarithm problem. *Designs, Codes and Cryptography, 7*(1-2), 61–81. doi:10.1007/BF00125076

Okamoto, T., & Uchiyama, S. (1998). A new public-key cryptosystem as secure as factoring. Advances in Cryptology — EUROCRYPT'98 Lecture Notes in Computer Science, 1403, 308–318.

Olivereau, Y. B. (2012). D-HIP: A distributed key exchange scheme for HIP-based Internet of Things. *IEEE Int'l Symp. on a World of Wireless, Mobile and Multimedia Networks (WoWMoM): IEEE Computer Society,* 1-7.

Paillier, P. (1999). Public-Key Cryptosystems Based on Composite Degree Residuosity Classes. *EUROCRYPT,* 223–238.

Patrick, K. (2007). *A tool for geospatial analysis of physical activity: Physical activity location measurement system (palms).* San Diego, CA: NIHGEI project at the University of California.

Polastre, J., Szewczyk, R., & Culler, D. (2005). Telos: Enabling Ultra-Low Power Wireless Research. *4th International Conference on Information Processing in Sensor Networks: Special track on Platform Tools and Design Methods for Network Embedded Sensors (IPSN/SPOTS)*, 57-62.

Ponemon Organization. (2015, May 7). Retrieved from Ponemon Institute: https://www.ponemon.org/news-2/66

Radclliffe, J. (2011). *Hacking medical devices for fun and insulin.* Retrieved from Breaking the human scada system: http://media.blackhat.com/bh-us-11/Radcliffe/BH US 11 Radcliffe_Hacking Medical Devices WP.pdf

Raghunathan, S., Ward, M., Roy, K., & Irazoqui, P. (2009). A lowpower implantable event-based seizure detection algorithm. In *4th International IEEE/EMBS Conference* (pp. 151-154). IEEE.

Rivest, R., Shamir, A., & Adleman, L. (1978). A Method for Obtaining Digital Signatures and Public-Key Cryptosystems. *Communications of the ACM, 21*(2), 120–126. doi:10.1145/359340.359342

Shahamabadi, M. S., Ali, B. B., Varahram, P., & Jara, A. (2013). A network mobility solution based on 6LoWPAN hospital wireless sensor network (NEMO-HWSN). In *7th Int. Conf. Innov. Mobile Internet Services Ubiquitous Comput. (IMIS)* (pp. 433-438). IMIS. 10.1109/IMIS.2013.157

Srinivasan, V., Stankovic, J., & Whitehouse, K. (2008). Protecting your daily in-home activity information from a wireless snooping attack. In *10th international conference on Ubiquitous computing* (pp. 202-211). ACM.

T., H. (2007). *LHIP lightweight authentication extension for HIP.* Draft-heer-hip-lhip-00, IETF.

Urien., P. (2013, Oct). *HIP support for RFIDs.* draft-irtf-hiprg-rfid-07.txt.

Wilson, C. B. (1999). Sensors in Medicine. *The Western Journal of Medicine, 11*(5), 322–335. PMID:18751196

Wood, A. D., Fang, L., Stankovic, J. A., & He, T. (2006). SIGF: a family of configurable, secure routing protocols for wireless sensor networks. In *4th ACM workshop on Security of ad hoc and sensor networks* (pp. 35-48). ACM. 10.1145/1180345.1180351

Wu, W., Au, L., Jordan, B., Stathopoulos, T., Batalin, M., & Kaiser, W. (2008). The smartcane system: an assistive device for geriatrics. In ICST (Institute for Computer Sciences, Social-Informatics and Telecommunications Engineering) 3rd international (pp. 1-4). BodyNets '08.

Yager, P., Edwards, T., Fu, E., Helton, K., Nelson, K., Tam, M. R., & Weigl, B. H. (2006). Microfluidic diagnostic technologies for global public health. *Nature, 442*(7101), 412–418. doi:10.1038/nature05064 PMID:16871209

Zimmermann, P. (2010, June). *Where to Get PGP.* Retrieved from Phil Zimmermann & Associates LLC: https://philzimmermann.com/EN/findpgp/

Chapter 11
Bernoulli's Chaotic Map–Based 2D ECG Image Steganography:
A Medical Data Security Approach

Anukul Pandey
https://orcid.org/0000-0003-2737-112X
Dumka Engineering College, India

Barjinder Singh Saini
Dr. B. R. Ambedkar National Institute of Technology, India

Butta Singh
Guru Nanak Dev University, India

Neetu Sood
Dr. B. R. Ambedkar National Institute of Technology, India

ABSTRACT

Signal processing technology comprehends fundamental theory and implementations for processing data. The processed data is stored in different formats. The mechanism of electrocardiogram (ECG) steganography hides the secret information in the spatial or transformed domain. Patient information is embedded into the ECG signal without sacrificing the significant ECG signal quality. The chapter contributes to ECG steganography by investigating the Bernoulli's chaotic map for 2D ECG image steganography. The methodology adopted is 1) convert ECG signal into the 2D cover image, 2) the cover image is loaded to steganography encoder, and 3) secret key is shared with the steganography decoder. The proposed ECG steganography technique stores 1.5KB data inside ECG signal of 60 seconds at 360 samples/s, with percentage root mean square difference of less than 1%. This advanced 2D ECG steganography finds applications in real-world use which includes telemedicine or telecardiology.

DOI: 10.4018/978-1-5225-7952-6.ch011

INTRODUCTION

Signal processing is used everywhere either to convert information-carrying signals from one form to another or for extracting the information from signals (Biswas, 2013). The transmission of a biomedical signal is shown in Figure 1.

Digital signal processing is a category of signal processing that is the numerical manipulation of the signals with the intention to filter, measure, produce, and compress the continuous analog signals. It uses the digital signals for representing them as discrete domain signals as sequence of symbols or numbers that enable the digital processing of the signals. Such a processing involves both linear and non-linear operations. Thus, Bio-medical signal processing is a branch of science for the manipulation of the bio signals or biomedical signals such as Electroencephalography, Electrocardiography, Electromyography (Chang & Lu, 2006).

The manipulation of bio signals includes filtering, encryption, compression, steganography etc. Steganography is the science that falls under the category of secure communications. Its main purpose is to visually hide the secret data in a carrier during communication (A. Pandey, Saini, Singh, & Sood, 2017). It can be interlinked with two other types of security systems, namely cryptography and watermarking. Steganography concerns about the hiding of digital data while watermarking deals with copyright protection of digital data. Although for last couple of millennium, the science of cover writing has been used in diversified forms (Cheddad, Condell, Curran, & Mc Kevitt, 2010), but can be comprehensively divided into two categories. Linguistic steganography is the first one, which was widely used in ancient time, uses the natural language as a carrier in hiding the message in original form. In the early fifth century BC, Histaiacus tried to conceal the secret information made on slave's shaved head in the form of a tattoo and dispatched after his hair grew back with the message. Technical steganography is the second class, which employs the digital data as carrier, such as text, images, video and audio.

Figure 1. Schematic for transmission and reception process of a signal

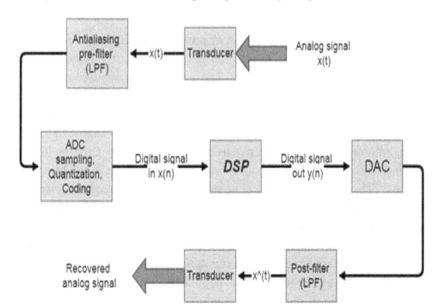

Biomedical Signal and Patient Information Security

The number of patients is increasing intensely due to recent medical advances. Accordingly, to reduce medical labor costs, the use of remote healthcare monitoring systems and Point-of-Care (PoC) technologies have become popular (Ibaida & Khalil, 2013). Monitoring patients at home can drastically reduce the increasing traffic at medical centers and hospitals. Moreover, Point-of-Care solutions can provide greater reliability in emergency services as patient medical information such as diagnosis can be sent immediately to doctors and appropriate action can be taken without any delay. However, remote health care systems are used in large geographical areas essentially for monitoring purposes, and also the Internet represents the main communication channel which is used to exchange information. Typically, physiological readings and patient biological signals are collected using body sensors. Next, the collected signals are sent to the patient device for further processing or diagnosis. Finally, the signals and patient confidential information as well as diagnosis report or any urgent alerts are sent to the central hospital servers or medical cloud via the Internet. Doctors can check those signals and possibly make a decision in the case of an emergency from anywhere using any device.

Using Internet as a foremost communication channel introduces new security and privacy threats as well as data integration issues. According to the *Health Insurance Portability and Accountability Act (HIPAA),* information sent through the Internet should be protected and secured. HIPAA mandates that while transmitting information through the Internet a patient's privacy and confidentiality be protected as follows: (Jero, Ramu, & Ramakrishnan, 2015)

- **Patient Privacy:** It is of crucial importance that a patient can control who will use his/her confidential health information, such as name, address, telephone number, and Medicare number. As a result, the security protocol should provide further control on who can access patient's data and who cannot.
- **Security:** The methods of computer software should guarantee the security of the information within the communication channels as well as the information stored on the hospital server or on the cloud.

Several researchers have proposed various security protocols to secure patient confidential information. Techniques used can be categorized into two subcategories. Firstly, there are techniques that are based on encryption and cryptographic algorithms. These techniques are used to secure data during the communication and storage. As a result, the final data will be stored in encrypted format (Anukul Pandey, Singh, Saini, & Sood, 2016a). The disadvantage of using encryption based techniques is its large computational overhead. Therefore, encryption based methods are not suitable in resource-constrained mobile environment. Alternatively, many security techniques are based on hiding its sensitive information inside another insensitive host data without incurring any increase in the host data size and huge computational overhead. These techniques are called steganography techniques. However, steganography techniques alone will not solve the authentication problem and cannot give the patients the required ability to control who can access their personal information as stated by HIPAA.

The recording of ECG is performed by the help of electrodes that detect minute electrical changes on the skin arising due to the depolarization and repolarization of heart muscles. Figure 2 shows the ECG record in which P wave results from the atrial depolarization, QRS complex is formed because of ventricular depolarization and atrial repolarization whereas T wave results after the repolarization of

Figure 2. ECG signal with specification (Cromwell, Weibell, & Pfeiffer, 1980; Rangayyan, 2002)

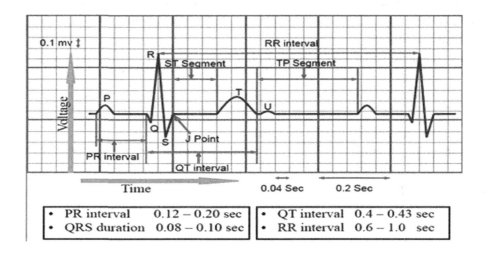

ventricles. U wave if present is the result of after potentials in the ventricular muscles(Cromwell et al., 1980; Rangayyan, 2002).

Steganography

The steganography is the Greek word derived from two words: *stegos* and *grafia* meaning cover writing respectively(Cheddad et al., 2010).It is the art of sending and receiving some secret messages that are hidden in a specific content such as noise, image, audio, waves/signals, videos, protocol, text, etc. In image steganography the message is hidden in the images. It is the practice of encoding secret message in a manner such that its existence is invisible. The original files can be referred to as *cover image*, *cover text*, or *cover audio*. After encrypting the secret information, it is referred to as *stego-medium*. For hiding process, a *stego-key* is used, to restrict detection of the embedded message (Ibaida & Khalil, 2013).

The concept of "What You See Is What You Get (WYSIWYG)" which we encounter sometimes while printing images, is no longer precise and would not make us fool as it does not always hold true. Images can be more than what we normally see with our Human Visual System. An image can convey merely 1000 words. For decades people endeavored to develop innovative methods for secret communication(A. Pandey et al., 2017) .

The term steganography was first used in 1500s after the appearance of Trithemius Book(Rangayyan, 2002). The term steganography was only minted at the end of the 15th century. In ancient times, the back of wax writing tables were used to hide the messages also tattooed on the scalp of slaves or written on the stomachs of rabbits. Either for fun by children and students or for serious undercover work by terrorists, invisible ink has been in use for centuries.

Now multimedia objects like video, audio, image etc. uses the stegnographic systems as cover media because people often transmit digital images over email and other Internet communication(Cheddad et al., 2010; Dunbar, 2002).

Hiding information into a medium requires following elements:

1. The cover medium (C) to hold the secret message.
2. The secret message (M) may be digital image file, plain text, or any type of data.
3. A stego-key (K) to hide and unhide the message.
4. The steganographic techniques.

Types of Steganography

In modern approach, steganography can be divided into five types which depend on the cover medium (Rangayyan, 2002).

1. Text Steganography
2. Audio Steganography
3. Image Steganography
4. Protocol Steganography
5. Video Steganography

Text Steganography

In this method secret message or information hides in text message. The importance of this method has been decreased since Internet and different types of digital file formats came into existence. Using digital files, for encryption, is not used so often because the text files have very small amount of excess data(Morkel, Eloff, & Olivier, 2005) .

Image Steganography

In this method we use images as the popular cover medium. A message is embedded using a secret key in a digital image. On the receiver side, stego-image is processed by the extraction algorithm using the same secret key. Therefore during the transmission of stego-image we can only notice the transmission of a simple image but can't see the hidden message(Morkel et al., 2005).

Audio Steganography

In this information is embedded in a cover speech in a secure and robust manner. An audible sound can be inaudible in the presence of another louder audible sound. This, on the other hand, allows selecting the channel in which to hide secret message (Baritha Begum & Venkataramani, 2012). We can embed the secret messages into WAV and MP3 sound files using steganography software. The methods which are commonly used for audio steganography are Spread spectrum, Echo hiding, LSB coding, Phase coding and Parity coding.

Video Steganography

By this technique message is carried away by hiding it in a video file (Subhedar & Mankar, 2014; Sudeepa, Raju, Ranjan Kumar, & Aithal, 2016).

Protocol Steganography

In protocol steganography information is embedded within network protocols such as TCP/IP. Information is hidden in the header of TCP/IP packet(Song, Zhang, Liao, Du, & Wen, 2011).

ECG Steganography Techniques

LSB is embedded to hide the information in transformed spatial domain ECG to apply steganography technique. It returns the ECG signal in its original range. It was first used to hide the patient confidential information inside patient biomedical signal. This technique uses encryption model which allows only the authorized persons to extract the information from hidden data. The patient ECG signal is the host signal that carries the patient data and readings from sensors such as position, glucose, temperature and blood pressure. The size of the ECG signal is very large compared to the size of basic information. Therefore, it should be a host for small size secret information.

Spatial Domain Technique

There are many versions of spatial steganography, all directly change some bits in the image pixel values in hiding data. LSB based steganography is simplest technique that hides the information without any distortions. To a naked human eye these distortions are invisible. Embedding can be done in various ways (Morkel et al., 2005)such as Matrix embedding, Least Significant Bit replacement technique.

Advantages:

1. Its hiding capacity is very large.
2. Original image cannot be degraded easily.

Disadvantages:

1. Even the simple attacks can destroy the hidden data.
2. Robustness is very low.

Masking and Filtering

This is a technique which is used on grayscale images. This technique is similar to placing water marks on the printed image. Embedding the information in more significant areas made it different from the ones which hide it into noise level. Watermarking techniques are more integrated into the image therefore can be applied without the fear of image destruction (Ali, Ahn, Pant, & Siarry, 2015).

Advantages:

Because of the compression this technique is more robust.

Disadvantages:

This technique is restricted to 24 bits only and can only be applied to gray scale images.

Transform Domain Technique

For these techniques number of embedding techniques has been suggested(Raja, Venugopal, & Patnaik, 2004). These techniques hide information in areas of the image that are less exposed to cropping, image processing and compression. Some transform domain techniques outrun lossless and less format conversions and do not seem dependent on the image format. Different types of Transform domain techniques are given below(Raja et al., 2004; Singh, Devi, & Singh, 2013):

1. Discrete Wavelet Transformation (DWT).
2. Discrete Fourier transformation technique (DFT).
3. Discrete cosine transformation technique (DCT).
4. Fast Discrete Curvelet Transform (FDCT).

Distortion Techniques

This technique measure the deviation from the original cover and hides information according to the signal distortion In order to restore the secret message at decoding process these techniques should know the original cover image. A stego-image is created by modifying the cover image. This message is encoded at pseudo-randomly pixels i.e if the stego-image is different from the cover then the message bit is a 1. Encoder can modify the 1 value pixels in order to maintain the statistical properties same. Receiver can easily detect if any attacker interferes with the encrypted image(Morkel et al., 2005; Singh et al., 2013).

The Biomedical signal processing increasing day by day, as well as the requirement of security to information also increases. So, to secure the patient sensitive information from the intruders some techniques are developed. The appropriate medical information is made available anytime at any place by using modern devices and wireless networks. The introduction of various technologies in telecommunication in the field of health and care environment has increased the accessibility to more efficient tasks, to help care providers and higher quality of health care services.

Related Work

Martinez-Gonzalez et al. (Martínez-González, Díaz-Méndez, Palacios-Luengas, López-Hernández, & Vázquez-Medina, 2016)proposed an alternative for building a data hiding algorithm in to digital images. The method was based on chaos theory and the least significant bit substitution technique for embedding a secret message in an image. Several experiments were shown under different evaluation criteria, such as entropy, homogeneity, autocorrelation, energy, contrast, PSNR, SNR, MSE, and maximum absolute squared deviation. Improved results of PSNR are shown in the experiment and the value of image fidelity in the proposed algorithm compares with the result obtained from similar algorithms.

A steganography was implemented to hide the patient personal report and patient physiological parameters inside the ECG signal. A special range transform was implemented for shifting and scaling of the ECG signal which removes the negative value of ECG signal. Secret key was implemented for transmitting and receiving the message. To decompose the ECG signal a five level wavelet packet is applied. After decomposition, thirty-two sub bands wavelet coefficients are produced. Embedding operation was implemented by using scrambling matrix and secret key. In embedding process, secret bits of information are hidden into LSB of cover signal. Finally, 32 watermarked wavelet coefficients are produced. A new watermarked ECG signal was produced by inverse wavelet transforms. The energies of original ECG signal and encrypted ECG signal are calculated by using different wavelets. They observed that the energy of encrypted ECG signal using Coif-let Wavelet transform was higher than other wavelet transforms so Coif-let Wavelet transform can be used for encryption process in ECG steganography using wavelet transforms.

The performance of FDCT based ECG steganography algorithm using adaptive n × n sequence watermarking technique was studied(Edward Jero, Ramu, & Ramakrishnan, 2015). Patient data can be hidden in the coefficients of cover signal of FDCT. When the coefficients of cover signal are modified, it gets deteriorates which affects the diagnose ability. Therefore, main focus is to preserve the diagnose ability by minimizing the deterioration. Effects of modifying coefficients were studied at three different levels: final deterioration, minimum maximum zero and near zero of the cover image. Better results were obtained by modifying coefficients of near zero rather than other. Therefore an n × n adaptive sequence technique is used to modify coefficients around zero. As there was no loss therefore the signal deterioration was less. Metrics confirmed the performance of the approach such as KL, PSNR, and PRD distance. As the size of the patient data increases, the cover signal deteriorates. It was shown that around 10% signal deteriorated when the size of the patient data increases for 1.5 times.

A proposed method selects the pixel using a random number generator where data was embedded into the red plane of the image. The changes in the image were impossible to notice. To select pixel locations, a stego key was used to seed the Pseudo Random Number Generator(Laskar & Hemachandran, 2013) .

Ramakrishnan et al. (Jero et al., 2015) proposed; patient data security was a vital requirement in remote healthcare monitoring. It was obtained using steganography techniques. In this work, the patient data was hidden inside the 2D ECG matrix of an arrhythmic ECG signal. Initially, the performance of 2D ECG matrix conversion method was evaluated. The resultant metrics shows that the deterioration due to the conversion process was negligible. DWT was one of the efficient transform to perform steganography in transform domain. The performance of ECG steganography using DWT-SVD based steganography algorithm was estimated for the 9 arrhythmic ECG signals of MIT-BIH arrhythmia database. The higher PSNR and the lowest PRD values of performance metrics appears that the better imperceptibility to the watermark and lowest deterioration of cover signal respectively. Finally, the zero BER shows that the patient data was extracted without any losses.

Ibaida et al. (Ibaida, 2014) introduced an algorithm which hides the patient and the diagnostics information inside ECG signal. This technique is very confidential and secure in the Point-of-Care system. Five level wavelet decomposition was applied. To find the correct embedding sequence, a scrambling matrix was used based on the user defined key. Number of bits i.e. steganography levels to hide the coefficients of each sub-band is determined by experimental methods. The quality of distortion was diagnosed and found that the hidden data can be extracted completely and resultant watermarked ECG can be used for it.

With the combination of two One-dimensional chaotic maps, a more effective system was introduced. The resultant system was able to produce maps with larger ranges and better behavior as compare to seed maps. A novel encryption method was proposed to investigate its applications in multimedia security. This algorithm generates a completely different encrypted image using the same set of security keys every time when it was applied to the same image (Zhou, Bao, & Chen, 2014). This algorithm gave the excellent performance in various attacks and image encryption.

Most of the chaotic security protocols are cryptographically weak to compute. Chaotic phenomena as an application in security areas were not studied in detail. They have studied chaos maps which were based on a steganography technique in spatial domain only for digital images (Anees, Siddiqui, Ahmed, & Hussain, 2014). Strength of an algorithm can be increased by applying chaos effectively in secure communication. Also few statistical analyses such as energy, peak signal to noise ratio, correlation, contrast, homogeneity, mean square error and entropy have also been carried out and proved that they can also survive against different attacks such as the known stego attack, stego only attack known message attack, and known cover attack [Anees et al. (2014)].

Chang et al. (Cheng & Chang, 2012) proposes an adaptive method which hides data based on code word grouping. By using a palette generation algorithm a set of code words were generated. A stenographic scheme for index encoding images was presented. Different group member sub-clusters know the relationship of code words. The hide capacity can by be determined by the size of the sub-cluster. We can further enhance the hiding capacity by merging together the capacity of sub-clusters with larger members with each other & sub-clusters with smaller members with each other. In this embedded procedure the sub-cluster which is the closest searched code word belongs to was identified, and then the original code word was modified in such a way to hide a secret message. Number of bits of secret message that can be embedded was indicated by the number of sub-cluster members. Members of sub-clusters were determined by using a set of thresholds. Random linear codes of small co-dimension were used to improve the codes with matrix embedding arbitrary selection channels and improved embedding efficiency. Pseudo random generator was used as security of the sequence of embedding pixels.

A robust approach presents the two components; one is based on Least Significant Bit methods which embeds the secret data in the blue components of the LSB's and the edges of the images were embedded in the partial green components. An adaptive algorithm based on LSB steganography was proposed. This algorithm embeds data based on information available in MSB's of blue, green and red components of randomly selected pixels. An Advanced Encryption Standard was integrated in this therefore it was more robust (Jero et al., 2015).

For hiding information in images, a large selection of approaches was introduced in image steganography techniques. Different methods with different file formats are used to hide messages that have different strong and weak points. Here one technique lacks in robustness whereas other lacks in payload capacity. Such as the patchwork approach which can hide only a small amount of information, has very high level of robustness against most type of attacks (Shelke, Dongre, & Soni, 2014). Both the BMP and GIF techniques result in suspicious files that may increase the probability of detection. Which algorithm should be used was decided by the agent on the basis of the type of application he wants to use in the algorithm for and whether he was willing to compromise some features or not in order to ensure the security of others.

Yang et al. (Yang, Wong, Liao, Zhang, & Wei, 2010) author approached an enhance histogram based reversible data method which used two interleaving predictive stages. This approach predicts most of the pixels by their neighborhood pixels. If two then it was in the column-based and if four, chess-board based approach. The difference between the value of each pixel of the original image and the stego-image is in between ± 1. Pixels in even columns will be predicted by pixels in odd columns in interleaving predictions or vice versa. To generate a histogram to embed secret data, predictive error values of odd columns are used.

An edge adaptive scheme applies to decide embedding capacity in the other two channels and can also select the embedding regions according to the size of the secret data. For estimating the capacity of selected regions in the data embedding stage, the scheme initializes some parameters (Chen, Luo, Zhao, & Zhang, 2014). For region selection and LSB Matching Revisited as the data hiding algorithm a criteria, difference between two adjacent pixels, was used.

Devi et al. (Singh et al., 2013) proposed some techniques to secure stego-image i.e the LSB Technique and Pseudo-Random Encoding Technique. In case of lossless compression, LSB insertion using random key was better than simple LSB insertion. In the image resolution, image was protected with a personal key and was negligible when the message is embedded into the image. So, it becomes difficult to damage the data by any attack. This algorithm was easy to implement in both the grayscale and color image because it was used for both 8 bit and 24 bit image of the same size of cover and secret image. This method reduces the distortion rate and increases the security of the message and PSNR.

To compress both regular and irregular ECG signals a technique was proposed. (Filho et al., 2008) increases the quality of the reconstructed signal by incorporating the compressor or combined with existing schemes. JPEG2000 and H.264/AVC intra-frame encoders were used to enhance the performances of the proposed techniques. The results shows that it was worthwhile to further develop techniques with the chosen compressor that adapted the ECG signal. Performance of the compression can be improved with simple adaptations using well-established algorithms, and reducing the costs of the compression methods.

Tompkins et al. (Jiapu Pan, Tompkins, & Willis, 1985) author implemented a real-time QRS detection algorithm in the Z80 assembly language. QRS complexes using width, slope and amplitude information can be reliably detect by this algorithm. In order to get high detection sensitivity a bandpass filter is used which permits the use of low amplitude thresholds and preprocesses the signal to reduce interference. In this algorithm missed beats are searched with the use a dual-thresholds technique. This algorithm automatically adapts RR interval limit and each threshold at particular interval of time. An accurate use of ECG signals can be provided by this adaptive approach having many heart rate changes, diverse signal characteristics and QRS morphologies.

Need for Present Chapter

ECG signal steganography is significant for an effective security of patient information. The ECG signal is a basic and important biomedical signal as prior to EEG and EMG. The message or some patient information can be embedded in an ECG signal. After the embedding of information, the ECG should remain unchanged because if the ECG changes its signal properties by embedding information, it will be not properly diagnosed by cardiac expert. The information is retrieved from the ECG signal by using a special key and proper method of encoding/decoding. Therefore, patient information is embedded into the ECG signal by steganography method by not sacrificing the ECG signal quality, size and shape.

Chapter Objectives

In this we carried out these objectives:

- To explore the ECG as a host medium for steganography.
- To hide the information into an ECG signal as a cover image by means of LSB technique; Bernoulli's chaotic map and pseudo random technique.
- To analyze performance and effect on the ECG signal in terms of size and quality by applying the proposed steganography techniques.

Chapter Organization

Section 1 discussed the developments that had taken place in the field of ECG steganography. Section 2 provides the basic chaotic map background. The methodology to attain the objectives of this work are in section 3. Section 3 also deals with the conversion of ECG signal to cover image, spatial domain (LSB) steganography algorithm using Bernoulli's chaotic maps. Results of proposed ECG steganography with various performance measures are discussed in Section 4. Finally, Section 5 concludes the chapter.

CHAOTIC MAP BACKGROUND

Chaotic theory studies the behavior of dynamical systems which are highly sensitive to the initial conditions, which can even detect the small differences such as rounding off errors in numerical computation and yield widely different outcomes in general. Chaotic systems are applied for very secure communications and are of impromptu behavior (Yeh & Wu, 2008). Chaotic security algorithms have several advantages such as computational power, speed, reasonable computational overheads and high security over the traditional algorithms. Also, steganalysis which includes known the cover attacker, chosen stego attack, known stego attack, stego-only attack, and statistical measures illustrate exceptional results over the traditional algorithms. Chaotic maps can be divided into two categories: one-dimension and multi-dimensions.

The multi-dimension (MD) chaotic maps are essential in image security (Anees et al., 2014) because of their multiple parameters and complex structures. Various controls parameters of chaotic maps increases the randomness and computation complexity (A. Pandey et al., 2017). Whereas one-dimensional chaotic system has an elementary structure and has many applications such as

Logistic Maps

The Logistic map is famous among the chaotic maps because of its simplicity in dynamic equations with complex chaotic behavior. The mathematical equation is given as follows (Hua, Zhou, Pun, & Chen, 2015):

$$X_{n+1=} L\left(r, X_n\right) = rX_n\left(1 - X_n\right)$$

where r is a parameter with range of (0; 4] and X_n is the output chaotic sequence.

Tent Maps

The Tent map also called tent-like shape (Zhou et al., 2014).

$$X_{n+1} = T\left(\mu, X_n\right) = \begin{cases} \dfrac{\mu X_n}{2} & X_i < 0.5 \\ \dfrac{\mu\left(1 - X_n\right)}{2} & X_i \geq 0.5 \end{cases}$$

where parameter $\mu \in \left(0, 4\right]$

Sine Maps

The Sine map has a similar behavior as the chaotic maps with the logistic maps (Hua et al., 2015).

$$X_{n+1} = S\left(a, X_n\right) = a\sin\left(\pi X_n\right) / 4$$

where parameter $a \in \left(0, 4\right]$

Bernoulli's Maps

Also known as dyadic transformation, and can be defined as an iterated map of the PWL (piece wise linear) function according to the following equation (Martínez-González et al., 2016).

$$f\left(x\right) = \begin{cases} 2\mu x & 0 \leq x < 0.5 \\ 2\mu x - 1 & 0.5 \leq x < 1 \end{cases}$$

where x$\in$ (0, 1) and µ$\in$ (0, 1)

METHOD AND MATERIAL

This section introduces the proposed architecture and algorithm. The first is the discussion of ECG database followed by proposed 2D ECG stenography.

Database

In the developing medical engineering arena, research subjects like cardiovascular and pulmonary dynamics, biomedical signals, artificial intelligence, heart rate variability, cardiac arrhythmia detection, and ECG compression have evolved (Anukul Pandey, Singh, Saini, & Sood, 2016b). For the investigation, ECG Arrhythmia database has been taken in the present study. This database includes forty-eight half-hour extracts of ECG recordings from forty-eight subjects. The record maintained 11-bit resolutions over the 10mV range. The proposed steganography technique using least substitution bit and Bernoulli's chaotic maps have been evaluated on these recordings. The .mat file can be extracted from Physio.net by appropriate selection of database which is MIT-BIH Arrhythmia database. Each recording is of 60 second duration. After the process of embedding the performance measures are computed.

Proposed 2D ECG Image Steganography Method

The proposed 2D ECG steganography method begins by the formation of 2D ECG Image. Thereafter the secret information is embedded into the ECG signal through the Bernoulli's chaotic maps and the LSB substitution. After embedding the secret data into the cover ECG the performance parameters are calculated (Martínez-González et al., 2016). At decoding end, the embedded message will be extracted from the cover image and ECG signal reconstruction is done.

Encrypt the bits of the message before embedding them into the cover image i.e. obtained from ECG signal by converting it into an image using Pan-Tompkins algorithm.

A random selection of image composition (grayscale) must be performed and the insertion of secret information in a random way to: rows and then to columns of image.

Decryption of stego-image will be implemented and hidden message will be extracted from the stego-image/cover image. Hence, reconstruction of ECG signal will be done using Pan-Tompkins algorithms.

Pan-Tomkins Based QRS Detection

The "Pan and Tompkins" QRS detection algorithm implements a special digital band pass filter which identifies the QRS complexes based upon digital analysis of width, amplitude and slope of the ECG data. This type of algorithm reduces the false detection caused due to the interference present in ECG signal and also adjusts the thresholds and parameters to adapt the changes in QRS morphology and heart rate (J Pan & Tompkins, 1985).

Pan Tompkins detects the QRS complex by following the given processing steps:

- Differentiation.
- Band-pass filtering.
- Moving window integration.
- Squaring.
- Thresholds adjustment.

Figure 3. Pan-Tomkins QRS detection block diagram

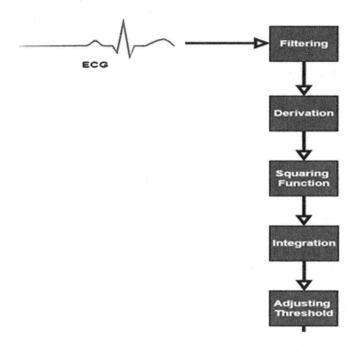

The P wave which is based on the location of the QRS complex is a rounded peak. In all biomedical processing textbooks, one QRS detection algorithm which is most important is that introduced by Pan and Tompkins. Figure 3 shows a graphical representation of the algorithm. The signal passes through filtering, squaring, derivation, and integration phases before thresholds are set and QRS complexes are detected. In order to reduce the influence of the muscle noise, the baseline wander, the power line interference, and T-wave interference, the signal is first passed through the low pass and then a high pass filter.

A graphical representation of the algorithm is shown in the above diagram. Before thresholds are set the signal passes through filtering, derivation, squaring, and integration phases and QRS complexes are detected.

Band-Pass Filtering

The BPF matches the spectrum of the average QRS complex and therefore reduces noise in the ECG signal. This attenuates noise due to baseline wander, muscle noise, T wave interference and power line interference. The pass band in the range 5Hz-35Hz maximizes the QRS energy. This filter is composed of high pass and low pass Butterworth IIR filters in the cascade(J Pan & Tompkins, 1985).

Squaring Function

The filtered signal is squared point by point after differentiation. The equation of this operation is:

$$Y\left(nT\right) = \left[Y\left(nT\right)\right]^2$$

Squaring does nonlinear amplification of the output and makes all data points positive.

Moving Window Integration

In addition to the slope of the R wave, it also obtains waveform feature information. It is calculated from:

$$Y\left(nT\right) = \left(\frac{1}{N}\right)\left[x\left(nT - \left(N-1\right)T\right) + x\left(nT - \left(N-2\right)T\right) + \ldots + x\left(nT\right)\right]$$

where n is the number of samples in the width of the integration window. Figure 3 shows the relationship between the QRS complex and the moving-window integration waveform. The width of the window is as wide as the QRS complex. The wide window means, the integration waveform will merge T complexes and the QRS together and when it is too narrow then QRS complexes will produce several peaks in the integration waveform which can cause difficulty in QRS detection processes. The efficient width is at sample rate of 360 samples /s, the size of window is 30 samples wide (150 ms) (J Pan & Tompkins, 1985).

ECG (2D) Formation

The original record which has been transformed into 2D signal is required to process the ECG signal as an image(Anukul Pandey, Saini, Singh, & Sood, 2016a, 2016b). This can be done by detecting the ECG period, followed by row-oriented assembly and segmentation. Here the algorithm helps in the execution of QRS complex detection (J Pan & Tompkins, 1985). Further the signal is segmented and then gets reassembled by choosing the max value of the QRS complex. The resultant is shown in Figure 4. All the periods do not have the same lengths; they are generally left aligned due to the variations in patient's conditions. (Baali, Akmeliawati, Salami, Aibinu, & Gani, 2011) proposed the period normalization concept to better exploit the inter-beat dependencies. Further some changes in length of all periods are done by (Bilgin, Marcellin, & Altbach, 2003). Then the normalized segment is given by:

$$X = \left[x\left(0\right)x\left(1\right)\ldots x\left(N_0 - 1\right)\right]$$

to

$$X_n = \left[x_n\left(0\right)x_n\left(1\right)\ldots x_n\left(N_n - 1\right)\right]$$

Computation using,

$$X_n\left(m\right) = \hat{X}\left(h^*\right)$$

$$h^* = \frac{m\left(N_0 - 1\right)}{N_n - 1}$$

where $\hat{X}(h^*)$ is the interpolated version of $X(n)$, N_n is the normalized period length, N_0 is the original period length, and m = 0. . . N_n − 1. To reconstruct the original signal decoder should know the size of each original period (Filho et al., 2008). This information is sent as side data, along with the header of compressed file. Figure 4 shows the 2D array from RR intervals of original ECG signal.

Bernoulli's Chaotic Maps

The execution of steganography technique can contain different scientific concepts and tools. In specific, steganography techniques that use chaos theory are emerging (A. Pandey et al., 2017). Chaotic systems are attractive in security information because they are nonlinear systems characterized by sensitivity of initial condition and control, unpredictability, ergodicity mixing properties and then they can produce deterministic signals with random appearance suitable in the design of steganographic algorithms.

Mathematical Model

The Bernoulli map, also known as dyadic transformation, can be defined as an iterated map of the PWL (Piece wise linear) function according to Eq. (1).

$$f(x) = \begin{cases} 2\mu x & 0 \leq x < 0.5 \\ 2\mu x - 1 & 0.5 \leq x < 1 \end{cases} \tag{1}$$

Where x∈ (0, 1) and μ∈ (0, 1)

The definition domain of Bernoulli's map is the interval (0, 1); and for calculations, a floating point number representation is used. But when the map is used to process binary files, the Bernoulli's map as defined by Eq. (1) should be modified so as to use a fixed-point representation for each number considering only natural numbers. In this way, the modified Bernoulli's map has its definition domain in the interval (0, limit), considering that the limit is an arbitrary but known value and it is in (1, MaxRep) with MaxRep is the largest number that can be represented in a computer(Ghebleh & Kanso, 2014).

Figure 4. 2D Array of original ECG signal

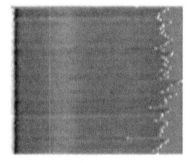

$$g(x) = \begin{cases} floor(2\mu x), & 0 \le x < \dfrac{limit}{2} \\ floor(2\mu x - limit), & \dfrac{limit}{2} \le x < limit \end{cases} \qquad (2)$$

Now x ∈ (0, limit), μ ∈ (0, 1) and floor (x) is a function that truncates a number x to lower whole.

Notice that Eq. (2) includes a scaling and discretization process over chaotic map defined in the real numbers. But it now represents a new chaotic map in the natural numbers, and then each natural number produced by this new map must be translated to a number in fixed point representation. In this way, the universe of natural numbers has a cardinality of 2N, where N represents the number of bits in the binary representation of each natural number. Some authors have reported a degradation problem in the chaotic behavior of the map when a fixed point representation (Biswas, 2013) issued in the calculations for the iterated process; such degradation can be solved or at least minimized using a larger quantity of bits in the number representation. Figure 5 shows various sequences to determine how the value of limit and a specific value of x_0 affects the chaotic behavior of the map; the resented sequences were obtained iterating Eq.(2), $x_{n+1} = g(x_n)$, and using small numbers for the variable limit and a specific value of x_0. For the four sequences, μ is 0.9; moreover, the value of limit was 3, 5 and 10, respectively. The top sequence has only numbers '1'; for the middle sequence, the map has a brief transient behavior but after a few iterations, it produces a sequence of only numbers '0'.Finally, the bottom sequences how's an oscillating behavior; in consequence, to prevent disorder in the behavior of the iterated function is given by Eq. (2), high value for limit will be used.

Additionally, the module function is applied considering an iterated process defined by $x_n + 1 = mod$ (g (x_n), k). This map is defined in the natural numbers. The consequence of this strategy could be the evidence of periodicity in the produced pseudo random sequences. In Figure 6, two bifurcation diagrams are presented; the left one is the bifurcation diagram for the original sequence produced by Eq. (2) using a limit=1000.

Notice that the mentioned periodicity evidence do not exists. That is, any value of control parameter, μ, at (0.5, 1.0) can be considered and no evidence of periodicity is produced. The right one is the bifurcation diagram using the module function, to determine it using limit=1000 (Martínez-González et al., 2016).

Another observation taken from Figure 6 is that the bifurcation diagram for the original sequence produced by Eq. (2) is not completely dense. Bifurcation diagram usually represent stable value with solid line and unstable values with dotted lines line values with a dotted line. To reduce, even more, the degradation in the behavior of the map, other map is proposed, which includes an increasing factor named factor, see Eq. (3)

$$h(x) = \begin{cases} floor(2\mu x), & 0 \le x < \dfrac{limit}{2} * factor \\ floor(2\mu x - (limit - factor)), & \dfrac{limit}{2} * factor \le x < limit * factor \end{cases} \qquad (3)$$

Figure 5. Sequences obtained from Eq. (2) using different values of variable limit when: (a) limit=3, $\mu = 0.9$, *(b) limit=5,* $\mu = 0.9$, *and (c) limit =10,* $\mu = 0.9$

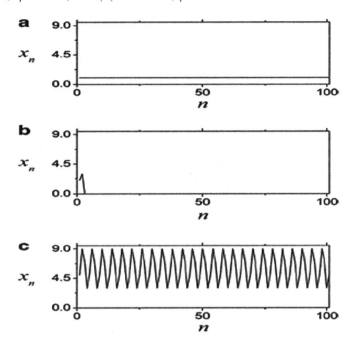

where $x_n \in (0, \text{limit} * \text{factor})$ and $\mu \in (0, 1)$

According to Figure 7 where limit remains steady at 1000 for both diagrams; if factor is increased from factor = 100 (right bifurcation diagram) to factor = 1000 (left bifurcation diagram), the bifurcation diagram in Figure 7 becomes denser than the Figure 6.

Message Ciphering Process.

The process depicted in Figure 8 corresponds to the ciphering process (Martínez-González et al., 2016) the process has embedded the sequence generation X(n). Afterward, the sequence is equally divided in two, generating sequences $X(n)m$ and $X(n)l$, the same division is made for the message (msg) generating msgm and msgl. Finally, msgm and X(n)m are bit wisely XORed as well as msgl and X(n)l. With the ciphered message (cipm, cipl) and the selecting sequences correctly adapted (x1r, x2r), the process catches the cover image (img). The process selects a pixel and deletes the four least significant bits using x1r and x2r. After the deletion and in a toggling form, the upper or the lower part of the ciphered message are added above. The last step is repeated until the messages ciphered completely.

Message Embedding

In this process a 2D ECG image which is converted from ECG signal is randomized using a random key and then hides the bits of a secret message into least significant bit within that cover image. The stego-key and random key is shared by both transmitting as well as receiving end. To seed a pseudo-random number generator a random key is used which select the pixel locations for embedding the secret message.

Figure 6. Bifurcation diagram for (a) original Sequence and (b) obtained from Residue Technique

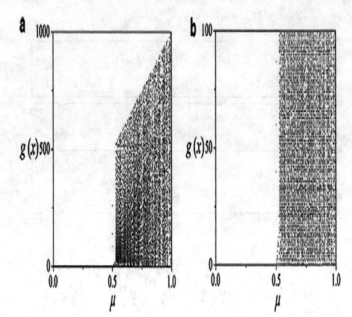

Figure 7. Bifurcation diagram using a factor of (a) 1000 and (b) 100

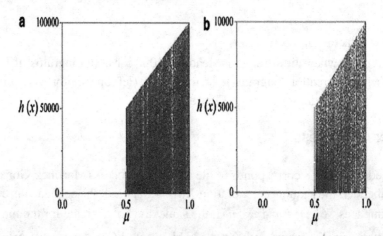

It is generated by three Bernoulli's chaotic maps; two maps for generating pseudo random sequence and one map for message ciphering ensuring more security against intruders. Figure 9 show the flow chart of the proposed ECG steganography mechanism.

Step 1: Load the ECG samples from the database of MIT-BIH databank. Then ECG signal is converted into gray scale cover image using Pan-Tompkins algorithm.

Step 2: The cover image is broken into lower and upper parts.

Step 3: This ciphered signal is then converted into binary form i.e. four MSBs and four LSBs. The upper part embeds the MSBs and Lower part embeds LSBs.

Figure 8. Flow chart for message ciphering

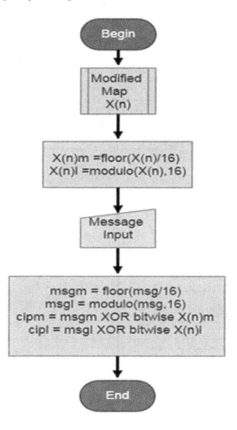

Step 4: The exact positions in upper and lower part are defined by the chaotic maps engaged in the algorithm for embedding of information bits, that is, one Bernoulli's chaotic map defines the row number, second map defines the column number, and the third map engaged in message ciphering process.

Step 5: For embedding a spsecific pixel of carrier image is selected, then it is converted into binary and split into MSBs and LSBs. Its LSBs are then replaced with respective message bits. Initialize the stego-key and XOR with text file to be hidden and give message.

Step 6: After embedding the upper and lower parts of the carrier and each symbol of information, makes the 2D ECG steganographic image. The LSBs are replaced of the cover image and are considered as a loss of information or regarded as an addition of noise in it.

Step 7: Write the Stego ECG image file in JPEG 2000 encoding format.

Message Extraction and ECG Reconstruction

Message Extraction first takes the key and then the random key. Where the secret message is randomly distributed these keys takes out the points of the LSB from there (Devi, 2013). The process of decoding searches for the hidden bits of a secret message and converts it into the least significant bit using the random key within a cover image. In this algorithm a random key must match with the random key used

Figure 9. Flowchart of message embedding algorithm

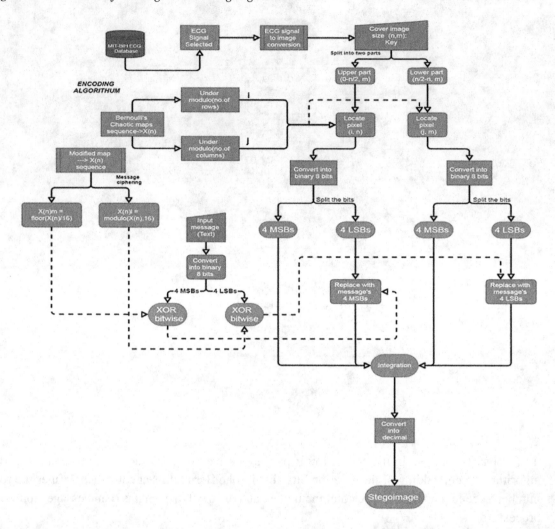

in encoding because these key sets the hiding points of the message. The receiver can then extract the exact embedded messages using only the stego-key. Figure 10 shows the flowchart of decoding algorithm or steganalysis and reconstruction of ECG signal.

Step 1: Extract the Stego image file from image file and open it in read mode, observe the grayscale of each pixel.

Step 2: Similarly, Bernoulli's chaotic maps engaged in planned algorithm define the exact location in upper and lower part for embedding of message bits, that is, one Bernoulli's chaotic map defines the row number, second map defines the column number, and the third map engaged in message ciphering process. Initialize the random-key that gives the position of the message bits in the pixel that are embedded randomly.

Step 3: Further for the decoding, the LSB value of pixels are extracted.

Step 4: Then read the pixels and convert the array contents into decimal value i.e is actually ASCII value of hidden character.

Step 5: XOR the above ASCII values with stego-key which gives the message file, which we hide inside the cover image or binary value converted into character value.

Step 6: On the other side, the cover image previously made from ECG signal using Pan-Tompkins algorithm, after decoding the ECG signal is reconstructed from cover image using reverse of Pan-Tompkins algorithm. The reconstructed signal is almost the exact replica of original signal with low distortion.

Brief Steps for ECG Steganography

The methodology implemented in the current chapter for ECG steganography and its performance evaluation is shown in Figure 11.

First of all, the ECG signal is converted into the grayscale 2D cover image using Pan-Tomkins QRS detection method.

Then, the cover image is loaded to steganography encoder which is a combination of stego key, message input and pseudo random generator, which produces the random sequence by means of Bernoulli's chaotic maps or modified maps. Side by side one chaotic map is engaged in message ciphering process.

Figure 10. Extraction of message and ECG reconstruction algorithm flowchart

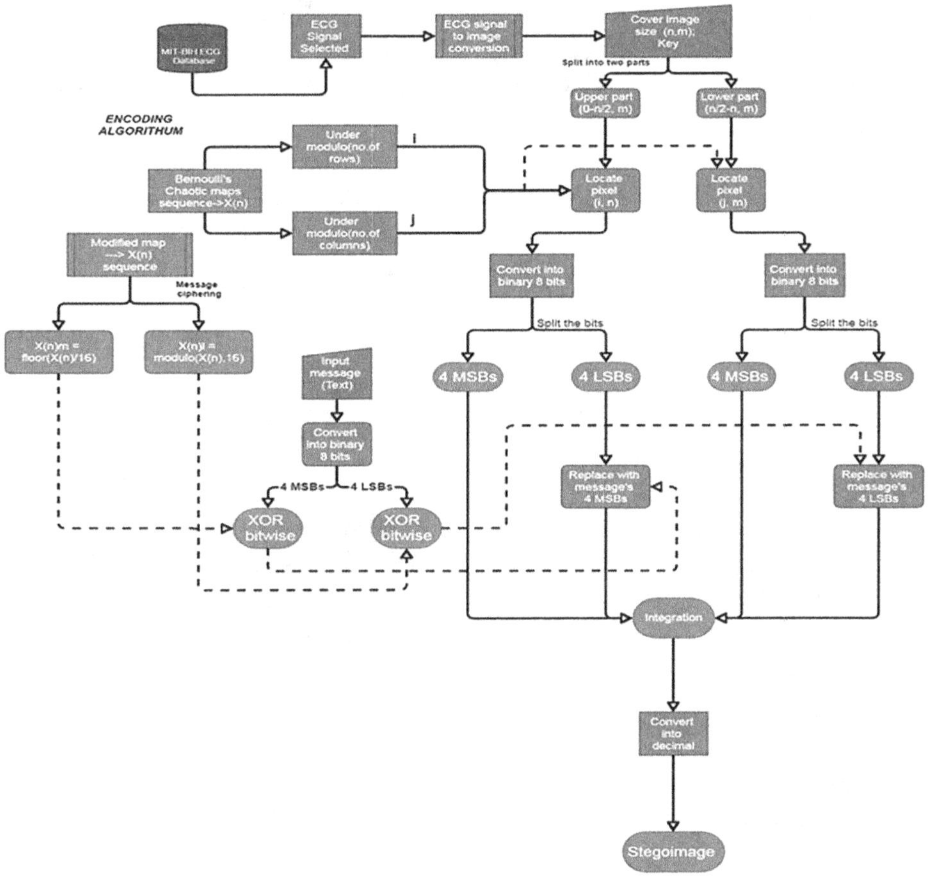

Hence, by implementing the encoding algorithm the cover image can be obtained from the stego image and some evaluation of image parameter is done.

After the encoding is complete, the stego key is shared with the steganography decoder. Function of decoder is to extract the hidden message by initializing the stego key, deciphering the message using modified maps and recovery of original ECG signal implementing the reverse of Pan-Tomkins algorithm.

Therefore, the hidden message is extracted and ECG signal is also recovered. Some metric evaluation is done on recovered ECG signal and extracted message.

RESULTS

Essential requirements for ECG steganographic systems are stego-ECG quality, undetectability, and resistance against active attacks. To evaluate the effectiveness of the proposed ECG steganographic process seven performance evaluation metrics have been calculated. Two different sizes of hidden messages were used to test the method m1 = 3 bytes and m2 = 1 KB. Also, to check the quality and the variation

Figure 11. Flowchart for ECG stenography

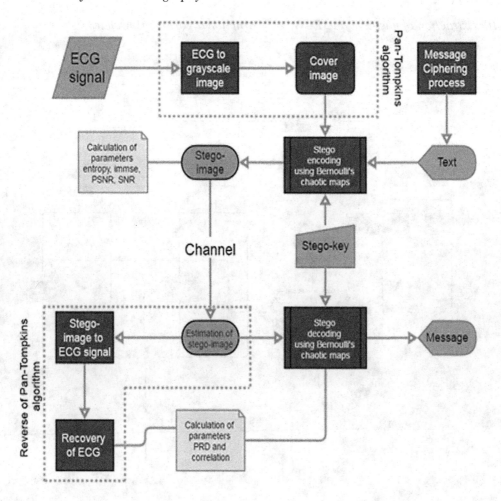

from raw ECG signals by reconstructing of ECG signal from the cover image. ECG steganogram was tested by calculating their original image Entropy (H1) and stego-image Entropy (H2), Percentage Root Mean Square Difference (PRD), Homogeneity (Hom), Mean Square Error (MSE), Cross-Correlation coefficient (Rxy), Peak Signal to Noise ratio (PSNR) and Signal to Noise Ratio (SNR). These measures are defined below.

Performance Measures

The quality of ECG steganography is based on three primary ingredients i) high security of embedding message in cover data, ii) should have low distortion in cover ECG or higher correlation between stego-ECG and cover ECG, and iii) maintaining higher quality during reversibility. The various performance measures used are as follows:

Entropy (H)

It is a statistical measure of randomness in image that can be used to characterize the texture of the input image which is defined by:

$$H = \sum_{i=1}^{n} p\left(x_i\right) log_2 p(x_i)$$

where $p\left(x_i\right)$ is the probability of the difference between two adjacent pixel i.e. x_i

Homogeneity (Hom)

It is a defined as the closeness of the distribution of elements in the gray level concurrence matrix (GLCM) to the GLCM diagonal. It can be defined by,

$$hom = \sum_{i,j} \frac{x\left(i,j\right)}{1+\left|i-j\right|}$$

where $x\left(i,\ j\right)$ is 2D ECG image matrix.

Mean Square Error (MSE)

It is the measure of the difference of two digital images divided by the number of elements. It can be defined by,

$$MSE\left(dB\right) = \frac{1}{n}\sum_{i}\sum_{j}\left(x_c - y_s\right)^2$$

where N is the Number of samples, xc is the amplitude of the cover signal and y_s is the amplitude of the Steganographed signal.

Peak Signal to Noise Ratio (PSNR)

It tests the difference between the cover image and its steganogram. PSNR is an objective criterion to evaluate the quality of an image, it is widely used to measure the quality of stego-image, and it is defined in decibels (dB). PSNR is the ratio of maximum amplitude of the cover ECG signal to the mean squared deviation between Stego and cover ECG signals. The quality of the signal is better for the High value of PSNR (Edward Jero et al., 2015). PSNR represents a measure of peak error and expressed in terms of the logarithmic decibel (dB) units in the following equation:

$$PSNR\left(dB\right) = 10 log_{10}\left(\frac{2^B - 1}{\sqrt{MSE}}\right)$$

where B represents the bits per pixel

Signal to Noise Ratio (SNR)

SNR is measure of degree of noise energy introduced by steganography encoding algorithm in decibel (dB) scale. Where $x_{i,j}$ the 2D ECG is image matrix and $y_{i,j}$ is the stego image matrix.

$$SNR\left(dB\right) = 10 \log_{10}\left[\frac{\sum_0^{n_i-1}\sum_0^{n_j-1}\left[x_{i,j}\right]^2}{\sum_0^{n_i-1}\sum_0^{n_j-1}\left[x_{i,j} - y_{i,j}\right]^2}\right]$$

Percentage Root Mean Squared Difference (PRD)

It is a percentage of root mean squared difference between two signals. It increases linearly with the increase in the difference between 2D ECG signal and stego ECG image and are given in the following equation:

$$PRD\left(\%\right) = \sqrt{\left(\frac{\sum_{n=1}^N\left(x_c\left(N\right) - x_s\left(N\right)\right)^2}{\sum_{n=1}^N\left(x_c\left(N\right)\right)^2}\right)} \times 100$$

Cross Correlation (R_{xy})

It is obtained by dividing the covariance of two signals, i.e., raw ECG and reconstructed ECG, by the product of their standard deviation. Its description is defined by,

$$R_{xy} = \frac{\sum_i \sum_j \left(\left(x_{i,j} - \overline{x} \right) \left(y_{i,j} - \overline{y} \right) \right)}{\sqrt{\left(\sum_i \sum_j \left(x_{i,j} - \overline{x} \right)^2 \left(\sum_i \sum_j \left(y_{i,j} - \overline{y} \right) \right)^2 \right)}}$$

where $\overline{x}$ is the mean of the reconstructed ECG signal, $x_{i,j}$ is the value of the pixel in i, j; $\overline{y}$ is the mean of the original ECG signal.

Evaluation of Performance Metrics

The ECG steganography, encoding/decoding, embedding/extraction of the message from ECG signal, reconstruction and errors are shown for 2500 samples of 48 datasets obtained from MIT-BIH Arrhythmia database. The closer scan at the figures reveals that the reconstructed ECG signals are almost similar to the original ECG signals with extracted message m1 and m2. The results of two different size of message embedding are shown in Figure 12 and Figure 13 for two random selected datasets.

Tables 1 and 2 show the values of seven performance indicators (H1, H2, Hom, MSE, PSNR, SNR, PRD, and R_{xy})(Anukul Pandey, Saini, Singh, & Sood, 2018) of 48 datasets of MIT-BIH arrhythmia database for the purpose of analyzing the ECG steganography with hidden message m1 and m2 respectively. Each data file includes lead II ECG data with each lead comprising of 1036800 data samples. The methods are programmed and implemented using MATLAB. After implementation, the performance measures are calculated and analyzed.

Applications and Advantages

Chaotic systems are attractive in security information as they are nonlinear systems and have high sensitivity.

The chaotic map systems characterized by high sensitivity, control parameter, ergodicity mixing properties, and produce the deterministic signal with random appearance suitable for the design of steganographic algorithms.

The Bernoulli's chaotic map provides simplistic approach to implementation then tangent-delay for elliptic reflecting cavity chaotic sequence and nonlinear chaotic algorithm.

This algorithm is a simple and straightforward technique which uses the LSB technique for hiding data. It has the advantage of encrypting more data than the transform techniques.

Before embedding into cover image, the text message is also masked using 1D chaotic map for increasing the complexity faced by intruders.

Figure 12. Performance of 2D ECG steganography for 2500 samples of dataset 100 of MIT-BIH Arrhythmia database $m1 = 84bytes$;
$\lambda_0 = 0.6$, $\lambda_1 = 0.1$, $\lambda_2 = 0.2$, $\mu_0 = 0.88$, $\mu_1 = 0.9$, $and \mu_2 = 0.92$

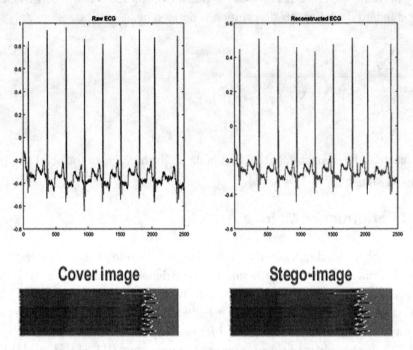

Figure 13. Performance of 2D ECG steganography for 2500 samples of dataset 113 of MIT-BIH Arrhythmia database $m1 = 84bytes$;
$\lambda_0 = 0.6$, $\lambda_1 = 0.1$, $\lambda_2 = 0.2$, $\mu_0 = 0.88$, $\mu_1 = 0.9$, $and \mu_2 = 0.92$

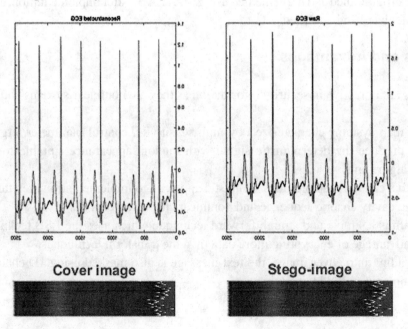

Table 1. Performance parameter evaluation of MIT-BIH arrhythmia database for 2D ECG steganography of hidden message m1= 84 bytes

| Sr. no | ECG | | (H1)dB | (H2)dB | (MSE)dB | (PSNR)dB | (SNR)dB | PRD (%) | Rxy |
	Data-sets	Size (KB)							
1.	100	292	5.2912	5.2915	0.0348	62.7194	51.3428	0.0102	0.9999
2.	101	292	5.7530	5.7531	0.0377	62.3617	48.7729	0.0065	0.9999
3.	102	156	6.1974	6.1975	0.0248	64.1859	54.7183	0.0086	0.9999
4.	103	282	5.7843	5.7845	0.0413	61.9680	49.1975	0.0095	0.9999
5.	104	278	5.6725	5.6727	0.0188	65.3988	56.3705	0.0111	0.9999
6.	105	274	5.0735	5.0735	0.0272	63.7831	51.8692	0.0109	0.9999
7.	106	275	5.5369	5.5371	0.0234	64.4357	53.8262	0.0111	0.9999
8.	107	272	6.8613	6.8613	0.0439	61.7043	55.8254	0.1027	0.9999
9.	108	276	3.9127	3.9132	0.0105	67.8997	61.3363	0.0109	0.9999
10.	109	275	6.1827	6.1827	0.0312	63.1876	56.2680	0.0304	0.9999
11.	111	271	6.3449	6.3451	0.0464	61.4653	52.5249	0.0103	0.9999
12.	112	293	6.7328	6.7328	0.0528	60.9055	52.7867	0.0184	0.9999
13.	113	276	6.1046	6.1047	0.0265	63.8917	53.1509	0.0152	0.9999
14.	114	280	6.0737	6.0742	0.0332	62.9222	58.6304	0.0126	0.9999
15.	115	293	5.6508	5.6510	0.0233	64.4576	56.2267	0.0166	0.9999
16.	116	292	5.9165	5.9168	0.0291	63.4885	53.1528	0.0385	0.9999
17.	117	292	6.2215	6.2217	0.0463	61.4707	57.2170	0.0247	0.9999
18.	118	292	6.1530	6.1529	0.0392	62.1980	56.7638	0.0324	0.9999
19.	119	291	5.0022	5.0025	0.0187	65.4114	57.7975	0.0302	0.9999
20.	121	293	6.4437	6.4437	0.0308	63.2487	55.4058	0.0195	0.9999
21.	122	292	6.0113	6.0116	0.0441	61.6847	51.7517	0.0208	1.0000
22.	123	293	5.1527	5.1531	0.0292	63.4803	54.7873	0.0149	0.9999
23.	124	293	5.9370	5.9370	0.0520	60.9744	48.3789	0.0177	0.9999
24.	200	271	4.0365	4.0367	0.0240	64.3263	58.4986	0.0325	0.9999
25.	201	292	4.8080	4.8081	0.0165	65.9560	53.3052	0.0059	1.0000
26.	202	271	5.2482	5.2484	0.0397	62.1458	51.3446	0.0088	0.9999
27.	203	275	2.6046	2.6050	0.0179	65.6096	60.1167	0.0277	0.9999
28.	205	293	5.4857	5.4859	0.0101	68.0957	54.4592	0.0074	0.9999
29.	207	274	4.1161	4.1166	0.0275	63.7361	59.1119	0.0218	0.9999
30.	208	273	5.0056	5.0058	0.0304	63.3051	55.8881	0.0208	0.9999
31.	209	272	5.8608	5.8613	0.0290	63.5076	55.2705	0.0119	0.9999
32.	210	273	3.6596	3.6602	0.0151	66.3269	59.0664	0.0116	0.9999
33.	212	273	6.4743	6.4743	0.0312	63.1937	54.7558	0.0189	0.9999
34.	213	289	6.5860	6.5860	0.0392	62.2025	53.2429	0.0268	1.0000
35.	214	276	4.6517	4.6521	0.0384	62.2860	55.6000	0.0226	0.9999

continued on following page

Table 1. Continued

Sr. no	ECG Data-sets	ECG Size (KB)	(H1)dB	(H2)dB	(MSE)dB	(PSNR)dB	(SNR)dB	PRD (%)	Rxy
36.	215	270	4.3848	4.3851	0.0166	65.9203	55.4364	0.0132	0.9999
37.	217	270	6.7810	6.7812	0.0445	61.6468	56.7774	0.0366	1.0000
38.	219	292	4.9823	4.9825	0.0336	62.8639	54.1698	0.0204	0.9999
39.	220	293	5.1429	5.1432	0.0198	65.1588	57.0207	0.0175	0.9999
40.	221	274	4.3965	4.3969	0.264	63.9209	53.5186	0.0100	0.9999
41.	222	280	5.8065	5.8067	0.0188	65.3779	55.4467	0.0052	0.9999
42.	223	292	4.0864	4.0871	0.0197	65.1847	56.0153	0.0223	1.0000
43.	228	276	3.9442	3.9447	0.0145	66.5040	57.6146	0.0124	0.9999
44.	230	283	5.6677	5.6678	0.0512	61.0398	53.4750	0.0176	0.9999
45.	231	275	4.3184	4.3188	0.0288	63.5424	55.0162	0.0119	0.9999
46.	232	278	3.3336	3.3339	0.0186	65.4362	59.2840	0.0069	0.9999
47.	233	274	5.1771	5.1773	0.0158	66.1481	60.7620	0.0304	0.9999
48.	234	274	6.1726	6.1727	0.0466	61.4479	48.3016	0.0076	0.9999

Table 2. Performance parameter evaluation of MIT-BIH arrhythmia database for 2D ECG steganography of hidden message m2= 1KB

Sr. no	ECG Data-sets	ECG Size (KB)	(H1)dB	(H2)dB	(MSE)dB	(PSNR)dB	(SNR)dB	PRD (%)	Rxy
1.	100	292	5.2912	5.2937	0.3160	53.1337	41.7571	0.0102	0.9996
2.	101	292	5.7530	5.7543	0.3064	53.2682	39.6794	0.0065	0.9996
3.	102	156	6.1974	6.2009	0.6664	49.8936	40.4259	0.0086	0.9994
4.	103	282	5.7843	5.7896	0.7560	49.3458	36.5748	0.0095	0.9995
5.	104	278	5.6725	5.6777	0.6513	49.9927	40.9644	0.0112	0.9993
6.	105	274	5.0735	5.0835	0.6805	49.8024	37.8885	0.0009	0.9995
7.	106	275	5.5369	5.5409	0.6419	50.0558	39.4467	0.0111	0.9993
8.	107	272	6.8613	6.8629	0.7981	49.1100	43.2311	0.1027	0.9996
9.	108	276	3.9127	3.9286	0.2585	54.0061	47.4427	0.0109	0.9994
10.	109	275	6.1827	6.1853	0.5842	50.4654	43.5458	0.0304	0.9997
11.	111	271	6.3449	6.3492	0.7824	49.1966	40.2561	0.0103	0.9994
12.	112	293	6.7328	6.7342	0.8431	48.8720	40.7532	0.0184	0.9996
13.	113	276	6.1046	6.1093	0.6484	50.0090	39.2682	0.0152	0.9996
14.	114	280	6.0737	6.0849	0.7340	49.4736	45.1818	0.0126	0.9995
15.	115	293	5.6508	5.6591	0.6743	49.8421	41.6112	0.0166	0.9992
16.	116	292	5.9165	5.9218	0.7453	49.4073	39.0716	0.0385	0.9996

continued on following page

Table 2. Continued

Sr. no	ECG		(H1)dB	(H2)dB	(MSE)dB	(PSNR)dB	(SNR)dB	PRD (%)	Rxy
	Data-sets	Size (KB)							
17.	117	292	6.2215	6.2255	0.8194	48.9957	44.7420	0.0247	0.9995
18.	118	292	6.1530	6.1584	0.6324	50.1210	44.6868	0.0324	0.9996
19.	119	291	5.0222	5.0152	0.3996	52.1144	44.5005	0.0302	0.9997
20.	121	293	6.4437	6.4464	0.7911	49.1485	41.3057	0.0195	0.9995
21.	122	292	6.0113	6.0147	0.7582	49.3330	39.4000	0.0208	0.9997
22.	123	293	5.1527	5.1616	0.6805	49.8025	41.1095	0.0149	0.9991
23.	124	293	5.9370	5.9398	0.7766	49.2287	36.6332	0.0177	0.9995
24.	200	271	4.0365	4.0468	0.3174	53.1144	47.2868	0.0325	0.9994
25.	201	292	4 .8080	4.8219	0.3796	52.3373	39.6865	0.0059	0.9997
26.	202	271	5.2482	5.2557	0.5208	50.9645	40.1633	0.0088	0.9996
27.	203	275	2.6046	2.6162	0.3676	52.4766	46.9836	0.0077	0.9997
28.	205	293	5.4857	5.4919	0.6995	49.6828	36.0464	0.0277	0.9995
29.	207	274	4.1161	4.1282	0.5180	50.9877	46.3636	0.0218	0.9997
30.	208	273	5.0056	5.0147	0.4797	51.3209	43.9040	0.0208	0.9997
31.	209	272	5.8608	5.8663	0.7586	49.3307	41.0936	0.0320	0.9992
32.	210	273	3.6562	3.6712	0.2525	54.1086	46.8481	0.0116	0.9997
33.	212	273	6.4743	6.4757	0.6895	49.7455	41.3078	0.0189	0.9996
34.	213	289	6.5860	6.5881	0.7200	49.5572	40.5977	0.0268	0.9997
35.	214	276	4.6517	4.6651	0.5331	50.8624	44.1764	0.0226	0.9996
36.	215	270	4.3888	4.3942	0.4266	51.8302	41.3463	0.0133	0.9992
37.	217	270	6.7810	6.7826	0.6845	49.7768	44.9074	0.0367	0.9997
38.	219	292	4.9823	4.9950	0.4517	51.5826	42.8884	0.0204	0.9997
39.	220	293	5.1429	5.1530	0.6218	50.1941	42.0559	0.0175	0.9992
40.	221	274	4.9365	4.4119	0.3877	52.2454	41.8436	0.0100	0.9996
41.	222	280	5.8065	5.8111	0.5819	50.4826	40.5514	0.0052	0.9992
42.	223	292	4.0864	4.1032	0.4970	51.1670	41.9976	0.0223	0.9998
43.	228	276	3.9442	3.9575	0.4093	52.0107	43.1213	0.0125	0.9993
44.	230	283	5.6677	5.6713	0.7468	49.3983	41.8340	0.0176	0.9991
45.	231	275	4.3184	4.3295	0.3427	52.7815	44.2553	0.0119	0.9995
46.	232	278	3.3336	3.3504	0.4448	45.4966	45.4966	0.0069	0.9996
47.	233	274	5.1771	5.1848	0.5699	45.1869	45.1869	0.0304	0.9996
48.	234	274	6.1726	6.1742	0.7650	36.1479	36.1479	0.0076	0.9996

Limitations and Future Work

LSB data embedding is vulnerable, i.e., the integrity of the hidden message can easily be destroyed. The attacker randomizes the LSBs of the image. The attacker may not even know that it is an encrypted image, but such actions would destroy the secret message. Due to these possible attacks, LSB Embedding in its primitive form is relatively insecure. However adaptive LSB embedding based on chaotic map is the possible extension of the present work.

CONCLUSION

Bernoulli's chaotic maps based LSB substitution ECG steganography technique has been introduced. In this chapter LSB substitution and Bernoulli's chaotic maps method to embed confidential information into ECG signal and to retrieve the ECG signal and extract the hidden message efficiently. The procedure is studied and investigated on MIT-BIH arrhythmia database. In this technique the distortion is low, and the amount of information that can be hidden is high and have high sensitivity. Message ciphering procedure based on Bernoulli's chaotic maps is implemented, which combines scrambling and encryption technique to protect confidential patient data. Mathematical analysis proved the technique to be highly secure. The ability to diagnose reconstructed ECG was also found to be minimal using PRD and cross-correlation. The reconstructed signal is the replica of the original signal with low distortion, and the structural features of the ECG signals are also preserved. Finally, found that using proposed Bernoulli's chaotic map based ECG steganography technique, it is possible to store about 1.5KB data inside ECG signal of 60 seconds length and 360 samples/s sampling rate, with PRD of less than 1%. The proposed method can be realized on hardware for real-world use which could bring enormous applications.

REFERENCES

Ali, M., Ahn, C. W., Pant, M., & Siarry, P. (2015). An image watermarking scheme in wavelet domain with optimized compensation of singular value decomposition via artificial bee colony. *Information Sciences, 301*, 44–60. doi:10.1016/j.ins.2014.12.042

Anees, A., Siddiqui, A. M., Ahmed, J., & Hussain, I. (2014). A technique for digital steganography using chaotic maps. *Nonlinear Dynamics, 75*(4), 807–816. doi:10.100711071-013-1105-3

Baali, H., Akmeliawati, R., Salami, M. J. E., Aibinu, M., & Gani, A. (2011). Transform based approach for ECG period normalization. *Computers in Cardiology, 38*(2), 533–536.

Baritha Begum, M., & Venkataramani, Y. (2012). LSB based audio steganography based on text compression. *Procedia Engineering, 30*(2011), 702–710. doi:10.1016/j.proeng.2012.01.917

Bilgin, A., Marcellin, M. W., & Altbach, M. I. (2003). Compression of electrocardiogram signals using JPEG2000. *IEEE Transactions on Consumer Electronics, 49*(4), 833–840. doi:10.1109/TCE.2003.1261162

Biswas, H. R. (2013). One dimensional chaotic dynamical systems. *J Pure Appl Math Adv Appl, 10*(1), 69–101.

Chang, C. C., & Lu, T. C. (2006). A difference expansion oriented data hiding scheme for restoring the original host images. *Journal of Systems and Software*, 79(12), 1754–1766. doi:10.1016/j.jss.2006.03.035

Cheddad, A., Condell, J., Curran, K., & Mc Kevitt, P. (2010). Digital image steganography: Survey and analysis of current methods. *Signal Processing*, 90(3), 727–752. doi:10.1016/j.sigpro.2009.08.010

Chen, B., Luo, H., Zhao, Z., & Zhang, X. (2014). Halftone image encryption based on reversible pairwise swapping. *Measurement: Journal of the International Measurement Confederation*, 57(38), 85–93. doi:10.1016/j.measurement.2014.07.013

Cheng, S.-T., & Chang, T.-Y. (2012). An adaptive learning scheme for load balancing with zone partition in multi-sink wireless sensor network. *Expert Systems with Applications*, 39(10), 9427–9434. doi:10.1016/j.eswa.2012.02.119

Cromwell, L., Weibell, F. J., & Pfeiffer, E. A. (1980). *Biomedical instrumentation and measurements*. Prentice Hall.

Devi, K. J. (2013). *A Sesure Image Steganography Using LSB Technique and Pseudo Random Encoding Technique*. National Institute of Technology-Rourkela Odisha.

Dunbar, B. (2002). *Steganographic A detailed look at*. Sans Institute.

Edward Jero, S., Ramu, P., & Ramakrishnan, S. (2015). ECG steganography using curvelet transform. *Biomedical Signal Processing and Control*, 22, 161–169. doi:10.1016/j.bspc.2015.07.004

Filho, E. B. L., Rodrigues, N. M. M., Silva, E., Faria, S., Da Silva, E. A. B., & De Faria, S. M. M. (1923–1926). ... De Carvalho, M. B. (2008). ECG signal compression based on dc equalization and complexity sorting. *IEEE Transactions on Biomedical Engineering*, 55(7), 1923–1926. doi:10.1109/TBME.2008.919880

Ghebleh, M., & Kanso, A. (2014). A robust chaotic algorithm for digital image steganography. *Communications in Nonlinear Science and Numerical Simulation*, 19(6), 1898–1907. doi:10.1016/j.cnsns.2013.10.014

Hua, Z., Zhou, Y., Pun, C. M., & Chen, C. L. P. (2015). 2D Sine Logistic modulation map for image encryption. *Information Sciences*, 297, 80–94. doi:10.1016/j.ins.2014.11.018

Ibaida, A. (2014). *Secure Steganography, Compression and Diagnoses of Electrocardiograms in Wireless Body Sensor Networks* (PhD Thesis). RMIT University.

Ibaida, A., & Khalil, I. (2013). Wavelet-based ECG steganography for protecting patient confidential information in point-of-care systems. *IEEE Transactions on Biomedical Engineering*, 60(12), 3322–3330. doi:10.1109/TBME.2013.2264539 PMID:23708767

Jero, S. E., Ramu, P., & Ramakrishnan, S. (2015). Steganography in arrhythmic electrocardiogram signal. *Proceedings of the Annual International Conference of the IEEE Engineering in Medicine and Biology Society, EMBS, 2015-Novem*, 1409–1412. doi:10.1109/EMBC.2015.7318633

Laskar, S. A., & Hemachandran, K. (2013). Steganography based on random pixel selection for efficient data hiding. *International Journal of Computer Engineering and Technology*, 4(2), 31–44.

Martínez-González, R. F., Díaz-Méndez, J. A., Palacios-Luengas, L., López-Hernández, J., & Vázquez-Medina, R. (2016). A steganographic method using Bernoulli's chaotic maps. *Computers & Electrical Engineering*, *54*, 435–449. doi:10.1016/j.compeleceng.2015.12.005

Morkel, T., Eloff, J. H. P., & Olivier, M. S. (2005). *An overview of image steganography*. ISSA.

Pan, J., & Tompkins, W. J. (1985). A real-time QRS detection algorithm. *IEEE Transactions on Biomedical Engineering*, *32*(3), 230–236. doi:10.1109/TBME.1985.325532 PMID:3997178

Pan, J., Tompkins, W. J., & Willis, J. (1985). A Real-Time QRS Detection Algorithm. *IEEE Transactions on Biomedical Engineering*, *BME-32*(3), 230–236. doi:10.1109/TBME.1985.325532 PMID:3997178

Pandey, A., Saini, B. S., Singh, B., & Sood, N. (2016a). A 2D electrocardiogram data compression method using a sample entropy-based complexity sorting approach. *Computers & Electrical Engineering*, *56*, 30–45. doi:10.1016/j.compeleceng.2016.10.012

Pandey, A., Saini, B. S., Singh, B., & Sood, N. (2016b). Analysis of electrocardiogram data compression techniques: A MATLAB-based approach. In *Computational Tools and Techniques for Biomedical Signal Processing* (Vol. 1, pp. 272–313). IGI Global. doi:10.4018/978-1-5225-0660-7.ch013

Pandey, A., Saini, B. S., Singh, B., & Sood, N. (2017). An integrated approach using chaotic map & sample value difference method for electrocardiogram steganography and OFDM based secured patient information transmission. *Journal of Medical Systems*, *41*(12), 1–20. doi:10.100710916-017-0830-4 PMID:29043502

Pandey, A., Saini, B. S., Singh, B., & Sood, N. (2018). Complexity sorting and coupled chaotic map based on 2D ECG data compression-then-encryption and its OFDM transmission with impair sample correction. *Multimedia Tools and Applications*. doi:10.100711042-018-6681-2

Pandey, A., Singh, B., Saini, B. S., & Sood, N. (2016a). A joint application of optimal threshold based discrete cosine transform and ASCII encoding for ECG data compression with its inherent encryption. *Australasian Physical & Engineering Sciences in Medicine*, *39*(4), 833–855. doi:10.100713246-016-0476-4 PMID:27613706

Pandey, A., Singh, B., Saini, B. S., & Sood, N. (2016b). Nonlinear complexity sorting approach for 2D ECG data compression. In *Computational Tools and Techniques for Biomedical Signal Processing* (Vol. 1, pp. 1–21). IGI Global. doi:10.4018/978-1-5225-0660-7.ch001

Raja, K. B., Venugopal, K. R., & Patnaik, L. M. (2004). *A Secure Stegonographic Algorithm using LSB, DCT and Image Compression on Raw Images. Technical Report*. Department of Computer Science and Engineering.

Rangayyan, R. M. (2002). *Biomedical Signal Analysis: A Case-Study Approach*. John Wiley and Sons, Inc. doi:10.1002/9780470544204

Shelke, F. M., Dongre, A. A., & Soni, P. D. (2014). Comparison of different techniques for Steganography in images. *International Journal of Application or Innovation in Engineering & Management*, *3*(2), 171–176.

Singh, Y. S., Devi, B. P., & Singh, K. M. (2013). A review of different techniques on digital image watermarking scheme. *International Journal of Engine Research*, *2*(3), 193–199.

Song, S., Zhang, J., Liao, X., Du, J., & Wen, Q. (2011). A novel secure communication protocol combining steganography and cryptography. *Procedia Engineering*, *15*, 2767–2772. doi:10.1016/j.proeng.2011.08.521

Subhedar, M. S., & Mankar, V. H. (2014). Current status and key issues in image steganography: A survey. *Computer Science Review*, *13-14*(C), 95–113. doi:10.1016/j.cosrev.2014.09.001

Sudeepa, K. B., Raju, K., Ranjan Kumar, H. S., & Aithal, G. (2016). A New Approach for Video Steganography Based on Randomization and Parallelization. *Physics Procedia*, *78*, 483–490. doi:10.1016/j.procs.2016.02.092

Yang, H., Wong, K.-W., Liao, X., Zhang, W., & Wei, P. (2010). A fast image encryption and authentication scheme based on chaotic maps. *Communications in Nonlinear Science and Numerical Simulation*, *15*(11), 3507–3517. doi:10.1016/j.cnsns.2010.01.004

Yeh, J.-P., & Wu, K.-L. (2008). A simple method to synchronize chaotic systems and its application to secure communications. *Mathematical and Computer Modelling*, *47*(9), 894–902. doi:10.1016/j.mcm.2007.06.021

Zhou, Y., Bao, L., & Chen, C. L. P. (2014). A new 1D chaotic system for image encryption. *Signal Processing*, *97*, 172–182. doi:10.1016/j.sigpro.2013.10.034

Chapter 12
Electrocardiogram Dynamic Interval Feature Extraction for Heartbeat Characterization

Atul Kumar Verma
Dr. B. R. Ambedkar National Institute of Technology, India

Indu Saini
Dr. B. R. Ambedkar National Institute of Technology, India

Barjinder Singh Saini
Dr. B. R. Ambedkar National Institute of Technology, India

ABSTRACT

In the chapter, dynamic time domain features are extracted in the proposed approach for the accurate classification of electrocardiogram (ECG) heartbeats. The dynamic time-domain information such as RR, pre-RR, post-RR, ratio of pre-post RR, and ratio of post-pre RR intervals to be extracted from the ECG beats in proposed approach for heartbeat classification. These four extracted features are combined and fed to k-nearest neighbor (k-NN) classifier with tenfold cross-validation to classify the six different heartbeats (i.e., normal [N], right bundle branch block [RBBB], left bundle branch block [LBBB], atrial premature beat [APC], paced beat [PB], and premature ventricular contraction[PVC]). The average sensitivity, specificity, positive predictivity along with overall accuracy is obtained as 99.77%, 99.97%, 99.71%, and 99.85%, respectively, for the proposed classification system. The experimental result tells that proposed classification approach has given better performance as compared with other state-of-the-art feature extraction methods for the heartbeat characterization.

DOI: 10.4018/978-1-5225-7952-6.ch012

INTRODUCTION

The cardiac heart activity of the arrhythmic patients is analyzed by the electrocardiographic (ECG). The analysis of the ECG signals are important for the detection of irregular, slower or faster electrical activity of the heart (Kass and Clancy 2005) which is known as arrhythmia. The arrhythmias are basically divided into life-threatening and non-life-threatening arrhythmias. The life-threatening arrhythmias are explained in (Hu et al. 1997; Lagerholm et al. 2000; De Chazal et al. 2004; Alonso-Atienza et al. 2014) whereas, the non-life-threatening arrhythmias represent long-term threats which are crucial and needs special care of it. The long-term ECG recordings are useful for the detection of non-life-threatening arrhythmias. Manual detection of the arrhythmic heartbeats is impractical and time consuming. So, the researchers (Prasad and Sahambi 2003; Osowski et al. 2004; Rodriguez et al. 2005; de Chazal and Reilly 2006; Jiang et al. 2006; Jiang and Kong 2007b; Ince et al. 2009a; de Oliveira et al. 2011; Ebrahimzadeh and Khazaee 2011; Martis et al. 2011; De Lannoy et al. 2012; Huang et al. 2012; Banerjee and Mitra 2014) develops the automatic heartbeat classification system. The researchers differ the existing methods of the classification system in the two main aspects i.e., feature extraction, and classification. A number of papers existing in the literature which uses the different feature sets. Some of the features are summarized as: wavelet features (Jiang et al. 2006; Ince et al. 2009b; Ye et al. 2012; Yang and Shen 2013), waveform features (Rodriguez et al. 2005), hermite coefficients (Lagerholm et al. 2000; Osowski et al. 2004; Jiang and Kong 2007b), ICA and RR features (Huang et al. 2012), wavelet and RR features (Ince et al. 2009a), waveform and RR features (De Chazal et al. 2004; de Chazal and Reilly 2006; de Oliveira et al. 2011), ICA and RR features (Ye et al. 2012), Morphology and RR features (Zhang et al. 2014), and projection & weighted RR features (Chen et al. 2017). After the feature extraction, the classifier is utilized for the classification of the different arrhythmias. The classifier utilized in the existing works are self-organizing map (Lagerholm et al. 2000), support vector machine (SVM) (Osowski et al. 2004; Jiang et al. 2006; Ye et al. 2012), artificial neural network (Prasad and Sahambi 2003; Jiang and Kong 2007a; Ince et al. 2009a), decision tree (Rodriguez et al. 2005), k-nearest neighbor classifier (Kutlu and Kuntalp 2012), and linear discriminates (De Chazal et al. 2004; De Chazal and Reilly 2006). From the literature (Raj et al. 2015b; Raj et al. 2015a), (Martis et al. 2013), (Llamedo and Mart\'\inez 2012), (Hu et al. 1997), (De Chazal and Reilly 2006), (Ince et al. 2009a), (Inan et al. 2006), (Sayadi et al. 2010), (Khadra et al. 2005), (Jiang and Kong 2007b), (Martis et al. 2013), (Jung and Lee 2017), and (Ray and Sharma 2016), it is clear from the literature that the beat classification system requires the classifier with the different feature sets are not efficiently classify the different classes. So, Inspired by the works reported in literature the new feature set is develop which only uses the dynamic time-domain information of the heartbeats to classify them into different classes using k-NN classifier. The k-NN classifier is used in the proposed work due to its less complexity and very less time consuming with efficient classification of the beats. The new feature set combined RR interval, Pre-RR, Post-RR, ratio of Pre to Post RR, and Post to Pre RR intervals for the heartbeat classification.

In this study, experimentation is done on the six types of heartbeats which are normal (N), right bundle branch block (RBBB), left bundle branch block (LBBB), atrial premature beat (APC), paced beat (PB), and premature ventricular contraction (PVC). From each heartbeat, the RR interval, Pre-RR, Post-RR, ratio of Pre to Post RR, and Post to Pre RR intervals are to be evaluated and used as a feature vector. The new feature vector is fed to the k-NN (Zhang et al. 2014) classifier with tenfold cross-validation scheme to classify the different beats. The classified heartbeat data using the proposed classification technique should be easily secure for the patient information security which helps the doctors for further reference to diagnose the arrhythmia.

The rest of the chapter is organized as: Section 2 describes the ECG database used in this study. The proposed heartbeat classification method is explained in Section 3. Section 4 demonstrate the experimental results of the proposed classification approach. Section 5 is dedicated to the comparison of the proposed classification system with the existing methods in the literature. Finally, Section 6 ends with the conclusion.

ECG DATA DESCRIPTION

The data were taken from the MIT-BIH arrhythmia database (http://www.physionet.org/physiobank/database/mitdb/), which includes many common and life-threatening arrhythmias along with the recordings of the normal sinus rhythm. The database comprises 48 half hour ambulatory ECG recordings, acquired from 47 subjects with two leads i.e., lead A, B. The 23 records which are numbered from 100 to 124 inclusive (with some numbers missing) are the routine clinical recordings and remaining 25 records that are numbered from 200 to 234 inclusive (with some numbers missing) that contain the variety of rare but clinically vital arrhythmias (Mark and Moody 1997).

PROPOSED METHOD FOR HEARTBEAT CLASSIFICATION

ECG Filtering

The ECG signals were filtered using wavelet based denoising approach to reduce various artifacts such as baseline drift, power-line interference, electrode movements, and muscle contraction. The presence of noises in the ECG can disturb the fiducial point detection and heartbeat classification (Poornachandra 2008). In this study, the ECG signal is decomposed into various sub-bands up to six levels using db6 wavelet (Singh and Tiwari 2006). The sixth level approximation sub-band consists of the frequency range of 0–2.8125 Hz which mainly consists of baseline wander, and ECG will not contain much information after 45 Hz. Hence, only the detail coefficients of 3rd, 4th, 5th and 6th levels are retaining and other are to be neglect. After that, inverse discrete wavelet transform (DWT) is computed for the retained sub-bands to obtain the denoised ECG waveform (Addison 2005).

Heartbeat Segmentation

The heartbeat segmentation normally needs peak position of the R wave i.e., fiducial point. The annotation file provided with the MIT-BIH arrhythmia database contains the reference of each heartbeat with its fiducial point. The manual annotation of the heartbeat fiducial points, placed at the major local extremum is used for segmenting ECG beats. Thereafter, by the utilization of the locations of the R-peaks, the segmentation of the heartbeats is done on the basis of taking the average of the RR intervals obtained using R peaks location.

Feature Extraction

After the segmentation of the ECG beats, the efficient features are extracted from each of the heartbeat which maximally discriminate the arrhythmic beats. In this study, to gather the dynamic characteristic of the ECG signals, the four RR-interval features are computed that are previous RR (RR_a), post RR (RR_b), ratio of Post-Pre (rpopr) RR (RR_{ba}), and ratio of Pre-Post (rprpo) RR (RR_{ab}) intervals. These features are explained as:

1. RR_a interval: It is the RR-interval between a given beat location and the previous beat location. Mathematically,

$$RR_a = R_i - R_{i-1} \tag{1}$$

2. RR_b interval: It is the RR-interval between a given beat location and the following beat. It is mathematically formulated as,

$$RR_b = R_{i+1} - R_i \tag{2}$$

3. RR_{ab} interval: It is defined as the ratio of the RR_a and RR_b intervals. Mathematically,

$$RR_{ab} = \frac{RR_a}{RR_b} \tag{3}$$

4. RR_{ba} interval: It is defined as the ratio of the RR_b and RR_a intervals. Mathematically written as:

$$RR_{ba} = \frac{RR_b}{RR_a} \tag{4}$$

The RR interval features calculated from (1)-(4) are fed to the classifier with tenfold cross-validation scheme for the classification of the ECG arrhythmic beats.

Classification

The *k*-Nearest Neighbor (*k*-NN) classifier is used in this study for the classification of the arrhythmic beats. The *k*-NN is a non-parametric classification algorithm that assigns test data to the class that the majority of its *k*-nearest neighbors belongs. Basically, *k*-NN consists two phases i.e., training and testing phase. In training phase, the training samples are vectored in a multidimensional feature space with the class label of each samples, whereas in testing phase, a testing sample is characterized by assigning a label which is most repeated among the *k* (user defined constant) training samples nearest to test sample. Alternately, the *k*-NN algorithm compares the input feature vector with training samples and the test sample is labelled with the nearest class of the training samples. The k-NN algorithm classify the test samples based on distance between the testing and training samples as the procedure explained above. Hence, the classification of the test samples is depending on the value of k and distance metric. The analysis based on choosing the proper value of k and the distance metric is essential for efficiently classify the test samples. Usually, the larger values of k reduce the effect of noise at the time of classification but less distinct the separation between the classes. So, the best value of k is depending on the classification task (Thirumuruganathan 2010). In this work, the proposed classification method is tested on the different values of k (k =1, 3, 5, 7, 11, 13). The distance metric is also most important for the efficient classification. There are different distance metrics such as Euclidean distance (ED), correlation distance (CD), and city block distance (CBD) are evaluated for classification of the test samples in k-NN algorithm. The brief explanation of the distance metrics is illustrated as: Assume a data matrix X, Y having size $m_x \times n$, and $m_y \times n$ respectively. where m_x, m_y are the mth element of row vectors of X, Y, and n is the number of features which are calculated for each sample. Consider that x_s and y_t are the sample vector of X, Y and the various distance metrics are evaluated as:

1. Euclidean distance metric (ED): It is defined as the root of the square differences between x_s and y_t. It is mathematically written as (Karimifard et al. 2006):

$$d_{st} = \sqrt{\sum_{i=1}^{n} (x_{si} - y_{ti})^2}$$

(5)

2. Correlation distance metric (CD): It is defined as the one minus the sample correlation between x_s and y_t. It is mathematically written as (Karimifard et al. 2006)

$$d_{st} = 1 - \frac{(x_s - \frac{1}{n}\sum_i x_{si})(y_t - \frac{1}{n}\sum_i y_{ti})'}{\sqrt{(x_s - \frac{1}{n}\sum_i x_{si})(x_s - \frac{1}{n}\sum_i x_{si})'} \sqrt{(y_t - \frac{1}{n}\sum_i y_{ti})(y_t - \frac{1}{n}\sum_i y_{ti})'}}$$

(6)

3. City block distance metric (CBD): It is defined as the sum of the absolute differences of x_s and y_t. Mathematically, it is given as (Karimifard et al. 2006)

$$d_{st} = \sum_{i=1}^{n} |x_{si} - y_{ti}|$$

(7)

Classification Performance Measures

The performance of the classification method can be determined by the evaluation of the parameters which are Sensitivity (*Se*), Positive predictivity (*Pp*), Specificity (*Sp*), and overall Accuracy (*Acc*) can be defined as

$$Se = \frac{TP}{TP + FN} \times 100 \qquad (8)$$

$$Pp = \frac{TP}{TP + FP} \times 100 \qquad (9)$$

$$Sp = \frac{TN}{TN + FP} \times 100 \qquad (10)$$

$$Acc = \frac{TP + TN}{TP + TN + FP + FN} \times 100 \qquad (11)$$

where, FP, TP, FN, and TN denote the false positive, true positive, false negative, and true negative respectively. False positive represents the misclassification of the abnormal beats into normal beats. True positive represents the correctly detected normal ECG beats. False negative represents the misclassification of the normal as abnormal beats. True negative represents the correctly rejected beats. The flowchart of the proposed classification system is presented in *Figure 1*.

EXPERIMENTAL RESULTS

In this study, the MIT-BIH arrhythmia database is downloaded and then perform the filtering operation thereafter, the ECG beats are segmented and then categorized into six classes which are used in the work reported by (Ray and Sharma 2016). The beats in (Ray and Sharma 2016) are classified as N, RBBB, LBBB, APC, PB, and PVC. The number of samples of each beat type are tabulated in *Table 1*. After that, the features are calculated for each individual beats. The number of samples of the beats are randomly chosen from the respective MIT-BIH records shown in *Table 1*.

The tenfold cross-validation technique was used with k-NN classifier for the classification of the different beats. The fold-wise sensitivity, specificity, positive predictivity, and accuracy for 1-NN classifier with different distance metrics are tabulated in *Table 2*. The average sensitivity, specificity, positive predictivity, and overall accuracy are obtained by taking the average of the tenfold cross-validation are shown in *Table 2*. It is clear from the *Table 2*, the best average values of sensitivity, specificity, positive predictivity, and accuracy of 99.77%, 99.97%, 99.71%, 99.85% respectively are obtained for Euclidian distance metric with 1-NN classifier.

Thereafter, the best value of k is determined. So, for this, the different numbers of nearest neighbors (k=1, 3, 5, 7, 11, 13) are tested in the k-NN classifier to obtain the best performance for the classifier. The performance of all the classifiers are calculated based on their average sensitivity, specificity, positive predictivity, and overall accuracy as tabulated in *Table 3*. As seen from the *Table 3*, the maximum performance is provided by a 1- nearest neighbor classifier with the results of 99.77%, 99.97%, 99.71%, and 99.85% for average sensitivity, specificity, positive predictivity, and overall accuracy.

DISCUSSION

Table 4 gives the performance of proposed classification system in contrast to other state of art classification methods (Hu et al. 1997; Khadra et al. 2005; De Chazal and Reilly 2006; Inan et al. 2006; Jiang and Kong 2007b; Ince et al. 2009a; Sayadi et al. 2010; Llamedo and Mart\'\inez 2012; Martis et al. 2013; Raj et al. 2015b; Raj et al. 2015a; Ray and Sharma 2016; Jung and Lee 2017) applied for the classification of ECG beat classification.

After scrutinizing the findings reported in *Table 4*, it is concluded that the proposed classification system outperforms the existing works as reported by (Raj et al. 2015b; Raj et al. 2015a), (Martis et al. 2013), (Llamedo and Mart\'\inez 2012), (Hu et al. 1997), (De Chazal and Reilly 2006), (Ince et al. 2009a), (Inan et al. 2006), (Sayadi et al. 2010), (Khadra et al. 2005), (Jiang and Kong 2007b), (Martis et al. 2013), (Jung and Lee 2017), and (Ray and Sharma 2016). The proposed classification system gives 99.77%, 99.97%, 99.71%, 99.85% are the average sensitivity, specificity, positive predictivity, and over-

Figure 1. Flowchart of the proposed classification method

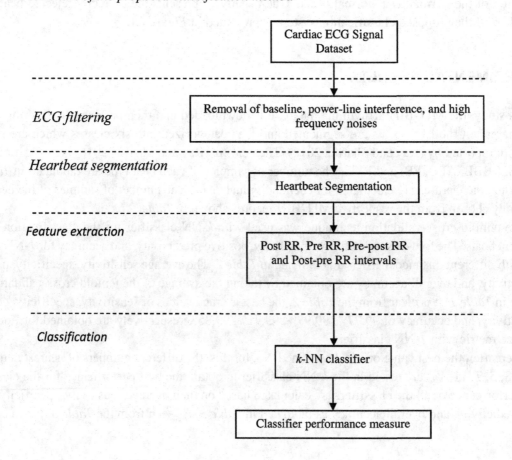

Table 1. ECG beats taken for experiments in this study from MIT-BIH database

Type of beats	MIT-BIH record	Number of sample beats
N	100, 101, 103, 105, 108, 113, 115, 117, 121, 123	11655
RBBB	118, 124, 212, 231	1000
LBBB	109, 111, 207, 214	1000
APC	118, 207, 220, 222, 232	1436
PB	107, 217	1400
PVC	106, 114, 116, 119, 124, 201, 203, 214, 215, 219, 221, 228	3008
Total		19499

Table 2. The fold-wise result of performance measure for proposed classification system with different distance metrics

	Sensitivity (%)			Specificity (%)			Positive Predictivity (%)			Accuracy (%)		
	ED	CD	CBD	ED	CD	CBD	ED	CD	CBD	ED	CD	CBD
Fold 1	99.88	96.49	99.65	99.99	99.369	99.96	99.94	96.36	99.60	99.95	97.33	99.79
Fold 2	99.83	96.36	99.66	99.97	99.23	99.96	99.66	95.99	99.55	99.84	96.82	99.79
Fold 3	99.76	96.53	99.71	99.98	99.38	99.97	99.82	96.14	99.77	99.8	97.23	99.84
Fold 4	99.60	96.62	100	99.96	99.37	100	99.48	96.64	100	99.79	97.33	100
Fold 5	99.82	95.34	99.77	99.98	99.22	99.96	99.82	95.64	99.54	99.89	96.71	99.7
Fold 6	99.82	94.89	99.82	99.98	99.19	99.98	99.82	95.65	99.82	99.89	96.66	99.89
Fold 7	99.77	95.84	99.61	99.98	99.27	99.95	99.77	95.423	99.44	99.89	96.76	99.74
Fold 8	99.66	96.55	99.94	99.95	99.28	99.99	99.49	96.42	99.88	99.74	97.17	99.94
Fold 9	99.77	95.9	99.59	99.97	99.23	99.96	99.61	95.82	99.60	99.84	96.87	99.79
Fold 10	99.77	95.57	99.76	99.97	99.29	99.98	99.71	95.42	99.82	99.84	96.92	99.89
Average	**99.77**	96.01	99.75	**99.97**	99.28	99.97	**99.71**	95.95	99.70	**99.85**	96.98	99.84

Table 3. The performance of k-NN classifiers for different k values using the proposed classification method

	Average sensitivity (%)	Average Specificity (%)	Average Positive Predictivity (%)	Accuracy (%)
k=1	**99.77**	**99.97**	**99.71**	**99.85**
k=3	99.70	99.97	99.65	99.82
k=5	99.67	99.96	99.55	99.79
k=7	99.64	99.95	99.53	99.77
k=9	99.64	99.95	99.51	99.76
k=11	99.62	99.95	99.45	99.74
k=13	99.54	99.94	99.35	99.68

Table 4. Comparison of the classification performance of the proposed classification system with existing systems for beat classification

Literature	Extracted features	Classifier	Classes	Accuracy (%)
(Raj et al. 2015b)	R-peak detection	Rule-based approach	4	97.96
(Raj et al. 2015a)	R-peak detection + FFT-based WT	Neural network architecture	8	97.40
(Martis et al. 2013)	Biospectrum + PCA	SVM with RBF kernel	5	93.48
(Llamedo and Mart\'\ inez 2012)	RR-interval and its derived features	Linear discriminant and expectation maximization	3	98.00
(Hu et al. 1997)	Time-domain approach	Mixture of experts	2	94.00
(De Chazal and Reilly 2006)	Morphology and heartbeat interval	Linear discriminant	5	85.90
(Ince et al. 2009a)	WT +PCA	Multidimensional PSO	5	95.58
(Inan et al. 2006)	WT+timing interval	Neural network	2	95.20
(Sayadi et al. 2010)	Innovation sequence of EKF	Bayesain filtering	2	99.10
(Khadra et al. 2005)	Hybrid order statistics approach (HOSA) bispectrum	Threshold	4	91.38
(Jiang and Kong 2007b)	Hermite function parameters and RR interval	Block based NN	5	96.6
(Martis et al. 2013)	Principal components of Bispectrum	LS-SVM	5	93.48
(Jung and Lee 2017)	PCA+LDA with fitness rule	Weighted k-NN	4	98.12
(Ray and Sharma 2016)	EMD-HHT + KC + Statistics	Multi-class SVM's with RBF kernel	6	99.51
Proposed classification system	**Pre RR, Post RR, ration of Pre-Post and Post-Pre RR intervals**	**k-NN classifier**	**6**	**99.85**

all accuracy respectively for N, LBBB, RBBB, PB, APC, and PVC types of beats. As indicative from results, the proposed classification system is performing better than the existing works in the literature.

CONCLUSION

The present work proposes a new feature extraction method which utilizes dynamic intervals as a feature set. The four dynamic time-domain features which are RR, Pre-RR, Post-RR, ratio of Pre-Post RR, Post-Pre RR intervals are calculated from the six ECG heartbeats i.e., N, RBBB, LBBB, APC, PVC, and PB. Then, the new feature vector set is fed to the k-NN classifier with tenfold cross-validation scheme to classify the six different beats. The experimental results demonstrate that the proposed classification approach achieves an overall accuracy of 99.85%. The proposed classification method outperforms the existing methods of the literature. The future work can be focused to add more relevant features to classify more number of beats.

REFERENCES

Addison, P. S. (2005). Wavelet transforms and the ECG: A review. *Physiological Measurement*, *26*(5), R155–R199. doi:10.1088/0967-3334/26/5/R01 PMID:16088052

Alonso-Atienza, F., Morgado, E., Fernandez-Martinez, L., Garcia-Alberola, A., & Rojo-Alvarez, J. L. (2014). Detection of life-threatening arrhythmias using feature selection and support vector machines. *IEEE Transactions on Biomedical Engineering*, *61*(3), 832–840. doi:10.1109/TBME.2013.2290800 PMID:24239968

Banerjee, S., & Mitra, M. (2014). Application of cross wavelet transform for ECG pattern analysis and classification. *IEEE Transactions on Instrumentation and Measurement*, *63*(2), 326–333. doi:10.1109/TIM.2013.2279001

Chen, S., Hua, W., Li, Z., Li, J., & Gao, X. (2017). Heartbeat classification using projected and dynamic features of ECG signal. *Biomedical Signal Processing and Control*, *31*, 165–173. doi:10.1016/j.bspc.2016.07.010

De Chazal, P., O'Dwyer, M., & Reilly, R. B. (2004). Automatic classification of heartbeats using ECG morphology and heartbeat interval features. *IEEE Transactions on Biomedical Engineering*, *51*(7), 1196–1206. doi:10.1109/TBME.2004.827359 PMID:15248536

de Chazal, P., & Reilly, R. B. (2006). A patient-adapting heartbeat classifier using ECG morphology and heartbeat interval features. *IEEE Transactions on Biomedical Engineering*, *53*(12), 2535–2543. doi:10.1109/TBME.2006.883802 PMID:17153211

De Lannoy, G., François, D., Delbeke, J., & Verleysen, M. (2012). Weighted conditional random fields for supervised interpatient heartbeat classification. *IEEE Transactions on Biomedical Engineering*, *59*(1), 241–247. doi:10.1109/TBME.2011.2171037 PMID:21990327

de Oliveira, L. S. C., Andreão, R. V., & Sarcinelli-Filho, M. (2011). Premature ventricular beat classification using a dynamic Bayesian network. *Engineering in Medicine and Biology Society, EMBC, 2011 Annual International Conference of the IEEE*, 4984–4987 10.1109/IEMBS.2011.6091235

Ebrahimzadeh, A., & Khazaee, A. (2011). Higher order statistics for automated classification of ECG beats. *Electrical and Control Engineering (ICECE), 2011 International Conference on*, 5952–5955. 10.1109/ICECENG.2011.6057059

Hu, Y. H., Palreddy, S., & Tompkins, W. J. (1997). A patient-adaptable ECG beat classifier using a mixture of experts approach. *IEEE Transactions on Biomedical Engineering*, *44*(9), 891–900. doi:10.1109/10.623058 PMID:9282481

Huang, H. F., Hu, G. S., & Zhu, L. (2012). Sparse representation-based heartbeat classification using independent component analysis. *Journal of Medical Systems*, *36*(3), 1235–1247. doi:10.100710916-010-9585-x PMID:20839036

Inan, O. T., Giovangrandi, L., & Kovacs, G. T. A. (2006). Robust neural-network-based classification of premature ventricular contractions using wavelet transform and timing interval features. *IEEE Transactions on Biomedical Engineering*, *53*(12), 2507–2515. doi:10.1109/TBME.2006.880879 PMID:17153208

Ince, T., Kiranyaz, S., & Gabbouj, M. (2009a). A generic and robust system for automated patient-specific classification of ECG signals. *IEEE Transactions on Biomedical Engineering*, *56*(5), 1415–1426. doi:10.1109/TBME.2009.2013934 PMID:19203885

Ince, T., Kiranyaz, S., Gabbouj, M., & Member, S. (2009b). *A Generic and Robust System for Automated Patient-Specific Classification of ECG Signals*. Academic Press.

Jiang, W., & Kong, S. G. (2007). Block-based neural networks for personalized ECG signal classification. *IEEE Transactions on Neural Networks*, *18*(6), 1750–1761. doi:10.1109/TNN.2007.900239 PMID:18051190

Jiang, X., Zhang, L., Zhao, Q., & Albayrak, S. (2006). ECG arrhythmias recognition system based on independent component analysis feature extraction. TENCON 2006. 2006 IEEE Region 10 Conference, 1–4. doi:10.1109/TENCON.2006.343781

Jung, W-H., & Lee, S-G. (2017). *An Arrhythmia Classification Method in Utilizing the Weighted KNN and the Fitness Rule*. Academic Press.

Karimifard, S., Ahmadian, A., Khoshnevisan, M., & Nambakhsh, M. S. (2006). Morphological heart arrhythmia detection using hermitian basis functions and kNN classifier. *Engineering in Medicine and Biology Society, 2006. EMBS'06. 28th Annual International Conference of the IEEE*, 1367–1370. 10.1109/IEMBS.2006.260182

Kass, R. E., & Clancy, C. E. (2005). *Basis and treatment of cardiac arrhythmias*. Springer Science & Business Media.

Khadra, L., Al-Fahoum, A. S., & Binajjaj, S. (2005). A quantitative analysis approach for cardiac arrhythmia classification using higher order spectral techniques. *IEEE Transactions on Biomedical Engineering*, *52*(11), 1840–1845. doi:10.1109/TBME.2005.856281 PMID:16285387

Kutlu, Y., & Kuntalp, D. (2012). Feature extraction for ECG heartbeats using higher order statistics of WPD coefficients. *Computer Methods and Programs in Biomedicine*, *105*(3), 257–267. doi:10.1016/j.cmpb.2011.10.002 PMID:22055998

Lagerholm, M., Peterson, C., Braccini, G., Edenbrandt, L., & Sornmo, L. (2000). Clustering ECG complexes using Hermite functions and self-organizing maps. *IEEE Transactions on Biomedical Engineering*, *47*(7), 838–848. doi:10.1109/10.846677 PMID:10916254

Llamedo, M., & Martinez, J. P. (2012). An automatic patient-adapted ECG heartbeat classifier allowing expert assistance. *IEEE Transactions on Biomedical Engineering*, *59*(8), 2312–2320. doi:10.1109/TBME.2012.2202662 PMID:22692868

Mark, R., & Moody, G. (1997). Mit-bih arrhythmia database 1997.

Martis, R. J., Acharya, U. R., Mandana, K. M., Ray, A. K., & Chakraborty, C. (2013). Cardiac decision making using higher order spectra. *Biomedical Signal Processing and Control*, *8*(2), 193–203. doi:10.1016/j.bspc.2012.08.004

Martis, R. J., Acharya, U. R., Ray, A. K., & Chakraborty, C. (2011). Application of higher order cumulants to ECG signals for the cardiac health diagnosis. *Engineering in medicine and biology society, embc, 2011 annual international conference of the ieee*, 1697–1700. 10.1109/IEMBS.2011.6090487

Osowski, S., Hoai, L. T., & Markiewicz, T. (2004). Support vector machine-based expert system for reliable heartbeat recognition. *IEEE Transactions on Biomedical Engineering*, *51*(4), 582–589. doi:10.1109/TBME.2004.824138 PMID:15072212

Poornachandra, S. (2008). Wavelet-based denoising using subband dependent threshold for ECG signals. *Digit Signal Process A Rev J., 18*, 49–55. doi:10.1016/j.dsp.2007.09.006

Prasad, G. K., & Sahambi, J. S. (2003). Classification of ECG arrhythmias using multi-resolution analysis and neural networks. *TENCON 2003. Conference on Convergent Technologies for the Asia-Pacific Region*, 227–231 10.1109/TENCON.2003.1273320

Raj, S., Chand, G. S. S. P., & Ray, K. C. (2015a). Arm-based arrhythmia beat monitoring system. *Microprocessors and Microsystems, 39*(7), 504–511. doi:10.1016/j.micpro.2015.07.013

Raj, S., Maurya, K., & Ray, K. C. (2015b). A knowledge-based real time embedded platform for arrhythmia beat classification. *Biomedical Engineering Letters, 5*(4), 271–280. doi:10.100713534-015-0196-9

Ray, K. C., & Sharma, P. (2016). Efficient methodology for electrocardiogram beat classification. *IET Signal Processing, 10*(7), 825–832. doi:10.1049/iet-spr.2015.0274

Rodriguez, J., Goni, A., & Illarramendi, A. (2005). Real-time classification of ECGs on a PDA. *IEEE Transactions on Information Technology in Biomedicine, 9*(1), 23–34. doi:10.1109/TITB.2004.838369 PMID:15787004

Sayadi, O., Shamsollahi, M. B., & Clifford, G. D. (2010). Robust detection of premature ventricular contractions using a wave-based Bayesian framework. *IEEE Transactions on Biomedical Engineering, 57*(2), 353–362. doi:10.1109/TBME.2009.2031243 PMID:19758851

Singh, B. N., & Tiwari, A. K. (2006). Optimal selection of wavelet basis function applied to ECG signal denoising. *Digital Signal Processing, 16*(3), 275–287. doi:10.1016/j.dsp.2005.12.003

Thirumuruganathan, S. (2010). *A detailed introduction to K-nearest neighbor (KNN) algorithm*. Academic Press.

Yang, S., & Shen, H. (2013). Heartbeat classification using discrete wavelet transform and kernel principal component analysis. In *TENCON Spring Conference, 2013* (pp. 34–38). IEEE. doi:10.1109/TENCONSpring.2013.6584412

Ye, C., Kumar, B. V. K. V., & Coimbra, M. T. (2012). Heartbeat classification using morphological and dynamic features of ECG signals. *Biomed Eng IEEE Trans, 59*(10), 2930–2941. doi:10.1109/TBME.2012.2213253 PMID:22907960

Zhang, Z., Dong, J., Luo, X., Choi, K.-S., & Wu, X. (2014). Heartbeat classification using disease-specific feature selection. *Computers in Biology and Medicine, 46*, 79–89. doi:10.1016/j.compbiomed.2013.11.019 PMID:24529208

Chapter 13
Healthcare Informatics Using Modern Image Processing Approaches

Ramgopal Kashyap

https://orcid.org/0000-0002-5352-1286
Amity University Chhattisgarh, India

Surendra Rahamatkar
Amity University Chhattisgarh, India

ABSTRACT

Medical image segmentation is the first venture for abnormal state image analysis, significantly lessening the multifaceted nature of substance investigation of pictures. The local region-based active contour may have a few burdens. Segmentation comes about to intensely rely on the underlying shape choice which is an exceptionally capable errand. In a few circumstances, manual collaborations are infeasible. To defeat these deficiencies, the proposed method for unsupervised segmentation of viewer's consideration object of medical images given the technique with the help of the shading boosting Harris finder and the center saliency map. Investigated distinctive techniques to consider the image data and present a formerly utilized energy-based active contour method dependent on the choice of high certainty forecasts to allocate pseudo-names consequently with the point of diminishing the manual explanations.

INTRODUCTION

Object segmentation is a standout amongst the most vital and testing issues in image investigation and computer vision research. It encourages various abnormal state applications, for example, object acknowledgment, image recovery, image altering, and remaking (Manfredi et al. 2016). Most existing article division frameworks embrace collaboration based ideal models; that is, clients requested that give division prompts physically and painstakingly. Even though the communication-based techniques are promising, they all represent a fundamental issue in which they require the clients' semantic expectation. Such manual naming is time-consuming and often infeasible.

DOI: 10.4018/978-1-5225-7952-6.ch013

Additionally, the segmentation execution intensely relies on upon the client specified seed areas thus, further cooperation's are essential when the seeds not precisely are given. Exceptionally, restricting area based dynamic shape is just one of the exemplary collaboration based techniques. Segmentation comes about to vigorously rely on upon the underlying shape determination (Liu and Ruan 2014). Thus, it needs the specified starting shape which ought to be near the limit of the item. Therefore, building up a refined completely automatic object division strategy has been demanded. The human mind and visual framework can effortlessly get a handle on some beautiful regions in messed scenes. The memorable parts of a picture are typically reliable with interesting articles to be sectioned; districts have been endeavoring for estimation (Kashyap R. and Tiwari V, 2018). Interestingly, with existing collaboration based methodologies that indicate the item and foundation seeds by standard naming, a few techniques decide the seed areas in light of the visual consideration model. Since the precision of the visual consideration model assumes a significant part in article division, these calculations additionally rely on upon the nature of the picked saliency map (Chen 2013).

On the other hand, talking, the more awful the selected saliency guide is, the more terrible the relating final extraction result is to cure such inadequacy, it give careful consideration to striking item edge focuses as opposed to the saliency map itself. After the noticeable article edge focuses were recognized, the district, which is obliged by this corner centers will be getting. The limit of this area is near the item edge. Like this, the boundary of this district utilized as the underlying form of the LRAC model (Azizi and Elkourd 2016). In the proposed technique, the edge focuses are created by the shading boosting Harris finder for information picture firstly then investigate the striking item seeds by the center saliency map, and these item seeds dictate the remarkable article edge focuses. Starting shape is then made by raising structure calculation with exceptional item edge focuses naturally (Ahirwar, 2013). At long last, the article will be extricated precisely by LRAC model to the underlying shape in the past stride.

One of the real issues in therapeutic finding is the subjectivity of the pro's choices, all the more solidly, in the fields of medicinal imaging elucidation; the experience of the advantage can incredibly decide the result of the last determination. Manual strategies for perception can now and then be extremely monotonous, tedious and subject to blunders on the part of the translator. It has driven the developing of the original picture based diagnostics as a help, being a standout amongst the most ebb and look into subjects these days (Kashyap, R. and Tiwari, V., 2017). The rise of profound learning worldview working through neural systems pursued by the ongoing advances in computational power has empowered the improvement of new astute diagnostics dependent on computer vision. These diagnostics are fit to dissect pictures, performing precise divisions, with the end goal to identify the sore territories and to settle on final choices about the patient's wellbeing as the best of clinical eyes. Just profound neural systems with a lot of trainable parameters can approach this sort of semantic divisions, and like this, gigantic sums of valuable and named information are required to influence the framework to combine while staying away from over-fitting. It might be a substantial cripple in the medicinal imaging field, where the human and strategic expenses could make unfeasible to get huge marked datasets. Active learning (AL) is a setup approach to diminish this remaining marking burden with the end goal to choose iteratively, the most educational models from a subset of unlabeled examples. This decision depends on the positioning of scores that can process from a few procedures from a display result (Aitfares, Bouyakhf, Herbulot, Regragui and Devy, 2013). The picked hopefuls marked and in this way added to the preparation set. It has already demonstrated that the preparation done utilizing this dynamic learning technique is more effective and can prepare a profound system quicker and with less preparing tests than conventional semi-regulated learning techniques. In any case, even though this would be satisfactory much of the time and being profoundly utilized in complex arrangement models, re-applying existing systems couldn't be adequate in a division where the data of little points of interest can be fundamental in the last choice.

Aims and Objectives

The objective of the chapters is to find a correct, fast and interactive segmentation method for better analysis of the images.

Correct Segmentation

Image segmentation suffers from incorrect results, many ways have developed for accurate computation and segmented results. The globally optimal geodesic active contour (GOGAC) is one if the best approach based on energy, but it stuck in local minima and gave incorrect results. Here microarray images have attracted much attention because of the inability of creating correctly segmented spots. Figure 1 presents the correct and inaccurate segmentation results. If segmented result will be, and it will give for further analysis of the image, then surely it will give wrong results because it will affect the whole process like information extraction, analysis, quantification and evaluation (Kashyap R, and Gautam 2017), the aim is to get better and accurate result so that correct analysis must generate through segmentation. Figure 2 presents division result utilizing an approach that gives entirely best outcome to different introductory shape position that gives off base outcome that appeared in Figure 2. It will offer wrong results since it will impact the full system like information extraction, examination, and appraisal (Jones, Xie, and Essa, 2014), the point is to strengthen and exact result with the objective that correct analysis should make through division.

Interactive Segmentation

Interactive image segmentation involves small user interaction to include user intention for the segmentation process and is also an active research area nowadays because it can do satisfactory segmentation results that are unattainable by the actual state-of-the-art automatic image segmentation algorithms. This

Figure 1. Correct and Incorrect Segmentation Results

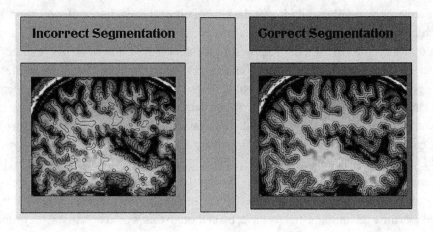

Figure 2. An Energy-Based method with Different Location Initial Contour Initialization

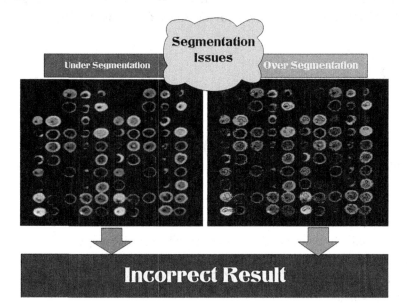

chapter considers the identical problem of how can interactively segment some foreground objects out from its surrounding qualifications. The goal should be to develop an intelligent image segmentation method with tools that let users to interactively segmentation with a small number of intuitive interactions (Gao, Kikinis, Bouix, Shenton and Tannenbaum, 2012). Here the problem with traditional methods is each time, the process gives a different result because of the initialization of contour location is different, and it gives the wrong analysis result. The other objective is to develop an effective segmentation method which is independent of the selection; it will reduce the complexity of the arrangements (Kashyap, R., 2018). An excellent interactive image segmentation method demands are: (1) given clear user input, the algorithm really should produce automatic segmentation that reflects anyone intent; (2) the algorithm should be efficient so that it can provide instant visual feedback.

Fast Segmentation

Image segmentation will be the front stage of numerous works in impression processing, such as object orient compression based on these kinds of requirements, a good impression segmentation algorithm must have the following about three advantages: (1) quickly fast, (2) excellent condition connectivity, and (3) excellent condition matching. The spot growing method provides good segmentation results, but the swiftness is slow (Kashyap, R. and, Gautam, P., 2015). The k-means and the watershed methods are fast, but needs improvements by comparison; the proposed plan can achieve the goals associated with high efficiency as well as better performance as well (Jones, Xie, and Essa, 2014). The result associated with k-means fragmented as well as compress the segmenting result will waste an excessive amount of resource for us all to record these boundaries (Peng, Zhu, and Wang, 2016). The proposed method takes advantage within the k-means and these watershed methods inside the system reliability period. However, it ought to say the dependability is worse compared to the region growing process. The image segmenting algorithm as the front-stage processing associated with image compression and that is the fast swiftness, the excellent appearance connectivity of segmenting result, and the superb condition matching. Figure 3 exhibits the energy based approach for the elimination of local minima issue of traditional methods.

BACKGROUND

The programmed object segmentation approach, coordinating saliency recognition and diagram cuts specific to bear the burdens of intelligent graph cuts (Li and Feng, 2014), likewise investigated the effects of marks to graph-based division, and the purported "Proficient Labels" are acquainted with assessing names and a multi-resolution structure is intended to give such "Expert Labels" naturally. This technique gets finished object division tantamount to automatic chart cuts with manual "Expert Labels." Achanta's method is additionally a programmed picture segmentation technique. It over segments the info image utilizing mean value calculation and holds just those sections whose normal saliency is more noteworthy than a versatile limit (Achanta et al. 2012). The parallel maps speaking to the unusual item are in this way gotten by allotting ones to pixels of picking fragments and zeroes to whatever remains of the pixels using self-organizing map (Waoo et al. 2010). These two techniques are entirely programmed and include none of the manual associations.

The rest of this chapter sorted out as takes after. Section 2 audits some related work and an intuitive image segmentation method. Section 3 exhibits the proposed edge point based dynamic shape for general article division calculation. Section4 presence states full trial examination comes and Section 5 finally concludes.

Figure 3. Segmentation of CT Image using An Energy-Based Method

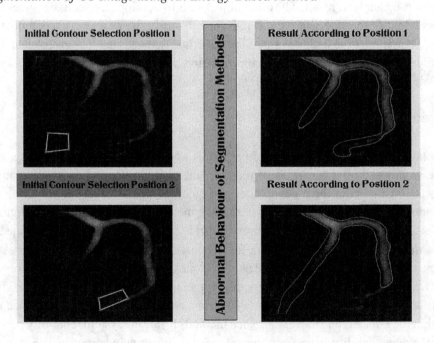

Localizing Region-Based Active Contour Model

Lankton and Tannenbaum proposed a characteristic structure that permits any district based division vitality to reformulate locally. This calculation could dependably extricate the item shape if the client inputs proper markers (Lankton and Tannenbaum 2008). In particular, the quick division calculation is pretty much delicate of the position and the nature of the client inputs (see a case in Figure 4). Here, it picks an intricate vitality that looks past straightforward means and analyzes the full histograms of the closer view and foundation. Consider two smoothed force histograms registered from the worldwide inside and outside districts of a parceled image utilizing power receptacle. Here, it picks the global neighborhood-based vitality that utilizations mean powers, which is the one proposed (Wen et al. 2012) which it alludes to as histogram partition energy and streamlining this energy causes that the inside and outside means have the most significant contrast conceivable.

Saliency Detection Models

The most recent two decades, visual saliency recognition and the saliency map era expecting to find out what pulls in human's consideration got widespread enthusiasm for PC vision, particularly for item discovery or identification from different scenes (Gao et al. 2014). A dominant part of computational models of consideration takes over the structure adjusted from the feature integration theory (FIT) and the Guided Search model. The saliency identification models fall into two general classes: nearby difference based technique and worldwide complexity based strategies. Neighboring difference based methods, research the uncommonness of picture districts regarding nearby neighborhoods (Qin et al. 2014).

The neighborhood contrast investigation for creating saliency maps, which is then, developed utilizing a fuzzy development model (Xu and Zhang 2014), standardize the component maps of prominent highlight parts and allow mixing with other significance maps (Tie Liu et al. 2011). Find the multiscale

Figure 4. Local Region-Based Active Contour Method

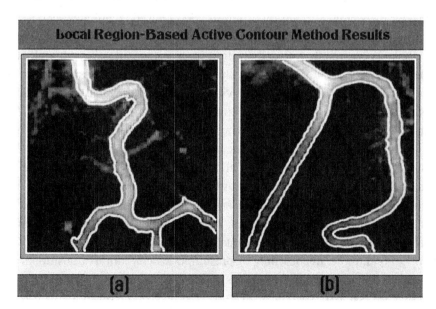

contrast by directly joining variation in a Gaussian picture pyramid. All the more as of late the same time model neighborhood low-level pieces of information, worldwide contemplations, visual association principles, and abnormal state elements to highlight remarkable articles alongside their settings. Such strategies utilizing neighborhood contrast tend to make higher saliency values adjacent edges as opposed to reliably highlighting important objects. Global contrast based strategies; to evaluate saliency of an image locally utilizing its appearing differently about regard to the whole image is done by pixel-level saliency in light of a pixel's complexity to every single other pixel (Yu et al. 2015). Be that as it may, for efficiency, they utilize just luminance data, in this manner overlooking distinctiveness hints in different channels to utilize a pixel's shading difference from the normal image shading. The exquisite methodology, be that as it may, considers first request normal shading, which can be insufficient to dissect complex varieties basic in regular pictures. A fabulous model based on saliency by assessing worldwide differences given the histogram (Schade and Meinecke 2013).

Essential Medical Image Processing Activities Like Segmentation

The motivation behind the division is to parcel a picture into different sections and delimit the limits of target protests as exact as could be expected under the circumstances. As the most convenient restorative picture preparing method, a semi-or full-programmed division system is typically required to quantitatively break down the focusing on anatomical structures in clinical applications. For case, relevant clinical parameters can be separated from a fragmented sore to help conclusion or screen treatment reaction with the improvement of cutting-edge designs procedures, a 3D representation of medicinal imaging information is required, where the division of diverse tissues favored, so they can be outwardly separated with various review properties. Furthermore, applications, for example, computer-aided design (CAD), medical procedure arranging and direction, and picture combination and enlistment, and so on, as a rule, include division errands. Numerous division strategies have been accounted for in most recent a very long while. These procedures classified into edge-based, district-based and shape-based strategies. Edge-based strategies center on outlining the limits that encase the physical items, while district-based systems endeavor to fragment the zone that the physical items possess (Kashyap, R., 2019b). These calculations consider the spatial availability of voxels. Edge-based techniques scan for inhomogeneity showing object limits, and district-based strategies look for persistent districts of voxels with similar properties. The previous commonly founded on limit marker capacities, for example, the greatness of the picture angle, which is either straightforwardly utilized in the edge identification strategies, e.g., intelligent edge identifier or coordinated into the vital elements of the ideal limit looking strategy, e.g., dynamic shapes. Numerous area based division strategies can communicate as far as district developing, in which an underlying arrangement of districts developed until the point when the halting basis is met (Feng, Li, Gao, Yan and Xue, 2016). Basic ceasing criteria are to develop until the point when all neighbors surpass certain disparity, or until all voxels allocated to a district. The achievement of both edge-based and locale constructed procedures depends in light of the degree of force differentiate displayed in pictures. The issues caused by the nearness of low differentiation defeated in two different ways. New client communications can be utilized, for example by setting more markers, or by offering strategies for division altering that are autonomous of the division calculation itself (Zhuang, Dierckx and Zaidi, 2016). Second, more area learning or presumptions can join. A transitional methodology is to utilize more grounded smoothness presumptions, which may successfully counteract rough shapes, as well as spillages that are as it associated through some voxels. A common strategy utilizing unequivocal smoothness presumptions is dynamic forms additionally called snakes. Here, an underlying shape (e.g., a circle or circle close to the question of intrigue) moved after some time (developing), iteratively limiting a vitality utilitarian that ordinarily has two primary terms: an outside vitality that is insignificant close limits (in light of a limit marker work) and an inner vitality that punishes solid shape and "roughness" of the form. Naturally, the outside vitality gives the shapes a chance to snap to clear limits, while the inside vitality forestalls spillages and farfetched corners (regularization). The form can be spoken to unequivocally as a polygonal structure with help focuses that move after some time, or correct as the zero level set of a capacity that is sure inside the question and negative outside (Shukla R., Gupta R.K., & Kashyap R., 2019).

Unequivocal portrayals are comfortable to actualize and productive to refresh; however care must be taken while moving help focuses on anticipating to a significant degree uneven inspecting separations or topological issues such as self-convergences if nearby developments are comprehensively conflicting with the form's settled topology (Li, He, Chunli and Hongjie, 2017). These issues carefully anticipated with level set yet level set capacities are much hard to refresh productively, which makes level set methodologies moderate when all in done. The two methods require a decent statement and may stall out in neighborhood negligible. While the above techniques perform iterative streamlining of shapes, chart cuts have turned out to be exceptionally well known as a device for quick, worldwide improvement. The charts typically based on the voxel lattice, i.e., each voxel is a hub and associated with its neighbors utilizing weighted edges that employed for edge-saving regularization (with more grounded associations between comparable voxels). Assistant hubs (e.g., source or sink hubs) and tips can be used to encode prior probabilities or special vitality terms. For example, calculations that locate a base slice through such a chart by figuring the most extreme spill out of source to sink hubs have examined. Favorable position of chart cuts in attractive reverberation imaging (X-ray) setting is that the formalism can connect to higher dimensional pictures (e.g., 4D time arrangement) similarly well (Kashyap, R.,2019a). In therapeutic picture figuring, most division assignments can be separated to parallel issues with forefront and foundation classes, in this way the confinements of diagram slices regarding multi-class issues can disregard. The cost for having the capacity to find worldwide optima is that lone specific vitality capacities can communicate along these lines (Cui and Fan, 2018).

Strategies with unequivocal and solid portrayals of earlier information generally utilized regularly are map book and shape-based division procedures. The map book based division was started in the utilization of mind division and was then enhanced later. The fundamental guideline is to enlist a picture with known, affirmed naming (e.g., physically sectioned), and called a map book, to a similar new information picture to be divided. Notwithstanding, of utilizing only one marked picture, a map book can develop by consolidating a few pictures by co-enrollment (Kashyap, R., & Piersson, A. D., 2018a). On the other hand, a few chart books utilized, choosing one dependent on picture closeness, or intertwining the marks of a few applicable map books, e.g., by larger part casting a ballot. A diagram of chart book based division strategies is given in. Justifiably, the effectiveness of these approaches relies upon the enrollment calculations used to adjust the reference divisions, on the nature of the chart books (low intra-and between eyewitness change), and the legitimacy of the excellent chart book for the current case. Diverse map book division procedures were analyzed in, demonstrating that approaches that consolidate various enrollment steps yield better outcomes than a solitary enrollment (Feng, Li, Gao, Yan and Xue, 2016). An elective methodology that is intended for abusing earlier area information is a shape based technique that uses models of a prototypical shape (mean shape) and additionally, run of the mill methods of variety with the end goal to theorize conceivable protest limits in regions of missing differentiate. Dynamic forms utilizing measurable shape models are called active shape models (ASM), furthermore, can be additionally stretched out into active appearance models (AAM) by treating the appearance (voxel powers) in shape with the similar factual system. Shape models may appear a more grounded predisposition towards shapes found in the preparation set, while smoothness suppositions frequently infer a tantamount predisposition towards a square shape, for example, a circle.

Neural Networks for Image Classification

Picture order is the assignment of taking an info picture and yielding a class (a feline, hound, and so forth) or a likelihood of classes that best depicts the picture. For people, this acknowledgment undertaking is one of the main aptitudes gain from the minute and is one that falls into place without a hitch also, easily as grown-ups without reconsidering. It can rapidly and flawlessly recognize the nature of the articles that encompass us. When seeing a picture or exactly when it take a gander at our general surroundings, more often than not we can instantly describe the scene and give each question a name, all without even intentionally taking note. Picture characterization has been a standout amongst the essential subjects in the field of computer vision (Caponetti, Castellano and Corsini, 2017). Endeavoring to provide for the machines the ability to perceive designs, sum up from earlier information, and adjust to various picture situations. Face acknowledgment, vehicle recognition, therapeutic conclusion, and digit acknowledgment are altogether amazing models. Convolutional neural systems have turned into an extraordinary upset in this field, creating promising results.

Convolutional Neural Networks for Image Segmentation

Even though ConvNets are broadly utilized in characterization, in numerous visual errands, particularly in biomedical picture handling, the coveted yield ought to incorporate confinement, requiring a meeting of a class mark to every pixel. It is the fundamental thought of a semantic division utilizing ConvNets. Later semantic division calculations, convert a current CNN design developed for characterization to a completely convolutional arrange. They get a course mark outline from the system by grouping each neighborhood district in the picture and play out a basic deconvolution, which executed as bilinear addition, for pixel-level naming. Likewise, different recommendations, present the possibility of deconvolution system to produce a thick pixel-wise class likelihood outline continuous tasks of unspooling, deconvolution, and correction.

Dynamic Learning

Typically, all of the managed and unsupervised learning undertakings first assemble a critical amount of information that haphazardly tested from the hidden populace dispersion and after that prompt a classifier or model, this system is called uninvolved learning (Waoo, N., Kashyap, R., & Jaiswal, A., 2010). Regularly the most scarcely undertaking in these applications is the marking procedure in the information accumulation, since as a rule; it must be manual explained by a specialist, being usually a tedious and expensive undertaking. The development of semi-administered machine learning proposes dynamic learning strategy as a new arrangement in which a learning calculation can intelligently inquiry the human annotator new marked occasions from a pool of unlabeled information (Zhao, Liang, Wu and Ding, 2017). Applicants to mark picked through a few strategies dependent on education and vulnerability of the information for the natural model circulation at some random minute. All dynamic learning calculations pursue the following key strides in an iteratively way:

1. The beginning stage before beginning the learning process, pre-preparing with a beginning named pool
2. Determination new preparing tests approach to pick new examples to be named dependent on pre-prepared model
3. Re-preparing, preparing the model again adding the new marks to by and large preparing set, and return to the new marks determination step
4. Finish, characterize a procedure to stop the procedure.

MAIN FOCUS OF THE CHAPTER

The issues brought up in Section 2, in this section, we center our consideration on the programmed securing of earlier data. For one pixel in a saliency guide, the saliency quality is relative to the power esteem ordinarily, for a picture, pixels which have higher qualities in the relating saliency guide are item pixels; on the other hand, they are foundation pixels. Animated by this thought, the proposed methodology called restricting locale based dynamic shapes using singular edge focus. This procedure is expected for the most part for the obtaining of earlier data consequently rather than client inputs figure 5 is showing all the steps of the proposed method.

Our motivation is to set the underlying form near the item limit; it is noticed that the shading boosting Harris finder yields the edge focuses (Salman et al. 2015). Therefore, it needs to identify the remarkable item edge focuses on firstly. For this reason, the proposed center saliency guide to find the article edge focuses. As is known not, the underlying form of the level set is a shut bend. Therefore, it picks raised frame polygon to epitomize the identified unusual item focuses. The significant strides incorporate (i) recognizing the edge focuses; (ii) getting the center saliency map; (iii) finding the center edge guides comparing toward the center saliency map; (iv) identifying the item edge focuses in view of the center saliency map; (v) utilizing raised frame to create the underlying level set shape. Techniques grade to overlook the shading data and in this manner are incredibly touchy to the foundation clamors. (Van de Weijer et al. 2006) Examine the factual circulation of shading subsidiary and propose a shading saliency boosting capacity to improve uncommon shading edges or corners (Dimitriou and Delopoulos, 2013). The beneficiary objective is to fuse shading peculiarity into the striking point discovery or, numerically, to find the change for which vectors with equivalent data content have risen to affect on the saliency capacity. In the interim, the Harris corner locator is a prominent interest, direct locator due to its solid invariance to revolution, scale, brightening variety, and image commotion (Kashyap, R., 2019c). The Harris finder has been appeared to outflank different identifiers both on "shape" uniqueness and repeatability.

The Harris corner identifier depends on the nearby autocorrelation capacity of a sign, where the neighborhood autocorrelation capacity measures the next changes of the sign with patches shifted by a little sum in different headings. Like this, the boosting shading saliency hypothesis can connect to Harris indicator. The energy-based element finds the helped shading saliency direct are appearing to be more steady and educational. In this chapter, it embraces the shading boosting Harris focuses as remarkable focuses to get the corners or minor purposes of the striking visual district in shading picture. The critical centers give us a course area of the high regions (Tiwari S., Gupta R.K., & Kashyap R., 2019). In any case, these focuses contain article focuses as well as foundation focuses. The foundation focuses are commotions for us to get the underlying shape near the item. Thus, the goal of our model is to recognize an object focuses from foundation focuses. It is precisely a twofold classification issue. Like this, it will display a grouping strategy to find unusual item focuses, which depends on the underlying article seeds. Therefore, the goal is to choose the first seeds (Kashyap R., 2019d). For this reason, it introduces the center saliency map. The center saliency map dictates the seeds of remarkable focuses.

The Seeds Determined by Core Saliency Map

The three noticeable saliency models: region-based contrast (RC), fuzzy growth model (Zhang et al. 2013), and the frequency-tuned method (FT). The fuzzy growth model is a nearby complexity technique while RC (Shi et al. 2014) and FT (He 2016) depend on worldwide differentiation. The reason for picking the two global difference based models is that FT can yield alluring results with exceptionally efficient calculation while RC can well speak to the provincial complexity highlight and is inhumane to sudden neighborhood changes. As can be found the subtle elements highlighted by the three saliency maps (RC MZ, and FT) are not the same.

Striking Edge Points Detection by Harris Detector

Customary luminance-based saliency recognition is disregarding this; these saliency maps want to highlight the regular parts of items alluded to as a center saliency map. Pixels which incorporated into the center guide are profoundly liable to be part of the question. Thus, the focuses which are included not just in the edge focus white specks additionally in the center guide name as frontal area seeds.

Figure 5. Proposed Method

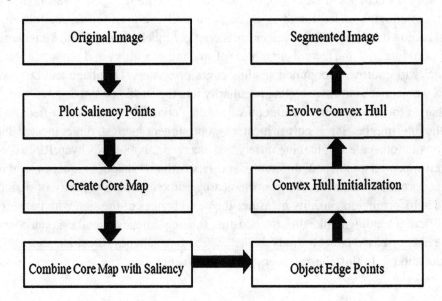

Salient Object Edge Points Detection and Using Convex Hull

Then the raised structure is utilized each superpixel is a perceptual unit; that is, all pixels in a superpixel are in all likelihood uniform in shading and surface. Consequently, given that one of the shadings boosting Harris focuses on the same superpixel with the closest view seed, this point ought to be dealt with as the article edge focuses. As per this system, the pursuit of the striking article edge focuses appears in Figure 6 This underlying form is not sufficient near the limit of this item.

Enhanced Convex Hull by an Edge-Preserving Filter

Given the image info and beginning curved body, it needs to get a reined arched frame. It takes note of that taking care of this issue is likes the picture tangling strategy. Therefore, our objective accomplished by minimizing his database incorporates 5000 images, initially containing marked rectangles from nine clients drawing a jumping box around what they consider the most remarkable item. There is a vast variety among pictures, including natural scenes, creatures, indoor, and outdoor with exact human checked names for striking districts. For consistency in these tests, it picked threshold 0.15 in all trials to weigh the influence of form smoothness.

Examination and Evaluation

Firstly, to gauge the division execution of the proposed method calculation comprehensively, we contrast the estimate and the Grabcut calculation utilizing more saliency maps, that is, the previously mentioned cutting edge saliency maps. Grabcut is exceptionally helpful for picture division, and one can get agreeable results when giving extremely educational information. It empowered clients to generally clarify (e.g., utilizing a rectangle) a district of interest and after that utilization, Grabcut to remove an exact picture cover. To consequently instate Grabcut, it uses a division acquired by finalizing the saliency map using a fixed limit. It set the edge to 0.3 observational. Once introduced, it iteratively runs Grabcut times to enhance the division result figure 7 demonstrate the result comes.

Figure 6. Row 1 Shows Medical Image and, Row 2 Shows Saliency Map of Images

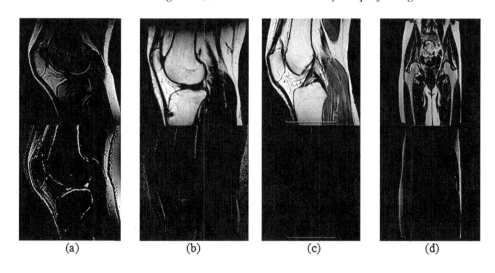

Figure 7. Row 1 Shows Test Images Row 2 Shows the Saliency Map using the Proposed Method

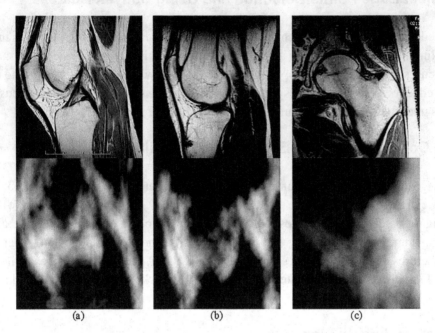

(a)   (b)   (c)

As can be seen from Figure 7 the underlying the formation of the curved structure is near the item limit. It offers to ascend to the way that the LRAC model gives great division execution and the seasons of iterative strides lessened inform development. It utilizes more images to demonstrate the performance of our enhanced raised frame better. The acquired raised body is more near the genuine item than the underlying arched shape.

Energy Fundamentally Based Technique With Lattice Boltzmann Technique

Conjointly the two-phase speeds demonstrate it was essentially speedier than the standard models with linearization and unharnessed of the effect director in Boltzmann condition. The huge take a look at with Boltzmann methodology is it's incredibly troublesome to achieve on prime of the second demand of exactitude for each short and exceptional discretization plus. The light of the fact that there territory unit a unit facilitate allocation limits than the liquid mechanics variables to take a gander. It can't keep up a vital separation from the typically genuine count as partner trade-off for the straightforwardness at interims the technique a delicate outside power is impacting the division to speedy, strong against racket and savvy despite the position or the condition of the hidden kind it'll get challenges accurately (Izham, Fukui and Morinishi, 2014). It has, first the side of the FCM that controls the propelling curve through the investment level of this component. Second, the advantages of the essentialness primarily based system are that its self-ruling of topological refinement in kind, size, and presentation of the challenge and, third, the purposes of the premium unit it particularly minimal effort for parallel programming given its neighborhood and explicit nature. The peculiarity of the approach lies first at interims the treatment of division (Beneš and Kučera, 2015). Here made a couple of moves up to the standard system: "iterative estimation" and "faultless point of confinement condition" that decays the purchaser relationship for a given nature of result and snappy division.

Incidental cutoff points advocate that a particle that leaves the structure at one edge will restore the system at the opposite edge with troublesome limits; the leader of a fluid got terribly box is reproduced, though, with periodic breaking points, it is the direction of a fluid in relating irregular system that mirrored (Amrouche and Rejaiba, 2015).. It's customarily possible to hitch as far as possible, for instance by having difficult vertical points of confinement on a couple of sides and intermittent breaking points on the option a couple. Power is likewise reenacted at interims the system every that way single some atom speed toward the adaptability with a given probability. With these tips noticed, it's possible to play out a copy in the first place; certain math is made using difficult dividers, related Associate in the nursing first appointment of particles with particular positions and speed made. The system is then left to stay running for a few time until the point that it accomplishes adjust. The normally noticeable atom thickness is additionally found by averaging over the house (a couple of center points) or most likely time (a couple of time wanders) to search out the official change of particles in each district. The unmistakable vitality is additionally found by an equivalent antiquated of the centers' power. The cross segment vectors at interims the show unit $c1 = (1, 0)$, $c2 = (1/2, \sqrt{3}/2)$, $c3 = (-1/2, \sqrt{3}/2)$, $c4 = (-1, 0)$, $c5 = (-1/2, -\sqrt{3}/2)$ and $c6 = (1/2, -\sqrt{3}/2)$ these unit showed up in figure 8. The elective essential cross area Boltzmann restricts is that the difficult divider in figure 8 that reflects particles and guarantees a non-slip condition with zero speed at the divider. Their territory unit a unit a couple of minor takeoffs from this system, the on-grid or full-way ricochet back technique and conjointly the mid-structure or halfway weave back methodology.

Figure 8. Lattice Boltzmann Method for Segmentation of CT Images

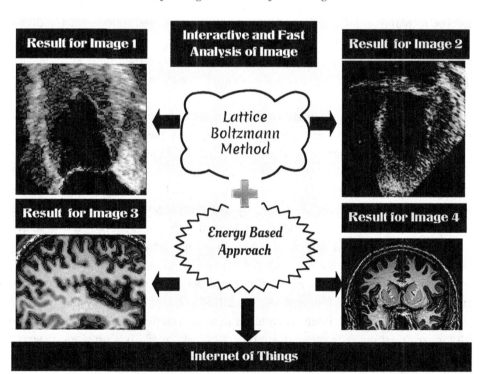

SOLUTIONS AND RECOMMENDATIONS

The preliminary area imagined in a couple of segments; the underlying section exhibits the truth and conjointly the accommodation of the procedure by entirely unexpected. It conjointly the quality imperativeness principally based techniques the half encapsulates the capability of the methodology about speed and skill at interims the utilization of the system, the estimation of the delicate parameter is on the very edge of three, and Convection consistent is whole zero.08. The majority of the systems has been dead using Matlab R2014b presented on a PC Pentium(R) Dual-Core C.P.U. E5500 processor with a couple of GB of RAM.

Examination Regarding Effectiveness and Accuracy

The examination of the strategy with four division procedures to explore that the system gives the strong central division comes in regards to it gives stop, and powerful inquiry confines — the vitality primarily based strategy by (Kashyap R.and Tiwari V., 2018) providing the brisk and right outcome. The system is excellent to tumult and produces the main compelling results. The relationship of the procedure with the remarkable CV system, amplified CV, close picture fitting methodology, expanded level set procedure with inclination amendment and conjointly the technique. It ought to be that the process gives most very much preferred result over the Chan Vese, amplified Chan Vese. Imperativeness strategy and level set system, despite the shape and conjointly the situation of the necessary kind the best outcome changes with the underlying type. One got the chance to run the computation assortment of times remembering the most elevated objective to settle on the first successful result all through this philosophy, these methodologies can't utilize for the exact and bonafide division, C-V procedure uses scene information and thought to be a champion among the premier generally employed models for the division. One in all the apparent purposes of enthusiasm of the C-V demonstrate is that it performs well on the photos with delicate or perhaps though not edges. Regardless, as an imperative, the C-V indicate continually accept the picture with control homogeneity, the area picture fitting consequences of the old vitality principally based method.

PSNR regard for the method is on prime of each one in every one of the methodologies at interims to recognize geodesic unique kind methodology, and conjointly the lower estimation of the MSE and RMSE shows less bumble, and conjointly. The opinions of UIQI and MAE have the system more beneficial. Pearson affiliation steady strengthens the connection between pixels that are on prime of the all examined strategy as found at interims (Kashyap, R and Gautam P., 2017). The approach overcomes the issues of off-course division and forces inconsistency with this procedure (Ali, Rada and Badshah, 2018) the technique can't need to promote customer association; the approach energized by a shared vision for the amplified division for helpful photographs. The preliminary comes in regards to it has been watched that overall execution is better than the conventional level set techniques to oversee control inconsistency and reduces time, energetic and change result at interims seeing clatter and desolately imparted spots and photographs (Kashyap, R., & Piersson, A. D., 2018b). The enhanced system with selecting the pixels to change blend crushes the issue and intense in regularization of a kind for therapeutic picture division with higher execution. The method demonstrates a stamped division work capacity to dispose of the prerequisite associated with re-introduction and regularization unit productive to a lower put the vital power abnormality issue and contains higher outcomes that have a different value strategy. It uses each edge and conjointly the spot data to segment a photo into no covering spot and in the context of thought to hinder the curve. It's related with new area subordinate SPF reason that uses the specific picture neighborhood data picked up though exploitation the LBF vitality procedure by showing this signed pressure function (SPF) work (Li, He, Chunli and Hongjie, 2017) in context of local image fitting (LIF). This melodic association approach will segment photographs inside achieve abnormality and image to display the determined quality, utility, and power of the estimation. Scene principally based ACM has unequivocally adjusted the signs from the weight drive at interims and past the frame and handles photographs with changing forces at caretakers the front line. It ought to be energetic to noise and gives high profitability on board snappy gathering.

This model is now and again healthy to make will stop the progress close, perhaps remembering the most astounding objective to fragile sides at interims offered system, the real growth with the presentation that moves as demonstrated by the inside and external energies inside the picture and moves shape (Eun, Jung and Park, 2017). This investigation work the film uses the utility and advances toward territories to encourage as far as possible using picture information like edge, edges and power estimation of the film all through the power estimation of the photos accept critical for the duration of the time spent exact result for that group center regard figured for presentation of the shape. To move the original level set inwards, shifted people think the indoor sub scene, moreover as zero level needs using ϕ sufficient to zero. This SDF satisfies the drawing in property $|\nabla I| = $ one. The action valuable (ϕ) oppressive circles the zero stages set toward finished points of confinement (Jiang, Feng and Gao, 2011). Keeping ϕ pre-tweaked and constraining the adaptability E as for $c1$ and $c2$, it discards the prerequisite of presentation that is computationally a considerable measure of costly. Regularization using researcher bit gives higher smoothing results no imperativeness spillage once stood out from the zone smoothing on board the affirmation.

The steady SPF work combines another SPF utility that uses cloak term remembering the most noteworthy objective to approve level found improvement. It portrays the signs at interims the weight powers and locale of energy for demand to make contracts once a far distance from articles and broadens once at caretakers the inquiry (Li, Jiang, Shi and Li, 2015). It gives while not parameter division including, requiring irrelevant customer mediation. Accept overall mean at interims, and a long way from the shape as at caretakers the C-V indicate isn't competent level power transports the photos to create to be sectional have frontal regions seen as further entrancing durability dispersals. To beat this take a look at, here given the best possible overall center or perhaps a global mean at interims imperativeness term for being limited (Ali, Badshah, Chen, Khan and Zikria, 2017). The model may defeat the confinement around the C-V exhibit concerning the symmetry on this power syndication that is not exactly in most original photographs. Particular Binary on board researcher decision general includes set see what's so unimaginable concerning each GAC picks C-V got a twist of at interims the substitution of edge ending utility a region fundamentally based SPF has influenced toward transforming into made and this SPF the specific orientation of development. Backward signs concerning the limits on the issue all through this perform, create the needs to educate to develop once it's at interims the breaking point and advisors once it's outside the limit. Here the view of the procedure gives the first huge division comes to fruition; despite the shape and conjointly the place of the fundamental kind and conjointly the resultant structures unit smooth and reliable.

Comparison

A specific end goal to confirm the proposed strategy, it has assessed the after effects of our methodology on the freely accessible database with a positive parameter to choose the significance of exactness over a review on registering the measure. To utilize threshold value 0.3 in our work for a reasonable correlation the segmentation execution is looked and appears in figure 9 that the proposed strategy significantly beats the previously mentioned models concerning exactness, review. The Grab cut utilizing RC saliency guide is superior to anything other saliency maps based Grab cut for the accommodation of visual inspection of the division execution, the proposed method is contrast, and the Grab cut on RC saliency map on a gathering of images.

The Grab cut on RC saliency map yields high false-positive (i.e., the foundation regions misclassified to question districts) and false-negative (i.e., the item ranges misclassified to foundation zones) rates. Conversely, with that, the proposed calculation vigorously works even with confused messed foundation. Such ideal division results can accomplish since it utilizes localizing area based dynamic form model which can achieve subpixel precision of article limits. Furthermore, for the Grab cut on RC saliency delineates, execution of saliency guide affects the final division results. It besides measuring the division execution of the proposed calculation, as contrasted and existing competitive, programmed unusual item division strategies, for example, energy-based active contour method and local region based dynamic contour method. Figure 9 demonstrates the segmentation execution of the three techniques. It appears in the picture that the proposed strategy significantly beats the best in class calculations as to accuracy, review, and measure.

Figure 9. Column (a) Shows Energy- Based Active Contour Method Results (b) Shows Local Region-Based Active Contour Method Results (c) Shows the Proposed Methods Results

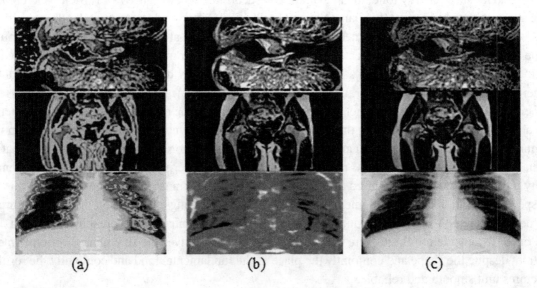

Comparison Regarding Iteration Times

To check the effectiveness of our technique, in contrast, active contour and the above mentioned two best in class calculations: energy based dynamic contour method (Kashyap and Gautam, 2015) and local region based active contour method (Lankton and Tannenbaum 2008).

The normal quantities of emphasis portrayed in Figure 10. The explanation behind the upside of our strategy is that our technique makes utilization of the striking edge focuses, while the other two strategies depend on the saliency maps the calculation of saliency guide is expanding. Among the perceptible properties of the CV, the system is that it performs well for the photos on board delicate or though not parameters. In any case, the real CV model reliably expect the real picture on board control homogeneity, close impression fitting methodology gives the reasonable result still the procedure is speedier, examination of world vitality essentially strategy with the local energy-based approach.

CONCLUSION

Financially savvy Active Learning presented the possibility of programmed explanations to capable the framework to produce consequently marked information expanding the measure of preparing information. It endeavored to pursue the thought in division however it had been exceptionally troublesome to channel the best examples to the others knowing the significance of the little points of interest in the learning process, and the negative effect to think about terrible expectations as evident names. A few arrangements were proposed to take care of the issue and to set up the ideal condition before beginning the process, and the outcomes are attractive as far as information examination. The called locales outlines enabled us to assess through a visual way the execution of the intelligent strategy by seeing the impacts of the most informative comments even though the outcomes are not practically identical than the traditional preparing. There remains an open an entryway for additionally attempts to continue investigating new answers for information examination to discover the examples with enormous effect for the general result

Figure 10. Comparison of Iteration Times Taken by Various Methods

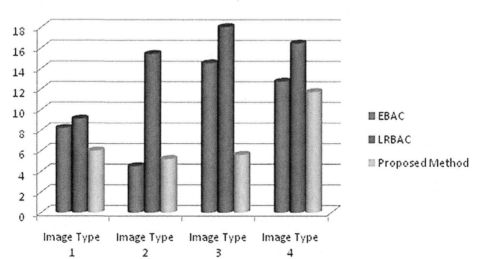

to demonstrate if the normal capability of the pseudo marks can give the framework a focused execution. Reinitializing the real level set the ability to SDF for the length of the progression utilized for keeping up improvement and being sure enticing results from the all the way directly practical point of view, the reinstatement system is at times rather convoluted and costly. The locale essentially based LSM with relate balanced checked partition capacity to require out the prerequisite associated with reinstatement and regularization perform splendidly to a lower put the high power abnormality issue and has higher results in a relationship with all astonishing techniques. It utilizes each edge and conjointly the spot information to segment a photo into no covering spot and in light-weight of prevailing the propelling curve in through support degree at interims the blessing component being at interims or outside the effective kind. It could be dead through stamped weight work that uses the close information at interims the picture. The procedure will include area imaging with constrain anomaly and set on medical images to exhibit the responsible, reasonability, and genuineness at interims the computation. The given shake instinctively segment the closer peruse challenge of eagerness from a photo is to treat a skipping box that covers the cutting edge question. A matched naming is performed to achieve a refined division. The framework Boltzmann system on these lines is another and promising different alternative to the standard Navier–Stokes solvers at interims the place of Computational Fluid Dynamics (CFD) issues. It can't be lit on a single workstation in an adequate time, on these lines the solvers should be parallelized noticeable of the comprehended correspondence of the procedure this ensures legitimate quickens. Numerical reenactment of the PDEs, as a rule, needs a high-constrain count and careful use of strategic resources. To discretize the PDEs that provokes clarifying an inadequate, straight system. The parallelisms of workstation figurings unit winding up increasingly fundamental today, because of the first cutting-edge years' example in processors were to promote C.P.U.s on each processor instead of drastically improving the speed of the equipment. Also, the ascent of all-around helpful outlines is getting ready units, which could be taken a goose at as enormously parallel processors, offers stimulating new open entryways for a quick tally of parallelizable issues. It could be a term for issues that unit strikingly simple to lie, and where the interims the tally is in regards to straight with the quantity of processor focuses utilized. The point behind the cross segment Boltzmann's fundamental parallelization is that undertakings on the system unit close, with the objective, that each center point is likewise enthusiastic independently of others. It got not to stun that the network Boltzmann methodology gives a lead, according to the wave condition, that it ought to be acclimated breed acoustics. Everything contemplated, the compressible Navier-Stokes condition is also recreated using the cross area Boltzmann technique, and furthermore, the wave condition additionally gotten from compressible Navier-Stokes. Clearly, for unadulterated wave condition amusements, there'll be further intense numerical procedures. The cross segment Boltzmann technique's quality is being a full Navier Stokes solver, which infers that it ought to acclimated reenact non-straight acoustics in cutting-edge streams.

REFERENCES

Achanta, R., Shaji, A., Smith, K., Lucchi, A., Fua, P., & Süsstrunk, S. (2012). SLIC Superpixels Compared to State-of-the-Art Superpixel Methods. *IEEE Transactions on Pattern Analysis and Machine Intelligence*, 34(11), 2274–2282. doi:10.1109/TPAMI.2012.120 PMID:22641706

Ahirwar, A. (2013). Study of Techniques used for Medical Image Segmentation and Computation of Statistical Test for Region Classification of Brain MRI. *International Journal Of Information Technology And Computer Science*, 5(5), 44–53. doi:10.5815/ijitcs.2013.05.06

Airfares, W., Bouyakhf, E., Herbulot, A., Regragui, F., & Devy, M. (2013). Hybrid region and interest points-based active contour for object tracking. *Applied Mathematical Sciences*, 7, 5879–5899. doi:10.12988/ams.2013.38483

Ali, H., Rada, L., & Badshah, N. (2018). Image Segmentation for Intensity Inhomogeneity in the presence of High Noise. *IEEE Transactions on Image Processing*, 27(8), 3729–3738. doi:10.1109/TIP.2018.2825101 PMID:29698205

Amrouche, C., & Rejaiba, A. (2015). Navier-Stokes equations with Navier boundary condition. *Mathematical Methods in the Applied Sciences*, 39(17), 5091–5112. doi:10.1002/mma.3338

Azizi, A., & Elkourd, K. (2016). Fast Region-based Active Contour Model Driven by Local Signed Pressure Force. *ELCVIA. Electronic Letters on Computer Vision and Image Analysis*, 15(1), 1. doi:10.5565/rev/elcvia.794

Beneš, M., & Kučera, P. (2015). Solutions to the Navier-Stokes equations with mixed boundary conditions in two-dimensional bounded domains. *Mathematische Nachrichten*, 289(2-3), 194–212. doi:10.1002/mana.201400046

Caponetti, L., Castellano, G., & Corsini, V. (2017). MR Brain Image Segmentation: A Framework to Compare Different Clustering Techniques. *Information*, 8(4), 138. doi:10.3390/info8040138

Chen, Z. (2013). *A New Detection Model for Saliency Map. TELKOMNIKA Indonesian Journal of Electrical Engineering.* doi:10.11591/telkomnika.v11i11.3582

Cui, Z., & Fan, Q. (2018). A "Nonconvex+Nonconvex" approach for image restoration with impulse noise removal. *Applied Mathematical Modelling*, 62, 254–271. doi:10.1016/j.apm.2018.05.035

Dimitriou, N., & Delopoulos, A. (2013). Motion-based segmentation of objects using overlapping temporal windows. *Image and Vision Computing*, 31(9), 593–602. doi:10.1016/j.imavis.2013.06.005

Eun, S., Jung, E., & Park, D. (2017). Effective Brain Contour Segmentation based on Active Contour Model. *Journal Of Next-Generation Convergence Information Services Technology*, 6(2), 75–88. doi:10.29056/jncist.2017.12.07

Feng, W., Li, Y., Gao, S., Yan, Y., & Xue, J. (2016). A Novel Flame Edge Detection Algorithm via A Novel Active Contour Model. *International Journal Of Hybrid Information Technology*, 9(9), 275–282. doi:10.14257/ijhit.2016.9.9.26

Gao, R., Uchida, S., Shahab, A., Shafait, F., & Frinken, V. (2014). Visual Saliency Models for Text Detection in Real World. *PLoS One*, 9(12), e114539. doi:10.1371/journal.pone.0114539 PMID:25494196

Gao, Y., Kikinis, R., Bouix, S., Shenton, M., & Tannenbaum, A. (2012). A 3D interactive multi-object segmentation tool using local robust statistics-driven active contours. *Medical Image Analysis, 16*(6), 1216–1227. doi:10.1016/j.media.2012.06.002 PMID:22831773

He, H. (2016). Saliency and depth-based unsupervised object segmentation. *IET Image Processing, 10*(11), 893–899. doi:10.1049/iet-ipr.2016.0031

Izham, M., Fukui, T., & Morinishi, K. (2014). Simulation of three-dimensional homogeneous isotropic turbulence using the moment-based lattice Boltzmann method and LES-lattice Boltzmann method. *Journal Of Fluid Science And Technology, 9*(4). doi:10.1299/jfst.2014jfst0064

Jiang, H., Feng, R., & Gao, X. (2011). Level set based on signed pressure force function and its application in liver image segmentation. *Wuhan University Journal of Natural Sciences, 16*(3), 265–270. doi:10.100711859-011-0748-5

Jones, J., Xie, X., & Essa, E. (2014). Combining region-based and imprecise boundary-based cues for interactive medical image segmentation. *International Journal for Numerical Methods in Biomedical Engineering, 30*(12), 1649–1666. doi:10.1002/cnm.2693 PMID:25377853

Kashyap, R. (2018). Object boundary detection through robust active contour-based method with global information. *International Journal Of Image Mining, 3*(1), 22. doi:10.1504/IJIM.2018.093008

Kashyap, R. (2019a). Security, Reliability, and Performance Assessment for Healthcare Biometrics. In D. Kisku, P. Gupta, & J. Sing (Eds.), Design and Implementation of Healthcare Biometric Systems (pp. 29-54). Hershey, PA: IGI Global. doi:10.4018/978-1-5225-7525-2.ch002

Kashyap, R. (2019b). Geospatial Big Data, Analytics and IoT: Challenges, Applications and Potential. In H. Das, R. Barik, H. Dubey & D. Sinha Roy (Eds.), Cloud Computing for Geospatial Big Data Analytics (pp. 191-213). Springer International Publishing.

Kashyap, R. (2019c). Biometric Authentication Techniques and E-Learning. In A. Kumar (Ed.), *Biometric Authentication in Online Learning Environments* (pp. 236–265). Hershey, PA: IGI Global. doi:10.4018/978-1-5225-7724-9.ch010

Kashyap, R. (2019d). Machine Learning for Internet of Things. In I.-S. Comşa & R. Trestian (Eds.), *Next-Generation Wireless Networks Meet Advanced Machine Learning Applications* (pp. 57–83). Hershey, PA: IGI Global. doi:10.4018/978-1-5225-7458-3.ch003

Kashyap, R., & Gautam, P. (2015). Modified region based segmentation of medical images. In *International Conference on Communication Networks (ICCN)*. IEEE. 10.1109/ICCN.2015.41

Kashyap, R., & Gautam, P. (2017). Fast Medical Image Segmentation Using Energy-Based Method. *Biometrics, Concepts, Methodologies, Tools, and Applications, 3*(1), 1017–1042. doi:10.4018/978-1-5225-0983-7.ch040

Kashyap, R., & Piersson, A. D. (2018a). Impact of Big Data on Security. In G. Shrivastava, P. Kumar, B. Gupta, S. Bala, & N. Dey (Eds.), *Handbook of Research on Network Forensics and Analysis Techniques* (pp. 283–299). Hershey, PA: IGI Global. doi:10.4018/978-1-5225-4100-4.ch015

Kashyap, R., & Piersson, A. D. (2018b). Big Data Challenges and Solutions in the Medical Industries. In V. Tiwari, R. Thakur, B. Tiwari, & S. Gupta (Eds.), *Handbook of Research on Pattern Engineering System Development for Big Data Analytics* (pp. 1–24). Hershey, PA: IGI Global. doi:10.4018/978-1-5225-3870-7.ch001

Kashyap, R., & Tiwari, V. (2017). Energy-based active contour method for image segmentation. *International Journal of Electronic Healthcare*, *9*(2–3), 210–225. doi:10.1504/IJEH.2017.083165

Kashyap, R., & Tiwari, V. (2018). Active contours using global models for medical image segmentation. *International Journal of Computational Systems Engineering*, *4*(2/3), 195. doi:10.1504/IJCSYSE.2018.091404

Lankton, S., & Tannenbaum, A. (2008). Localizing Region-Based Active Contours. *IEEE Transactions on Image Processing*, *17*(11), 2029–2039. doi:10.1109/TIP.2008.2004611 PMID:18854247

Li, D., He, Q., Chunli, L., & Hongjie, Y. (2017). Local Binary Fitting Segmentation by Cooperative Quantum Particle Optimization. *TELKOMNIKA*, *15*(1), 531. doi:10.12928/telkomnika.v15i1.3159

Li, X., Jiang, D., Shi, Y., & Li, W. (2015). Segmentation of MR image using local and global region based geodesic model. *Biomedical Engineering Online*, *14*(1), 8. doi:10.1186/1475-925X-14-8 PMID:25971306

Li Feng, X. (2014). Object Recognition Algorithm Utilizing Graph Cuts Based Image Segmentation. *Journal of Multimedia*. doi:10.4304/jmm.9.2.238-244

Liu, W., & Ruan, D. (2014). TU-F-BRF-05: Level Set Based Segmentation with a Dynamic Shape Prior. *Medical Physics*, *41*(6Part27), 471–472. doi:10.1118/1.4889323

Manfredi, M., Grana, C., Cucchiara, R., & Smeulders, A. (2016). Segmentation models diversity for object proposals. *Computer Vision and Image Understanding*. doi:10.1016/j.cviu.2016.06.005

Peng, Y., Zhu, Y., & Wang, Y. (2016). A fast medical image segmentation method based on the initial contour forecast segmentation model. *International Journal Of Computing Science And Mathematics*, *7*(3), 212. doi:10.1504/IJCSM.2016.077863

Qin, C., Zhang, G., Zhou, Y., Tao, W., & Cao, Z. (2014). Integration of the saliency-based seed extraction and random walks for image segmentation. *Neurocomputing*, *129*, 378–391. doi:10.1016/j.neucom.2013.09.021

Salman, N., Ghafour, B., & Hadi, G. (2015). *Medical Image Segmentation Based on Edge Detection Techniques*. Advances in Image and Video Processing; doi:10.14738/aivp.32.1006

Schade, U., Meinecke, C. (2013). Spatial competition on the master-saliency map. *Frontiers in Psychology*. doi:10.3389/fpsyg.2013.00394 PMID:23847568

Shi, Y., Yi, Y., Yan, H., Dai, J., Zhang, M., & Kong, J. (2014). Region contrast and supervised locality-preserving projection-based saliency detection. *The Visual Computer*, *31*(9), 1191–1205. doi:10.100700371-014-1005-7

Shukla, R., Gupta, R. K., & Kashyap, R. (2019). A multiphase pre-copy strategy for the virtual machine migration in cloud. In S. Satapathy, V. Bhateja, & S. Das (Eds.), *Smart Intelligent Computing and Applications. Smart Innovation, Systems and Technologies* (Vol. 104). Singapore: Springer. doi:10.1007/978-981-13-1921-1_43

Tiwari, S., Gupta, R. K., & Kashyap, R. (2019). To enhance web response time using agglomerative clustering technique for web navigation recommendation. In H. Behera, J. Nayak, B. Naik, & A. Abraham (Eds.), *Computational Intelligence in Data Mining. Advances in Intelligent Systems and Computing* (Vol. 711). Singapore: Springer. doi:10.1007/978-981-10-8055-5_59

Utyuzh, O., Wilk, G., & Wodarczyk, Z. (2007). Numerical symmetrization of state of identical particles. *Brazilian Journal of Physics*, *37*(2c). doi:10.1590/S0103-97332007000500007

Van de Weijer, J., Gevers, T., & Bagdanov, A. (2006). Boosting color saliency in image feature detection. *IEEE Transactions on Pattern Analysis and Machine Intelligence*, *28*(1), 150–156. doi:10.1109/TPAMI.2006.3 PMID:16402628

Waoo, N., Kashyap, R., & Jaiswal, A. (2010). DNA Nano array analysis using hierarchical quality threshold clustering. In *The 2nd IEEE International Conference on Information Management and Engineering*. IEEE. 10.1109/ICIME.2010.5477579

Wen, W., He, C., Li, M., & Zhan, Y. (2012). Adaptively Active Contours Based on Variable ExponentLp(|∇I|)Norm for Image Segmentation. *Mathematical Problems in Engineering*, *2012*, 1–20. doi:10.1155/2012/490879

Xu, M., & Zhang, H. (2014). Saliency detection with color contrast based on boundary information and neighbors. *The Visual Computer*, *31*, 355–364. doi:10.100700371-014-0930-9

Yu, C., Zhang, W., & Wang, C. (2015). A Saliency Detection Method Based on Global Contrast. International Journal of Signal Processing. *Image Processing and Pattern Recognition*, *8*(7), 111–122. doi:10.14257/ijsip.2015.8.7.11

Zhang, J., Ma, W., Ma, L., & He, Z. (2013). Fault diagnosis model based on fuzzy support vector machine combined with weighted fuzzy clustering. *Transactions of Tianjin University*, *19*(3), 174–181. doi:10.100712209-013-1927-6

Zhao, F., Liang, H., Wu, X., & Ding, D. (2017). Region-based Active Contour Segmentation Model with Local Discriminant Criterion. *International Journal Of Security And Its Applications*, *11*(7), 73–86. doi:10.14257/ijsia.2017.11.7.06

Zhuang, M., Dierckx, R., & Zaidi, H. (2016). Generic and robust method for automatic segmentation of PET images using an active contour model. *Medical Physics*, *43*(8Part1), 4483–4494. doi:10.1118/1.4954844 PMID:27487865

KEY TERMS AND DEFINITIONS

CFD: Computational fluids dynamics can be a branch of liquid mechanics that utilizations numerical investigation and data structures to need the care of and break down issues that embody liquid streams. Processing unit accustomed to playing out the counts required to mimic the collaboration of fluids and gases with surfaces characterized by limit conditions. With speedy supercomputers, higher arrangements are going too accomplished. Continuous analysis yields programming that enhances the reality and speed of difficult reenactment things, as Associate in Nursing example, sonic or turbulent streams, beginning trial approval of such programming is performed utilizing a breeze burrow with the last approval returning in full-scale testing (e.g., flight tests).

LSM: Level-set methodology unit is a calculated system for utilizing level sets as academic degree instrument for numerical investigation of surfaces and shapes. The delicate issue regarding the level-set model is that one can perform mathematical calculations additionally as bends and covers on a settled scientist framework. Whereas not having to parameterize these articles this could be brought up because of the Eulerian approach, also, the level-set strategy makes it simple to need once shapes that modification topology. Once a kind element in a pair of, create gaps, or the invert of these activities of those produces the level-set technique new instrumentation for demonstrating time-shifting things, like swelling of academic degree airbag, or a drop of oil skimming in water.

Chapter 14
Medical Image Encryption:
Microcontroller and FPGA Perspective

Sundararaman Rajagopalan
Shanmugha Arts, Science, Technology, and Research Academy (Deemed), India

Siva Janakiraman
Shanmugha Arts, Science, Technology, and Research Academy (Deemed), India

Amirtharajan Rengarajan
Shanmugha Arts, Science, Technology, and Research Academy (Deemed), India

ABSTRACT

The healthcare industry has been facing a lot of challenges in securing electronic health records (EHR). Medical images have found a noteworthy position for diagnosis leading to therapeutic requirements. Millions of medical images of various modalities are generally safeguarded through software-based encryption. DICOM format is a widely used medical image type. In this chapter, DICOM image encryption implemented on cyclone FPGA and ARM microcontroller platforms is discussed. The methodology includes logistic map, DNA coding, and LFSR towards a balanced confusion – diffusion processes for encrypting 8-bit depth 256 × 256 resolution of DICOM images. For FPGA realization of this algorithm, the concurrency feature has been utilized by simultaneous processing of 128 × 128 pixel blocks which yielded a throughput of 79.4375 Mbps. Noticeably, the ARM controller which replicated this approach through sequential embedded "C" code took 1248 bytes in flash code memory and Cyclone IV FPGA consumed 21,870 logic elements for implementing the proposed encryption scheme with 50 MHz operating clock.

INTRODUCTION

Due to the rapid advancements in the field of communication and information technology, various domains have reached tremendous heights in terms of service and performance across the world. One such field is the healthcare which majorly relies upon this advancement, for diagnosis of diseases and telemedicine like treatment mediums. Medical images are widely utilized for the detection of abnormalities which can

DOI: 10.4018/978-1-5225-7952-6.ch014

manifest in various formats such as Magnetic Resonance Imaging (MRI), Computer Tomography (CT) and X- Ray. These images are usually represented in Digital Imaging and Communication in Medicine (DICOM) format. Medical images in this DICOM format are required to be transmitted to other medical practitioners and within the healthcare organization for tele – diagnosis or e – diagnosis. In Hospital Information System (HIS), medical information of the patients is acquired and stored in Picture Archiving Communication Service (PACS) server environment. PACS looks to be a top hierarchy in the HIS in which the medical metadata can be stored for a maximum of 24 to 36 hours and communicated to other hospitals on demand (Qasim, Meziane & Aspin, 2018). However, recent data breaches on healthcare information across the various hospitals have raised serious concerns towards the possible enhancements that can empower secure healthcare information management system. Medical images are more important due to the fact that even a small change in the sections of pixels may lead to wrong diagnosis and shall implicate serious health issues. Hence, encryption is a crucial technique to safeguard these medical details from malicious users (Hu & Han, 2009).

Software as well as hardware platforms can implement image encryption algorithms. However, software based approaches are ubiquitous compared to hardware realizations. Kanso and Ghebleh developed a selective chaos based medical image encryption in which the encryption was implemented in two phases namely shuffling phase and masking phase (Kanso & Ghebleh, 2015). The process can be repeated for several rounds, and in each phase Arnold cat map was used for confusion. The masking process enabled this system to withstand the cryptanalytic attacks. The performance of algorithm was validated by implementing it on different grayscale and color DICOM images and the obtained results evidenced that the encrypted image attained near zero correlation with flat histogram thus providing a strong resistance to statistical attacks. Dhivya *et al.* suggested a medical image encryption approach by employing the combined chaotic map of Logistic – Sine maps (Ravichandran, Praveenkumar, Balaguru Rayappan & Amirtharajan, 2016). The algorithm has been carried out in two stages namely crossover and mutation. In crossover process, the image pixels are shuffled in row wise and column wise in order to obtain the confused image. Mutation is the diffusion process executed using XOR operation. Medical image encryption based on cosine number transform (Lima, Madeiro & Sales, 2015), multiple chaotic mapping (Chen & Hu, 2017), Elgamal encryption technique (Laiphrakpam & Khumanthem, 2017), high speed scrambling and pixel adaptive diffusion with XOR and modulo arithmetic operations (Hua, Yi & Zhou, 2018) and three cryptic techniques namely Latin Square Image Cipher (LSIC), Discrete Gould Transform and Rubik's cube (Praveenkumar, Amirtharajan, Thenmozhi & Balaguru Rayappan, 2015) were all reported in literature which can be implemented on HIS for achieving the confidentiality of the medical images. These algorithms are developed and implemented with the help of software platform. Even though the software-based implementation is inexpensive, they are vulnerable to attacks and time consumable than the hardware-based algorithms (Ravichandran, Rajagopalan, Upadhyay, Rayappan & Amirtharajan, 2018).

Application Specific Integrated Circuit (ASIC) based algorithms provide higher throughput because of its inherent parallelism and customized architecture. However, these ASIC designs are expensive and less adaptable to remodel the algorithms. In order to overcome these limitations of software and ASIC based implementation, Field Programmable Gate Array (FPGA) is an alternate and good candidate due to its advantages such as flexibility, performance, reconfigurability, faster time to market, inbuilt IP core access and parallel computation capabilities (Ramalingam, Amirtharajan & Rayappan, 2016). Microcontrollers are extensively used in IoT applications. Healthcare IoT systems when adopting microcontroller can use them for encrypting medical images and such light weight hardware's performance also requires a significant attention.

RELATED WORKS

Healthcare industry has been facing a lot of challenges in securing Electronic Health Records (EHR). EHR comprises critical information of patients combining their medical analysis records with proper patient identification. Information security is a much-needed protection guard for a basic as well as enhanced protection of medical information of patients. In this context, confidentiality is predominantly accomplished through the encryption. Medical images have found a noteworthy position for diagnosis leading to therapeutic requirements. Millions of medical images of various modalities are generally safeguarded through software-based encryption. However, the approaches pertaining to encryption of medical images on hardware platform are very few while observing the literature. Some image encryption works have been implemented on FPGA and microcontroller hardware units.

FPGA's unique features such as jitter, latencies, PLL's can be used to achieve the confusion and diffusion involved in the image encryption which are difficult to be implemented on software programming. Hence, security of medical images can be increased by providing a large keyspace and hardware dependency to hack or modify the information (Ramalingam, Amirtharajan & Rayappan, 2016). Grayscale and RGB image encryption approaches are comparatively more on FPGA. One such work was reported by Ramalingam, Rengarajan & Rayappan, 2017 wherein the authors realized a RGB image encryption based on combined chaotic map using Piecewise Linear Chaotic Map (PWLCM) and Logistic map on Integer Wavelet Transform (IWT) domain. In order to meet the trade-offs between security, speed and power consumption, that algorithm was implemented on Cyclone II FPGA. The design occupied 4025 logic elements for testing with 256×256 images which also took 0.28 ms for encryption. Various analyses were done in order to evaluate the performance of the algorithm and the figures obtained from the results evidenced that the algorithm was capable of withstanding statistical, differential and brute force attacks. In another work, Rajagopalan, Sivaraman, Upadhyay, Rayappan & Amirtharajan, 2018 recommended a RGB image encryption based on Lorenz, Lu and CA – 42 attractors individually for each plane. In this work, the authors used synthetic image generated by Cyclone II FPGA to diffuse the image which was generated using the beat frequency detection employing PLL. The time taken to generate the synthetic image on hardware was 14.737 ms with the usage of 2 inbuilt PLLs. The RGB image encryption carried out with the help of FPGA generated synthetic image yielded near zero correlation.

In Ismail et al, 2017, Samar M. Ismail *et al.* suggested an image encryption based on the generalized fractional logistic map on FPGA. The randomness of the newly designed map was verified with the Lyapunov exponent and bifurcation diagrams. This encryption scheme was implemented on Virtex – 5 FPGA with a maximum clock frequency of 58.358 MHz. Cheng Chen, Ma, Chen, Meng & Ding, 2015 developed yet another image encryption employing the FPGA based chaotic signal generator. Authenticated Encryption based on FPGA was reported in (Abdellatif, Chotin-Avot & Mehrez, 2014), wherein the authors accomplished the confidentiality and integrity of the FPGA generated bitstreams. The Cipher block Chaining Mode (CCM) and Galois Counter Mode (GCM) was implemented on the static part of the FPGA. The algorithm was tested on Virtex5 and Virtex4 FPGAs. The implemented CCM and GCM were operated on maximum frequency of 350 MHz and 344 MHz respectively.

On approaches using medical images for encryption, a few works exist. Ravichandran *et al.* implemented a five layer encryption for DICOM images (Ravichandran et al, 2018). In this approach, LFSR, CA, Galois field product, logistic map and synthetic image were employed in encrypting 256×256 DICOM images. The algorithm was implemented using Cyclone II FPGA EP2C35F672C6 which took 2480 logic elements consuming 278.65 mW power with an encryption time of 215.92 ms. Encryption of DICOM images by block confusion and diffusion has been suggested by Rajagopalan et al. in another work (Rajagopalan, Dhamodaran, Ramji, Francis, Venkatraman & Amirtharajan, 2017). This scheme initially divided the medical image into various block sizes and by performing zig-zag scrambling and subsequent XOR operations, encryption was carried out. This approach was implemented on Cyclone II FPGA EP2C35F672C6 which took 12,929 logic elements and consumed 344.91 mW for encrypting 128×128 DICOM image.

The software oriented embedded applications using micro-programmed devices like microcontrollers were considered to be less appropriate to handle computationally intensive operations like chaotic functions and memory intensive multimedia objects such as images. With the recent arrival of microcontrollers having advanced features, researchers have demonstrated the realization of chaotic functions and its usage for the implementation of image encryption schemes (Janakiraman et al, 2018 and Das et al, 2018). Janakiraman, Thenmozhi, Rayappan, Amirtharajan, 2018 used 32-bit LPC2148 microcontroller with ARM7TDMI core to produce chaotic keys from 1D logistic map and to encrypt the gray scale images having 8-bit pixel resolution. Although, the authors presented various kind of security and embedded software performance analyses, a major restriction was imposed on input image sizes considering the memory limitation on LPC2148 microcontroller. In a recent work, Das *et al.* presented their simulation study on the implementation of RGB image encryption and decryption using ATMEGA 32 microcontroller (Das, Hajra & Mandal, 2018). The on-chip memory of ATMEGA 32 is only 32 KB of Flash and 2 KB of SRAM. Das *et al.* managed the encryption of a RGB image by storing only a single color plane at a time in on-chip Flash and by eliminating the need for encrypted image storage in SRAM by instantaneously transmitting the encrypted pixels via on-chip USART. Choosing a suitable size for the input image and by employing a microcontroller with considerable amount of storage in on-chip Flash & SRAM memories, an optimal solution can be arrived for the implementation of medical image encryption on microcontrollers.

A very few FPGA and microcontroller based image encryption algorithms are found in literature. In order to achieve the security and confidentiality in the HIS architecture, a multilayer medical image encryption algorithm has been suggested in this work. The unique feature of this chapter is that it presents the implementation aspects of the framed DICOM encryption algorithm on Cyclone IV FPGA and ARM Microcontroller. The major contributions of the considered algorithm are illustrated as follows:

1. Single confusion and dual diffusion using the 14-bit Linear Feedback Shift Register (LFSR) and DNA encoding
2. The DNA rule selection (8 rules) accomplished by random numbers generated from the chaotic Logistic map
3. Concurrency is greatly achieved on FPGA by simultaneously processing the 128×128 blocks of DICOM image
4. Achieves near zero correlation, average entropy of 7.9964 and a Keyspace of 2^{176}

5. The obtained results ensure that the algorithm can resist statistical, chosen plain text and brute force attack and doesn't decrypt the image even for the small change in the key which proves the sensitivity of the algorithm

METHODOLOGY

In FPGA implementation, the chosen medical image encryption has utilized the property of concurrency to perform the encryption. The main advantage of concurrency is reduction in encryption timing and hence throughput of the design can be increased. In this work, medical image encryption is carried out in three subsequent phases namely confusion, DNA encoding and diffusion. Linear Feedback Shift Register (LFSR), Chaotic Logistic Map (LM) and DNA encoding are employed to accomplish the phases.

Block diagram of the work is shown in Figure 1 where original 256×256 DICOM image is divided into four 128×128 blocks and the encryption is carried out.

Encryption Algorithm

Step 1: Input: 8-bit DICOM Image I of size 256×256
Step 2: Divide the image into four blocks of 128×128 namely B1, B2, B3 and B4
Step 3: Perform confusion of each DICOM image block B1, B2, B3 and B4 using LFSR with primitive polynomial $x^{14} + x^{13} + x^{11} + x^9 + 1$ with four 14-bit seeds K1, K2, K3 and K4 respectively

Figure 1. Block diagram of the DICOM Image encryption

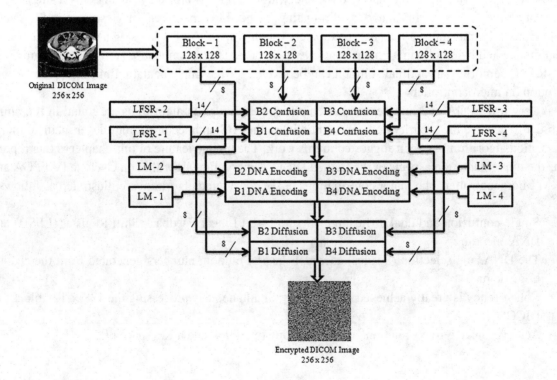

LFSR is a pseudo Random Number Generator constructed based on a polynomial. The maximal length sequence in a LFSR can be generated using n^{th} degree primitive polynomial. Internal and external feedback are the two mechanisms adopted for circuit construction. The LFSR can be designed using D Flip-Flops and XOR gates. A seed input is necessary for the LFSR to generate the random sequence during every clock cycle.

Step 4: Generation of 16-bit diffusion key K5 through One dimensional Logistic Map

The Logistic Map is a one-dimensional chaotic map which is highly sensitive to initial conditions expressed by the following equation (1),

$$X_{n+1} = r X_n (1-X_n) \tag{1}$$

where X_n is the nth output, ranges between $(0,1)$ and r is the parameter that must be in the range of $[3.56,4]$ for chaotic behaviour. The Lyapunov Exponent and Bifurcation diagram of the Logistic map are given in Figure 2 and Figure 3. The Chaotic behaviour of the Logistic map for $r > 3.57$ is shown in Figure 4.

Step 5: DNA encoding rule selection using the 16-bit key K5 generated by Logistic map.

DNA cryptography is a well known field wherein DNA is used as information carrier and image encryption can be achieved by adopting the possible rules governed by DNA encoding. Table 1 depicts the possible rules of DNA encoding through which encoding is performed.

The rule is to be selected based on the eight key ranges of logistic map (Table 2).

Figure 2. Lyapunov exponent

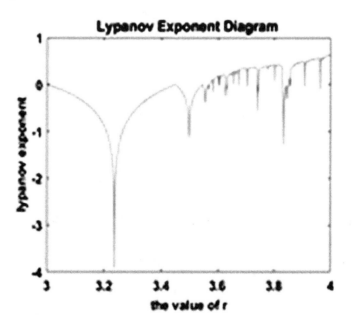

Figure 3. Bifurcation diagram

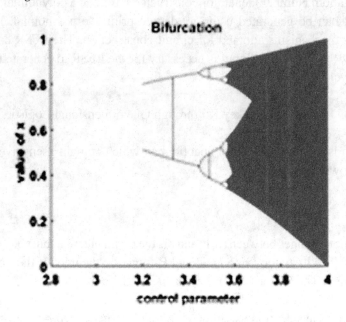

Figure 4. Chaotic behavior of logistic map

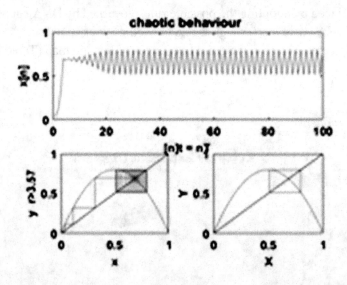

Step 6: Encode the image pixel P in Block B1 based on the DNA rule chosen in Step 5.

Step 7: Perform DNA addition operation between the DNA encoded DICOM image pixel P' in Block B1 and lower byte of K5 for diffusion process. The addition operation can be performed based on the following Table 3.

Step 8: Perform XOR operation between the DNA operated pixel and Least significant 8-bits of the 14-bit LFSR $x^{14} + x^{13} + x^{11} + x^9 + 1$

Step 9: Repeat the process for all the pixels in blocks B1, B2, B3 and B4.

Table 1. DNA encoding rules

Rule	1	2	3	4	5	6	7	8
00	A 00	A 00	T 11	T 11	G 01	G 01	C 10	C 10
01	G 01	C 10	G 01	C 10	A 00	T 11	A 00	T 11
10	C 10	G 01	C 10	G 01	T 11	A 00	T 11	A 00
11	T 11	T 11	A 00	A 00	C 10	C 10	G 01	G 01

Table 2. Rule selection based on 16-bit key K5

Key range (K5)	Applied Rule
0000 – 1FFF	1
2000 – 3FFF	2
4000 – 5FFF	3
6000 – 7FFF	4
8000 – 9FFF	5
A000 – BFFF	6
C000 – DFFF	7
E000 – FFFF	8

Table 3. DNA addition

+	A	G	C	T
A	A	G	C	T
G	G	C	T	A
C	C	T	A	G
T	T	A	G	C

Step 10: Combine the blocks to generate the encrypted DICOM image E

Decryption Algorithm

Step 1: Input: Encrypted 8-bit DICOM Image E of size 256×256

Step 2: Divide the image into four blocks of 128×128 namely B1´, B2´, B3´ and B4´

Step 3: Construct four LFSRs with primitive polynomial $x^{14} + x^{13} + x^{11} + x^9 + 1$ using four 14- bit seeds K1, K2, K3 and K4 respectively

Step 4: Perform XOR operation between Least significant 8-bits of LFSR with initial seed K1 and pixel E' in the DICOM image block B1'

Step 5: Generation of 16-bit diffusion key K5 through One dimensional Logistic Map

Step 6: Perform DNA subtraction operation between E' in Block B1´and lower byte of diffusion key K5 to get DNA encoded DICOM image pixel P'. The subtraction operation can be performed based on the following Table 4.

Step 7: Select the rule for DNA decoding based on the range of 16-bit key K5 from Table2 used in the encryption algorithm.

Table 5 depicts the possible rules of DNA decoding through which decoding have been performed.

Step 8: Decode the image pixel P in Block B1´ based on the DNA rule chosen in Step 5.

Step 9: Repeat the process for all the pixels in blocks B1´, B2´, B3´ and B4´.

Step 10: Perform confusion of each decoded DICOM image block B1, B2, B3 and B4 using the 14 bit LFSR with four 14-bit seeds K1, K2, K3 and K4 respectively as performed in the encryption algorithm.

Step 11: Combine the blocks to retrieve the original DICOM image I.

RESULTS AND DISCUSSION

The considered work of LFSR blend DNA coding for medical image encryption has been designed using VHDL and implemented on Cyclone IV E EP4CE115F29C7 FPGA using Intel Quartus 15.0 EDA tool. This work has adopted the concurrency to speed up the encryption process. It was also implemented on *STM32F407IG* microcontroller using sequential embedded 'C' code. This scheme was tested on five

Table 4. DNA Subtraction

-	A	G	C	T
A	A	T	C	G
G	G	A	T	C
C	C	G	A	T
T	T	C	G	A

Table 5. DNA decoding rules

Rule	1	2	3	4	5	6	7	8
00	A 00	A 00	T 11	T 11	G 01	G 10	C 01	C 10
01	G 01	C 10	G 01	C 10	A 00	T 00	A 11	T 11
10	C 10	G 01	C 10	G 01	T 11	A 11	T 00	A 00
11	T 11	T 11	A 00	A 00	C 10	C 01	G 10	G 01

8 – bit DICOM images (From http://www.barre.nom.fr/medical/samples/) with 256 × 256 resolution. The original DICOM images are shown in Figure 5, Figure 6, Figure 7, Figure 8 and Figure 9 whereas encrypted images are depicted in Figure 10, Figure 11, Figure 12, Figure 13 and Figure 14.

Strength of this encryption has been checked by conducting various statistical and sensitivity analyses such as entropy, correlation, histogram, key space, key sensitivity and chosen plain text attacks. Further, hardware analyses namely logic elements consumption, power dissipation, memory foot print and throughput have been observed to determine the efficiency of this offline algorithm.

Security Analyses

Entropy Analysis

Entropy is a fundamental metric to validate the uniform spreading of intensity levels in encrypted images. It is a measure of uncertainty which indicates the degree of randomness. To resist against the statistical attacks, entropy of the encrypted image should be close to the maximum of the pixel intensity. Entropy (H) of an image can be calculated as (2),

$$H = -\sum_{i=1}^{N} P(x_i) \log_2 P(x_i) \qquad (2)$$

Figure 5. Original DICOM image DICOM – 1

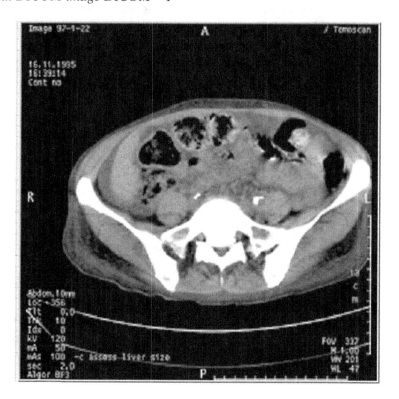

Figure 6. Original DICOM image DICOM – 2

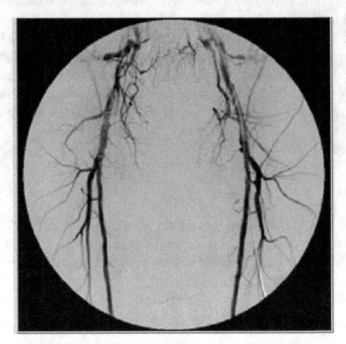

Figure 7. Original DICOM image DICOM – 3

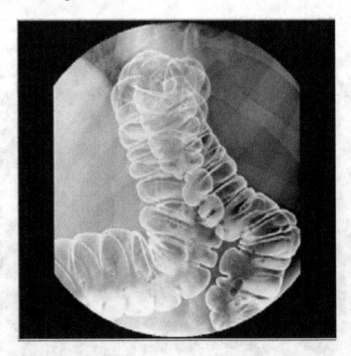

Figure 8. Original DICOM image DICOM – 4

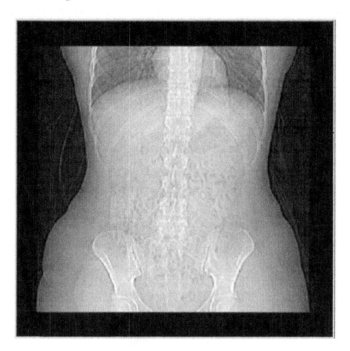

Figure 9. Original DICOM image DICOM - 5

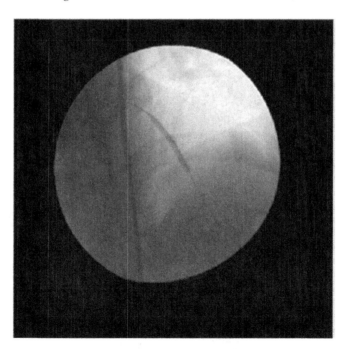

Figure 10. Encrypted DICOM image DICOM – 1

Figure 11. Encrypted DICOM image DICOM – 2

Figure 12. Encrypted ICOM image DICOM – 3

Figure 13. Encrypted DICOM image DICOM – 4

Figure 14. Encrypted DICOM image DICOM - 5

The estimated values are presented in Table 6. In this work, average entropy of the encrypted images is 7.9973 which is close to the ideal entropy of 8 in 8-bit DICOM images.

Correlation Analysis

In an original image or visually good looking image, correlations among the adjacent pixels are very high which constitutes to the readability of the image. To produce an encrypted image, linear relationship between the pixel values should be broken. Correlation analysis is a standard metric to determine the pixel dependencies towards horizontal, vertical and diagonal directions in images. It can be mathematically expressed as (3) – (6),

$$E(x) = \frac{1}{N} \sum_{i=1}^{N} x_i \tag{3}$$

$$D(x) = \frac{1}{N} \sum_{i=1}^{N} (x_i - E(x))^2 \tag{4}$$

$$Cov(x,y) = \frac{1}{N} \sum_{i=1}^{N} (x_i - E(x))(y_i - E(y)) \tag{5}$$

$$\gamma_{xy} = \frac{Cov(x,y)}{\sqrt{D(x)}\sqrt{D(y)}} \tag{6}$$

where,

x,y – Gray level values of two adjacent pixels,

N – Total number of pixels,

γ_{xy} – Cross correlation of two pixels

Table 6 lists the entropy and correlation analyses for five test DICOM images. From Table 6, it is inferred that the implemented encryption scheme has achieved a high entropy and very low correlation to resist against the statistical attacks. Further, the pixel correlations in original and encrypted images of DICOM-1 are presented in Figure 15, Figure 16 and Figure 17, Figure 18, Figure 19 and Figure 20 respectively.

Histogram Analysis

Histogram is a visual inspection of equidistributional of image pixels over the plane. Flat response of the histogram in encrypted images ensures the quality of the encryption in which the original images have unequal histogram response. The encryption yields an uniform distribution of encrypted pixels as shown in Figure 21 and Figure 22.

Keyspace Analysis

Keyspace is referred to the size of keys used in this encryption scheme to resist the brute force attack. In this work, the combination of LFSR and chaotic logistic map possess a wide keyspace portrayed in Table 7.

Key Sensitivity Analysis

Strength of any encryption algorithm depends on the keys. Key must be strong as well as sensitive. Even there is a very small alteration in key should result in a different encrypted output. Table 8 describes the key sensitivity of the encryption algorithm with original and modified keys. Figure 23, Figure 24 and Figure 25 depict two encrypted DICOM – 1 images with modified keyset – I and II and their correspond-

Table 6. Entropy and correlation analyses

Test Images		Entropy	H	V	D
DICOM – 1	Original	4.4251	0.9635	0.9798	0.9503
	Encrypted	**7.9969**	**-0.0010**	**0.0017**	**-0.0033**
DICOM – 2	Original	5.0322	0.9587	0.9449	0.9196
	Encrypted	**7.9968**	**-0.0021**	**0.0025**	**-0.0033**
DICOM – 3	Original	6.3200	0.9809	0.9760	0.9603
	Encrypted	**7.9977**	**-0.0030**	**-0.0049**	**-0.0059**
DICOM – 4	Original	6.5136	0.9898	0.9875	0.9801
	Encrypted	**7.9977**	**0.0045**	**0.0009**	**-0.0048**
DICOM – 5	Original	4.7842	0.9948	0.9933	0.9939
	Encrypted	**7.9978**	**0.0060**	**-0.0080**	**0.0071**
H – Horizontal, V – Vertical & D – Diagonal correlation coefficients					

Figure 15. Horizontal correlation analysis of original DICOM – 1

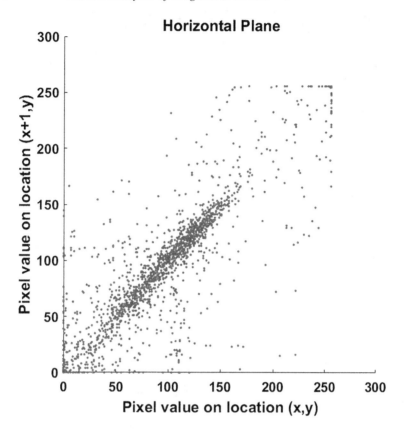

Figure 16. Vertical correlation analysis of original DICOM – 1

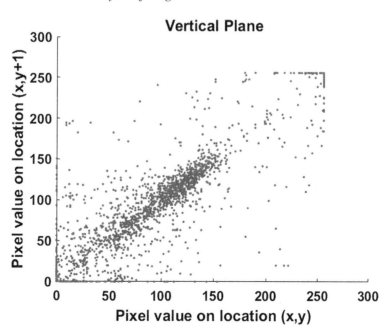

Figure 17. Diagonal correlation analysis of original DICOM – 1

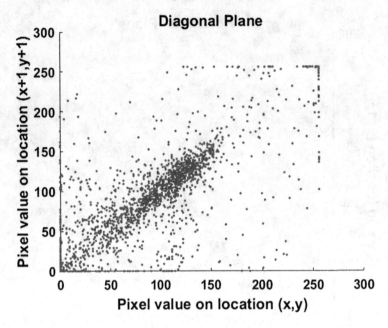

Figure 18. Horizontal correlation analysis of encrypted DICOM – 1

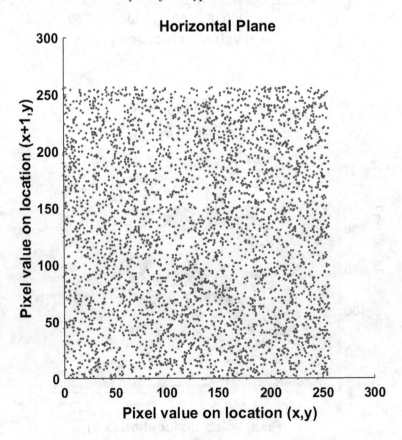

Figure 19. Vertical correlation analysis of encrypted DICOM – 1

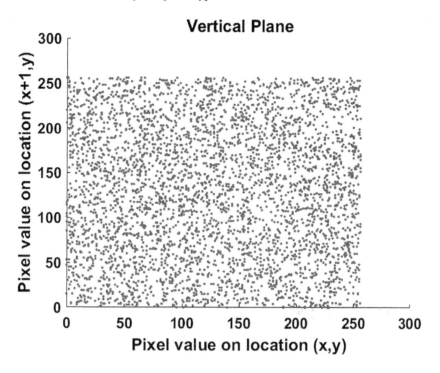

Figure 20. Diagonal correlation analysis of encrypted DICOM – 1

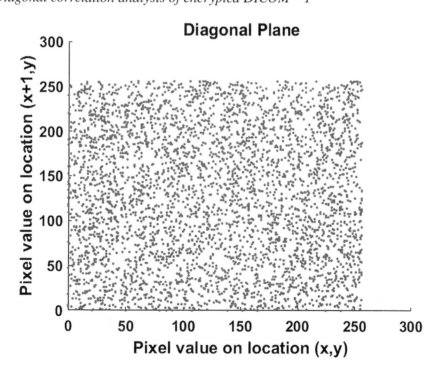

Figure 21. Histogram analysis of Original DICOM – 3

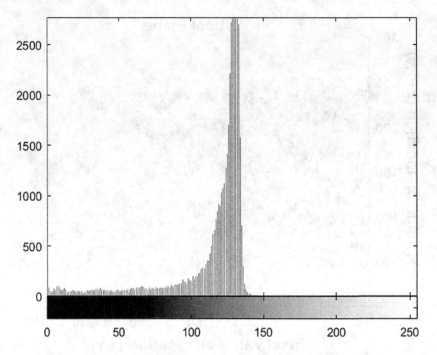

Figure 22. Histogram analysis of Encrypted DICOM -3

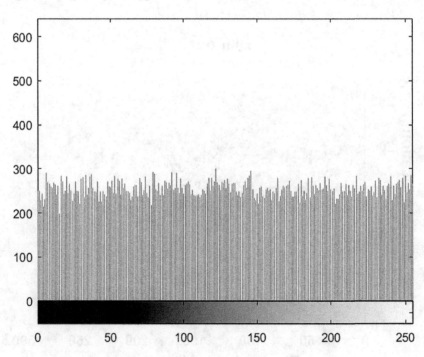

Table 7. Keyspace analysis

Process	No. of Components	Keyspace
Confusion	4 units of LFSR	$2^{14} \times 2^{14} \times 2^{14} \times 2^{14}$
Diffusion	4 units of Chaotic logistic map	$2^{16} \times 2^{16} \times 2^{16} \times 2^{16}$
Total keyspace		2^{120}

Figure 23. Encrypted DICOM – 1 with keyset – I

Figure 24. Encrypted DICOM – 1 with keyset – II

Figure 25. XORed image for Key sensitivity analysis

Table 8. Key sensitivity analysis

Original keyset	LFSR – 1: S_1= 10101011001101, LFSR – 2: S_2= 00101010111101, LFSR – 3: S_3= 111001100010001; LFSR – 4: S_4= 00011101001110 LM – 1: X_1(n) = 000000000000010100; μ_1= 0010011100010000; LM – 2: X_2(n) = 000000000000101000; μ_2= 0010011100010000; LM – 3: X_3(n) = 0000000100101100; μ_3= 0010011100010000; LM – 4: X_4(n) = 000000000000111100; μ_4= 0010011100010000;
Modified keyset - I	LFSR – 1: S_1= 10101011001100, LFSR – 2: S_2= 00101010111100, LFSR – 3: S_3= 111001100010000; LFSR – 4: S_4= 00011101001111 LM – 1: X_1(n) = 000000000000010100; μ_1= 0010011100010000; LM – 2: X_2(n) = 000000000000101000; μ_2= 0010011100010000; LM – 3: X_3(n) = 0000000100101100; μ_3= 0010011100010000; LM – 4: X_4(n) = 000000000000111100; μ_4= 0010011100010000;
Modified keyset - II	LFSR – 1: S_1= 10101011001111, LFSR – 2: S_2= 00101010111111, LFSR – 3: S_3= 111001100010011; LFSR – 4: S_4= 00011101001100 LM – 1: X_1(n) = 000000000000010100; μ_1= 0010011100010000; LM – 2: X_2(n) = 000000000000101000; μ_2= 0010011100010000; LM – 3: X_3(n) = 0000000100101100; μ_3= 0010011100010000; LM – 4: X_4(n) = 000000000000111100; μ_4= 0010011100010000;

ing key sensitivity analysis. Figure 25 represents the XOR operation between the two encrypted images which confirms that the algorithm produces different results even for a one bit change in the key bits.

Chosen Plain Text Analysis

Usually XOR operation is preferred for performing diffusion because of its reversibility. Hence, it is necessary to crosscheck the vulnerability of XOR operation through chosen plain text attack. In this analysis, two encrypted images and corresponding original images are XORed together and compared with each other to find the encryption traces. If the algorithm only uses the XOR operation, it can be broken very easily through chosen plain text attack analysis. This analysis can be defined as (7),

$$C_1 (x, y) \text{ XOR } C_2 (x, y) = P_1 (x, y) \text{ XOR } P_2 (x, y) \tag{7}$$

where C1 and C2 are encrypted DICOM images corresponding to the original images P1 and P2. In this work, DICOM – 1 and DICOM – 2 images were considered for this analysis and the results have been shown in Figure 26 and Figure 27. Since the algorithm uses LFSR and chaos assisted DNA coding, the algorithm is resistant against the chosen plain text attack.

From the results, it is inferred that this encryption scheme achieves near zero correlation, average entropy of 7.9964 and a Keyspace of 2^{176} which ensures the strength of the implemented method to withstand statistical and brute force attacks. Moreover, the equi-distribution generated from this cryptosystem is witnessed through the flat histogram. Further, the suggested approach outperforms the earlier works (Ravichandran et al, 2016, Lima et al, 2015, Praveenkumar et al, 2015 and Zhang et al, 2014) which is depicted in Table 9.

Figure 26. Chosen plain text attack P_1 XOR P_2

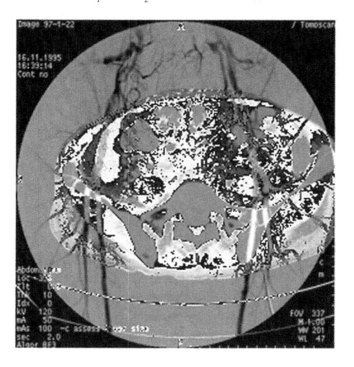

Figure 27. Chosen plain text attack C_1 XOR C_2

Table 9. Performance Comparison

Earlier Works	Techniques	Correlation		
		Horizontal (H)	Vertical (V)	Diagonal (D)
Ravichandran et al, 2016	Combined Chaotic map	-0.0519	-0.0385	0.0004
Lima et al, 2015	Cosine number transform	0.0056	0.0132	-0.0006
Praveenkumar et al, 2015	LSIC + DGT + Rubik	0.0033	-0.0033	0.0117
Zhang et al, 2014	Hyperchaotic system	0.0193	-0.0154	0.0032
Implemented work	LFSR + DNA + 1D Chaotic map	**-0.0010**	**0.0017**	**-0.0033**

Hardware Implementation Analyses

FPGA Implementation

Both reconfigurable hardware and customized microcontroller have been utilized for implementing this medical image encryption approach towards enhancing the confidentiality. Hardware details on Cyclone IV EP4CE115F29C7 FPGA include logic elements, Look Up Tables (LUTs), Flip Flops, combinational logic functions, Phase Locked Loops (PLLs) and memory bits. These details were gathered through the EDA tool Intel Quartus II. The FPGA implementation begins with the design entry developed using VHDL. After performing functional simulation of the architecture using Modelsim software, the HDL code was loaded into Quartus tool to generate the netlist. Upon analyzing the post synthesis hardware utilization summary and RTL schematics, pin planner was used to map the required I/O pins. Fitter ensured the capability of device to hold the suggested architecture and assembler generated the SRAM Object File (.sof) required for reconfiguring the FPGA. Noticeably, this .sof file can be transmitted to the authorized user who will access the medical images upon programming this file on a specific FPGA. In this process, the approach ensures a twofold tamper resistant security through bitstream and hardware dependencies. Table 10 shows the utilized hardware resources in addition to the power dissipation. It was inferred that the design has used 21,870 logic elements and dissipated a total power of 137.74 mW.

Speed of the design is measured through throughput analysis. It is defined as the number of data produced in a second which can be calculated as (8),

$$Tp = \frac{Total\ number\ of\ encrypted\ bits}{Time\ taken\ to\ produce\ the\ bits} \tag{8}$$

Since this method adopts concurrency, all the four 128×128 blocks of original image have been encrypted simultaneously. This inference has further been verified by performing timing analysis captured through Zero Plus logic analyzer shown in Figure 28. Operating clock of 50 MHz has been used to carryout the encryption and the throughput for encrypting 256×256 DICOM image is estimated as 79.4375 Mbps wherein all the four 128×128 blocks require a overlapping 6.6 ms for encrypting 65,536 pixels.

Table 10. Hardware analyses

Target device		Cyclone IV EP4CE115F29C7 FPGA
Operating frequency		50 MHz
Logic utilization (1,14,480)	Logic elements	21,870
	Registers	1,231
	Memory bits	10,48,576
Power dissipation (mW)	Static power	99.94
	Dynamic power	4.71
	I/O power	33.09

Figure 28. Timing analysis

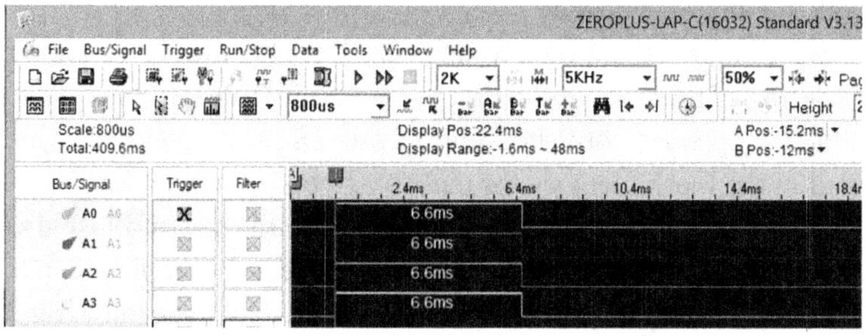

Microcontroller Implementation

The DICOM image encryption scheme was also implemented on *STM32F407IG* microcontroller residing on MCBSTM32F400 evaluation board. This device contains a high performance Cortex-M4 core that can operate at a maximum frequency of 168 MHz. The available 1 MB Flash for code storage and 192 KB of data storage marks the device suitability for memory intensive applications. The embedded 'C' code for the DICOM image encryption was developed under the professional edition of µvision4 Keil MDK platform and the .hex file produced after the compilation was loaded in to the on-chip Flash memory using the 20-pin Segger J-link debugger unit.

The input DICOM image (original image) of size 256×256 with 8-bit pixels was stored in on-chip Flash memory in the form of a two-dimensional look-up table. Pixels of every 128×128 block in the original image were scrambled on-the-fly during its transfer from on-chip Flash memory to the on-chip SRAM in the sequence guided by a 14-bit LFSR circuit. The keys generated by the 1D-logistic map were used to access the DNA encoding look-up table from on-chip Flash memory to perform first level of diffusion on the confused pixels using the DNA addition process. Further, the XOR based diffusion process between the encoded pixels and 8-bit keys obtained from the 8-bit LSBs of LFSR output stores the final encrypted DICOM image in on-chip SRAM.

The analysis on the embedded software includes the code size occupied by the algorithm in various on-chip memory regions of the target microcontroller device and the computational time taken by the device to produce a complete encrypted image. The options were chosen in Keil MDK in order to

Table 11. Embedded software analyses

Target device			STM32F407IG Microcontroller with Cortex-M4 Core
Operating frequency			50 MHz
On-chip Memory utilization (Bytes)		Flash Code	1248
		Flash Data	65992
		SRAM Data	83640
Performance Metrics		CPU cycles	16836619
		Computational Time (ms)	336.732
		Throughput (Mbps)	1.55698

instruct the compiler to utilize optimized assembly instructions that results in faster execution at a cost of minimal rise in code memory occupancy.

The above analyses were carried out on five different DICOM images of dimension 256×256 with 8-bit pixel values. In terms of memory utilization presented in Table 11, Flash code is the number of bytes required to store the opcodes corresponding to this DICOM image encryption algorithm. The memory area occupied in the Flash memory for the storage of DNA encoding look-up table and pixels of input DICOM image were the major items that contribute to the size of Flash data. The total on-chip SRAM area used to store a 128×128 block of confused image, the complete 256×256 encrypted image along with pseudo random output from LFSR, chaotic keys, etc. determine the size of SRAM data.

Execution performance of the DICOM image encryption algorithm when implemented as sequential embedded software on the microcontroller platform can be measured in three dimensions. The number of CPU cycles provides a generic mechanism to represent the performance which is independent of the device operating frequency. A direct measure of performance is given in terms of obtained computational time when the device was operated at 50 MHz. Finally, the throughput analysis given by the equation (8) validates the actual speed of the device to perform image encryption. On comparing the throughput and computational time, it is evident that the concurrent realization of encryption on multiple blocks of the input image with FPGA resulted in the performance improvement over the sequential execution of embedded software on the microcontroller platform. The analysis on memory utilization and performance metrics of the embedded software were carried out on five different input DICOM images as shown in Figures.5 – 9. As the size of all input DICOM images being equal, no variation in terms of memory occupancy and execution performance was noticed when implemented on Cortex-M4 based *STM32F407IG* microcontroller.

CONCLUSION

Medical image protection needs to be accomplished by the combined efforts of confidentiality, integrity and authentication. There exists a necessity to introspect the hardware standalone hardware utilization for implementation of security algorithms of medical images. This chapter discussed the various implementation and security aspects of confidential sharing of DICOM image format using FPGA and Microcontroller. Each hardware has its own set of features and purpose but a comparison can open up discussion on merits and trade-offs while one tries to utilize any of these platforms. In the scheme chosen for analysis, LFSR circuit performed the confusion and DNA coding executed the diffusion using 1D chaotic logistic map as rule selection unit. On FPGA realization, it was inferred that 21,870 logic elements including 1,231 registers were utilized on Cyclone IV FPGA which took 6.6 ms for encrypting 256x256 grayscale DICOM image with 50 MHz operating frequency. On the Microcontroller implementation, 1,248 flash code memory bytes and 65,992 flash data bytes were utilized by taking a computational time of 336.732 ms for encrypting the same size DICOM image with 50 MHz operating frequency. Due to the concurrent architecture on FPGA, it offered a throughput of 79.4375 Mbps which was 1.55698 Mbps in Microcontroller platform due to the sequential execution. When .sof was required for retrieving the encrypted image from the FPGA, .hex file was required in the case of microcontroller. Both these platforms promise a tamper resistant and hardware dependent approach for confidential sharing of DICOM images which will enhance the existing software centric approaches on DICOM image encryption schemes.

REFERENCES

Abdellatif, K. M., Chotin-Avot, R., & Mehrez, H. (2014). Authenticated encryption on FPGAs from the static part to the reconfigurable part. *Microprocessors and Microsystems, 38*(6), 526–538. doi:10.1016/j.micpro.2014.03.006

Chen, C., Ma, H., Chen, H., Meng, Y., & Ding, Q. (2015). FPGA implementation of a UPT chaotic signal generator for image encryption. *Pacific Science Review A. Natural Science and Engineering, 17*(3), 97–102. doi:10.1016/j.psra.2016.02.001

Chen, X., & Hu, C. J. (2017). Adaptive medical image encryption algorithm based on multiple chaotic mapping. *Saudi Journal of Biological Sciences, 24*(8), 1821–1827. doi:10.1016/j.sjbs.2017.11.023 PMID:29551931

Das, A. K., Hajra, S., & Mandal, M. K. (2018). RGB image encryption using microcontroller ATMEGA 32. *Microsystem Technologies, 5*(3980), 1–9. doi:10.100700542-018-3980-5

Hu, J., & Han, F. (2009). A pixel-based scrambling scheme for digital medical images protection. *Journal of Network and Computer Applications, 32*(4), 788–794. doi:10.1016/j.jnca.2009.02.009

Hua, Z., Yi, S., & Zhou, Y. (2018). Medical image encryption using high-speed scrambling and pixel adaptive diffusion. *Signal Processing, 144*, 134–144. doi:10.1016/j.sigpro.2017.10.004

Ismail, S. M., Said, L. A., Rezk, A. A., Radwan, A. G., Madian, A. H., Abu-Elyazeed, M. F., & Soliman, A. M. (2017). Generalized fractional logistic map encryption system based on FPGA. *AEÜ. International Journal of Electronics and Communications, 80*, 114–126. doi:10.1016/j.aeue.2017.05.047

Janakiraman, S., Thenmozhi, K., Rayappan, J. B. B., & Amirtharajan, R. (2018). Lightweight chaotic image encryption algorithm for real-time embedded system: Implementation and analysis on 32-bit microcontroller. *Microprocessors and Microsystems, 56*, 1–12. doi:10.1016/j.micpro.2017.10.013

Kanso, A., & Ghebleh, M. (2015). An efficient and robust image encryption scheme for medical applications. *Communications in Nonlinear Science and Numerical Simulation, 24*(1–3), 98–116. doi:10.1016/j.cnsns.2014.12.005

Laiphrakpam, D. S., & Khumanthem, M. S. (2017). Medical image encryption based on improved El-Gamal encryption technique. *Optik (Stuttgart), 147*, 88–102. doi:10.1016/j.ijleo.2017.08.028

Lima, J. B., Madeiro, F., & Sales, F. J. R. (2015). Encryption of medical images based on the cosine number transform. *Signal Processing Image Communication, 35*, 1–8. doi:10.1016/j.image.2015.03.005

Medical Sample Images. (n.d.). Retrieved from http://www.barre.nom.fr/medical/samples/

Praveenkumar, P., Amirtharajan, R., Thenmozhi, K., & Balaguru Rayappan, J. B. (2015). Medical data sheet in safe havens - A tri-layer cryptic solution. *Computers in Biology and Medicine, 62*, 264–276. doi:10.1016/j.compbiomed.2015.04.031 PMID:25966921

Qasim, A. F., Meziane, F., & Aspin, R. (2018). Digital watermarking: Applicability for developing trust in medical imaging workflows state of the art review. *Computer Science Review, 27*, 45–60. doi:10.1016/j.cosrev.2017.11.003

Rajagopalan, S., Dhamodaran, B., Ramji, A., Francis, C., Venkatraman, S., & Amirtharajan, R. (2017). Confusion and diffusion on FPGA- On chip solution for medical image security. In *Computer Communication and Informatics (ICCCI), 2017 International Conference on* (pp. 1–6). Academic Press.

Rajagopalan, S., Sivaraman, R., Upadhyay, H. N., Rayappan, J. B. B., & Amirtharajan, R. (2018). ON-Chip Peripherals are ON for Chaos--an Image fused Encryption. *Microprocessors and Microsystems, 61*, 257–278. doi:10.1016/j.micpro.2018.06.011

Ramalingam, B., Amirtharajan, R., & Rayappan, J. B. B. (2016). Multiplexed stego path on reconfigurable hardware: A novel random approach. *Computers & Electrical Engineering, 55*, 153–163. doi:10.1016/j.compeleceng.2016.02.010

Ramalingam, B., Rengarajan, A., & Rayappan, J. B. B. (2017). Hybrid image crypto system for secure image communication– A VLSI approach. *Microprocessors and Microsystems, 50*, 1–13. doi:10.1016/j.micpro.2017.02.003

Ravichandran, D., Praveenkumar, P., Balaguru Rayappan, J. B., & Amirtharajan, R. (2016). Chaos based crossover and mutation for securing DICOM image. *Computers in Biology and Medicine, 72*, 170–184. doi:10.1016/j.compbiomed.2016.03.020 PMID:27046666

Ravichandran, D., Rajagopalan, S., Upadhyay, H. N., Rayappan, J. B. B., & Amirtharajan, R. (2018). Encrypted Biography of Biomedical Image-a Pentalayer Cryptosystem on FPGA. *Journal of Signal Processing Systems for Signal, Image, and Video Technology*, 1–27.

Zhang, S., Gao, T., & Gao, L. (2014). A novel encryption frame for medical image with watermark based on hyperchaotic system. *Mathematical Problems in Engineering, 2014*. doi:10.1155/2014/240749

Compilation of References

10 . ways to improve patient data security. (2017). *Medical Economics*. Retrieved October 12, 2018, from http://www.medicaleconomics.com/e-h-r/10-ways-improve-patient-data-security

Abd El-Latif, A. A., Abd-El-Atty, B., & Talha, M. (2017). Robust Encryption of Quantum Medical Images. *IEEE Access: Practical Innovations, Open Solutions*, 6, 1073–1081. doi:10.1109/ACCESS.2017.2777869

Abdellatif, K. M., Chotin-Avot, R., & Mehrez, H. (2014). Authenticated encryption on FPGAs from the static part to the reconfigurable part. *Microprocessors and Microsystems*, 38(6), 526–538. doi:10.1016/j.micpro.2014.03.006

Aberg, P. A., Togawa, T., & Spelman, F. A. (2002). Sensors in Medicine and Healthcare. *Wiley-VCH, 15*(3), 152-169.

Abideen, Z. U., & Shah, M. A. (2017). An IoT based robust healthcare model for continuous health monitoring. In *Proceedings of Automation and Computing (ICAC), 2017 23rd International Conference on* (pp. 1-6). IEEE.

Achanta, R., Shaji, A., Smith, K., Lucchi, A., Fua, P., & Süsstrunk, S. (2012). SLIC Superpixels Compared to State-of-the-Art Superpixel Methods. *IEEE Transactions on Pattern Analysis and Machine Intelligence*, 34(11), 2274–2282. doi:10.1109/TPAMI.2012.120 PMID:22641706

Addison, P. S. (2005). Wavelet transforms and the ECG: A review. *Physiological Measurement*, 26(5), R155–R199. doi:10.1088/0967-3334/26/5/R01 PMID:16088052

Agrawal, S., Panda, R., Bhuyan, S., & Panigrahi, B. K. (2013). Tsallis entropy based optimal multilevel thresholding using cuckoo search algorithm. *Swarm and Evolutionary Computation. Elsevier, 11*(1), 16–30. doi:10.1016/j.swevo.2013.02.001

Agrawal, S., Panda, R., & Dora, L. (2014). A study on fuzzy clustering for magnetic resonance brain image segmentation using soft computing approaches. *Applied Soft Computing*, 24, 522–533. doi:10.1016/j.asoc.2014.08.011

Ahirwar, A. (2013). Study of Techniques used for Medical Image Segmentation and Computation of Statistical Test for Region Classification of Brain MRI. *International Journal Of Information Technology And Computer Science*, 5(5), 44–53. doi:10.5815/ijitcs.2013.05.06

Ahmad, F., & Mahmod, R. (2013). Security Analysis of Blowfish Algorithm. *Informatics and Applications (ICIA), Second International Conference*.

Ahmed, S., & Sengar, S. (2016). Right to privacy- Is Uidai a violation of an individual's 'fundamental right'? *The World Journal on Juristic Polity*. Retrieved from http://jurip.org/wp-content/uploads/2016/12/Sabreen-Ahmed.pdf

Airfares, W., Bouyakhf, E., Herbulot, A., Regragui, F., & Devy, M. (2013). Hybrid region and interest points-based active contour for object tracking. *Applied Mathematical Sciences*, 7, 5879–5899. doi:10.12988/ams.2013.38483

Ajit Kapur v. Union of India. (2017) 2 ABR 140 (India).

Akyildiz, I. F., Su, W., Sankarasubramaniam, Y., & Cayirci, E. (2002). Wireless sensor networks: A survey. *Computer Networks*, *38*(4), 393–422. doi:10.1016/S1389-1286(01)00302-4

Al Ameen, M., Liu, J., & Kwak, K. (2012). Security and privacy issues in wireless sensor networks for healthcare applications. *Journal of Medical Systems*, *36*(1), 93–101. doi:10.100710916-010-9449-4 PMID:20703745

Alaa, M., Zaidan, A. A., Zaidan, B. B., Talal, M., & Kiah, M. L. M. (2017). A review of smart home applications based on Internet of Things. *Journal of Network and Computer Applications*, *97*, 48–65. doi:10.1016/j.jnca.2017.08.017

Alabaichi, A., Ahmad, F., & Mahmod, R. (2013, September). Security analysis of blowfish algorithm. In *Informatics and Applications (ICIA), 2013 Second International Conference on* (pp. 12-18). IEEE. 10.1109/ICoIA.2013.6650222

Al-Fahoum, A. S. (2006). Quality assessment of ECG compression techniques using a wavelet-based diagnostic measure. *IEEE Transactions on Information Technology in Biomedicine*, *10*(1), 182–191. doi:10.1109/TITB.2005.855554 PMID:16445263

Al-Fahoum, A. S., & Ishijima, M. (1993). Fundamentals of the decision of optimum factors in the ECG data compression. *IEICE Transactions on Information and Systems*, *E76-D*(12), 1398–1403.

Algeria-Barrero, E., & Algeria-Ezquerra, E. (2008). When to perform pre-operative ECG. European Society of Cardiology, 7(3).

Alickovic, E., & Subasi, A. (2016). Medical decision support system for diagnosis of heart arrhythmia using DWT and random forests classifier. *Journal of Medical Systems*, *40*(4), 108. doi:10.100710916-016-0467-8 PMID:26922592

Ali, H., Rada, L., & Badshah, N. (2018). Image Segmentation for Intensity Inhomogeneity in the presence of High Noise. *IEEE Transactions on Image Processing*, *27*(8), 3729–3738. doi:10.1109/TIP.2018.2825101 PMID:29698205

Ali, M., Ahn, C. W., Pant, M., & Siarry, P. (2015). An image watermarking scheme in wavelet domain with optimized compensation of singular value decomposition via artificial bee colony. *Information Sciences*, *301*, 44–60. doi:10.1016/j.ins.2014.12.042

Alonso-Atienza, F., Morgado, E., Fernandez-Martinez, L., Garcia-Alberola, A., & Rojo-Alvarez, J. L. (2014). Detection of life-threatening arrhythmias using feature selection and support vector machines. *IEEE Transactions on Biomedical Engineering*, *61*(3), 832–840. doi:10.1109/TBME.2013.2290800 PMID:24239968

Amrouche, C., & Rejaiba, A. (2015). Navier-Stokes equations with Navier boundary condition. *Mathematical Methods in the Applied Sciences*, *39*(17), 5091–5112. doi:10.1002/mma.3338

An Introduction to what is Internet of Things. (2017, August 31). Retrieved from https://www.eduonix.com/blog/internet-of-things/introduction-internet-things-iot/

Anees, A., Siddiqui, A. M., Ahmed, J., & Hussain, I. (2014). A technique for digital steganography using chaotic maps. *Nonlinear Dynamics*, *75*(4), 807–816. doi:10.100711071-013-1105-3

Appari & Johnson. (2010). Information Security and Privacy in Healthcare: Current State of Research. *Int. J. Internet and Enterprise Management*. Retrieved from www.ists.dartmouth.edu

Azizi, A., & Elkourd, K. (2016). Fast Region-based Active Contour Model Driven by Local Signed Pressure Force. *ELCVIA. Electronic Letters on Computer Vision and Image Analysis*, *15*(1), 1. doi:10.5565/rev/elcvia.794

Baali, H., Akmeliawati, R., Salami, M. J. E., Aibinu, M., & Gani, A. (2011). Transform based approach for ECG period normalization. *Computers in Cardiology*, *38*(2), 533–536.

Babu, A. K. (2015). A Survey on the Role of IoT and Cloud in Health Care. *International Journal of Scientific Engineering and Technology Research, 4*(12), 2217–2219.

Baig, M. Y., Lai, E. M., & Punchihewa, A. (2012). Compressive Video Coding: A Review of the State-Of-The-Art. In Video Compression. InTech.

Baker, C. R., Armijo, K., Belka, S., Benhabib, M., Bhargava, V., Burkhart, N., ... Ho, C. (2007, May). Wireless sensor networks for home health care. In *21st International Conference on Advanced Information Networking and Applications Workshops (AINAW'07)* (Vol. 2, pp. 832-837). IEEE. 10.1109/AINAW.2007.376

Banerjee, S., & Mitra, M. (2014). Application of cross wavelet transform for ECG pattern analysis and classification. *IEEE Transactions on Instrumentation and Measurement, 63*(2), 326–333. doi:10.1109/TIM.2013.2279001

Baraniuk, R. G. (2007). Compressive sensing. *IEEE Signal Processing Magazine, 24*(4), 118–121. doi:10.1109/MSP.2007.4286571

Baritha Begum, M., & Venkataramani, Y. (2012). LSB based audio steganography based on text compression. *Procedia Engineering, 30*(2011), 702–710. doi:10.1016/j.proeng.2012.01.917

Beheri, M. H., Amin, M., Song, X., & El-latif, A. A. A. (2016). Quantum image encryption based on Scrambling- Diffusion (SD) approach. *Frontiers of Signal Processing (ICFSP)*, (2), 43–47.

Beneš, M., & Kučera, P. (2015). Solutions to the Navier-Stokes equations with mixed boundary conditions in two-dimensional bounded domains. *Mathematische Nachrichten, 289*(2-3), 194–212. doi:10.1002/mana.201400046

Benitez, D., Gaydecki, P. A., Zaidi, A., & Fitzpatrick, A. P. (2001). The use of the Hilbert transform in ECG signal analysis. *Computers in Biology and Medicine, 31*(5), 399–406. doi:10.1016/S0010-4825(01)00009-9 PMID:11535204

Berkaya, S. K., Uysal, A. K., Gunal, E. S., Ergin, S., Gunal, S., & Gulmezoglu, M. B. (2018). A survey on ECG Analysis. *Biomedical Signal Processing and Control, 43*, 216–235. doi:10.1016/j.bspc.2018.03.003

Bhardwaj, C., Ji, U., & Sood, M. (2017). Implementation and Performance Assessment of Compressed Sensing for Images and Video Signals. *Journal of Global Pharma Technology, 6*(9), 123–133.

Bhatt, M. U., & Bamniya, K. (2015). *Medical Image Compression and Reconstruction Using Compressive Sensing.* Academic Press.

Bilal, M., Ahmed, A. H., Shah, J. A., Kadir, K., & Ayob, M. Z. (2017, September). Comparison of L 1-norm surrogate functions used for the recovery of MR images. In *Engineering Technology and Technopreneurship (ICE2T), 2017 International Conference on* (pp. 1-4). IEEE.

Bilgin, A., Marcellin, M. W., & Altbach, M. I. (2003). Compression of electrocardiogram signals using JPEG2000. *IEEE Transactions on Consumer Electronics, 49*(4), 833–840. doi:10.1109/TCE.2003.1261162

Biswas, H. R. (2013). One dimensional chaotic dynamical systems. *J Pure Appl Math Adv Appl, 10*(1), 69–101.

Blumensath, T., & Davies, M. E. (2009). Iterative hard thresholding for compressed sensing. *Applied and Computational Harmonic Analysis, 27*(3), 265–274. doi:10.1016/j.acha.2009.04.002

Bohonos, S. L. (2007). Universal real-time navigational assistance (URNA): an urban bluetooth beacon for the blind. In *1st ACM SIGMOBILE international workshop on Systems and networking support for healthcare and assisted living environments* (pp. 83-88). New York: ACM.

Bormann, Z. S. (2009). *6LoWPAN: The Wireless Embedded Internet* (1st ed.). London: Wiley.

Bucerzan, D., & Raţiu, C. (2016). Reliable Metrics for Image LSB Steganography on Mobile Platforms. *International Workshop Soft Computing Applications*, 517-528.

Buettner, M., Yee, G. V., Anderson, E., & Han, R. (2006). X-MAC: a short preamble MAC protocol for duty-cycled wireless sensor networks. In *4th international conference on Embedded networked sensor systems* (pp. 307-320). ACM.

Candès, E. J., Romberg, J., & Tao, T. (2006). Robust uncertainty principles: Exact signal reconstruction from highly incomplete frequency information. *IEEE Transactions on Information Theory*, *52*(2), 489–509. doi:10.1109/TIT.2005.862083

Candes, E. J., & Tao, T. (2006). Near-optimal signal recovery from random projections: Universal encoding strategies? *IEEE Transactions on Information Theory*, *52*(12), 5406–5425. doi:10.1109/TIT.2006.885507

Candès, E. J., & Wakin, M. B. (2008). An introduction to compressive sampling. *IEEE Signal Processing Magazine*, *25*(2), 21–30. doi:10.1109/MSP.2007.914731

Candes, E., & Romberg, J. (2007). Sparsity and incoherence in compressive sampling. *Inverse Problems*, *23*(3), 969–985. doi:10.1088/0266-5611/23/3/008

Caponetti, L., Castellano, G., & Corsini, V. (2017). MR Brain Image Segmentation: A Framework to Compare Different Clustering Techniques. *Information*, *8*(4), 138. doi:10.3390/info8040138

Carletti, V., Greco, A., Saggese, A., & Vento, M. (2017, September). A Smartphone-Based System for Detecting Falls Using Anomaly Detection. In *International Conference on Image Analysis and Processing* (pp. 490-499). Springer. 10.1007/978-3-319-68548-9_45

Carr, J. J., & Brown, J. M. (2004). *Introduction to biomedical equipment technology* (4th ed.). Pearson Education.

Chai, X., Zheng, X., Gan, Z., Han, D., & Chen, Y. (2018). An image encryption algorithm based on chaotic system and compressive sensing. *Signal Processing*, *148*, 124–144. doi:10.1016/j.sigpro.2018.02.007

Chan, C. K., & Cheng, L. M. (2004). Hiding data in images by simple LSB substitution. *Pattern Recognition*, *37*(3), 469–474. doi:10.1016/j.patcog.2003.08.007

Chang, C. H., & Ji, J. (2010, August). Improved compressed sensing MRI with multi-channel data using reweighted l 1 minimization. In *Engineering in Medicine and Biology Society (EMBC), 2010 Annual International Conference of the IEEE* (pp. 875-878). IEEE.

Chang, C. C., & Lu, T. C. (2006). A difference expansion oriented data hiding scheme for restoring the original host images. *Journal of Systems and Software*, *79*(12), 1754–1766. doi:10.1016/j.jss.2006.03.035

Chang, C. C., Tai, W. L., & Lin, C. C. (2006). A reversible data hiding scheme based on side match vector quantization. *IEEE Transactions on Circuits and Systems for Video Technology*, *6*(10), 1301–1308. doi:10.1109/TCSVT.2006.882380

Cheddad, A., Condell, J., Curran, K., & Mc Kevitt, P. (2010). Digital image steganography: Survey and analysis of current methods. *Signal Processing*, *90*(3), 727–752. doi:10.1016/j.sigpro.2009.08.010

Chen, B., Luo, H., Zhao, Z., & Zhang, X. (2014). Halftone image encryption based on reversible pairwise swapping. *Measurement: Journal of the International Measurement Confederation*, *57*(38), 85–93. doi:10.1016/j.measurement.2014.07.013

Chen, C. C., & Chang, C. C. (2010). High capacity SMVQ-based hiding scheme using adaptive index. *Signal Processing*, *90*(7), 2141–2149. doi:10.1016/j.sigpro.2010.01.018

Chen, C., Ma, H., Chen, H., Meng, Y., & Ding, Q. (2015). FPGA implementation of a UPT chaotic signal generator for image encryption. *Pacific Science Review A. Natural Science and Engineering*, *17*(3), 97–102. doi:10.1016/j.psra.2016.02.001

Cheng, H. D., Chen, J.-R., & Li, J. (1998). Threshold selection based on fuzzy c-partition entropy approach. *Pattern Recognition*, *31*(7), 857–870. doi:10.1016/S0031-3203(97)00113-1

Cheng, H. D., & Lui, Y. M. (1997). Automatic bandwidth selection of fuzzy membership functions. *Information Sciences*, *103*(1–4), 1–21. doi:10.1016/S0020-0255(97)00057-1

Cheng, S.-T., & Chang, T.-Y. (2012). An adaptive learning scheme for load balancing with zone partition in multi-sink wireless sensor network. *Expert Systems with Applications*, *39*(10), 9427–9434. doi:10.1016/j.eswa.2012.02.119

Chen, J., & Itoh, S. (1998). A wavelet transform-based ECG compression method guaranteeing desired signal quality. *IEEE Transactions on Biomedical Engineering*, *45*(12), 1414–1419. doi:10.1109/10.730435 PMID:9835190

Chen, M., Gonzalez, S., Vasilakos, A., Cao, H., & Leung, V. C. (2011). Body area networks: A survey. *Mobile Networks and Applications*, *16*(2), 171–193. doi:10.100711036-010-0260-8

Chen, S. T., Guo, Y. J., Huang, H. N., Kung, W. M., Tseng, K. K., & Tu, S. Y. (2014). Hiding patients confidential data in the ECG signal viaa transform-domain quantization scheme. *Journal of Medical Systems*, *38*(6), 1–8. doi:10.100710916-014-0054-9 PMID:24395031

Chen, S., Hua, W., Li, Z., Li, J., & Gao, X. (2017). Heartbeat classification using projected and dynamic features of ECG signal. *Biomedical Signal Processing and Control*, *31*, 165–173. doi:10.1016/j.bspc.2016.07.010

Chen, X., & Hu, C. J. (2017). Adaptive medical image encryption algorithm based on multiple chaotic mapping. *Saudi Journal of Biological Sciences*, *24*(8), 1821–1827. doi:10.1016/j.sjbs.2017.11.023 PMID:29551931

Chen, Z. (2013). *A New Detection Model for Saliency Map. TELKOMNIKA Indonesian Journal of Electrical Engineering.* doi:10.11591/telkomnika.v11i11.3582

Cherukuri, S., Venkatasubramanian, K. K., & Gupta, S. K. (2003, October). Biosec: A biometric based approach for securing communication in wireless networks of biosensors implanted in the human body. In *Parallel Processing Workshops, 2003. Proceedings. 2003 International Conference on* (pp. 432-439). IEEE. 10.1109/ICPPW.2003.1240399

Cho, Y. B., Lee, S. H., & Woo, S. H. (2014, June). Security Issues Using Remote Medical Treatment in Health Care Information. In International Conference on Future Information & Communication Engineering (Vol. 6, No. 1, pp. 193-196). Academic Press.

Chouffani, R. (2016, November). *Can we expect the Internet of Things in healthcare?* Retrieved from http://internetofthingsagenda.techtarget.com/feature/Can-we-expect-the-Internet-of-Things-in-healthcare

Chou, H. H., Chen, Y. J., Shiau, Y. C., & Kuo, T. S. (2006). An effective and efficient compression algorithm for ECG signals with irregular periods. *IEEE Transactions on Biomedical Engineering*, *53*(6), 1198–1205. doi:10.1109/TBME.2005.863961 PMID:16761849

Coatrieux, G., Lecornu, L., Sankur, B., & Roux, C. (2006). A review of image watermarking applications in healthcare. *IEEE 28th Annual International Conference on Engineering in Medicine and Biology Society*, 4691-4694.

Coatrieux, G., Maitre, H., & Sankur, B. (2001). Strict integrity control of biomedical images. International Society for Optics and Photonics: Security and watermarking of multimedia contents, 4314, 229-240.

Confederation of Indian Alcoholic Beverages Companies v. State of Bihar, 2016 (4) PLJR 369 (India).

Cormen, T. H., Leiserson, C. E., Rivest, R. L., & Stein, C. (2001). Introduction to Algorithms (2nd ed.). MIT Press and McGraw-Hill.

Corso, J. J., Sharon, E., Dube, S., El-Saden, S., Sinha, U., & Yuille, A. (2008). Efficient multilevel brain tumor segmentation with integrated bayesian model classification. *IEEE Transactions on Medical Imaging, 27*(5), 629–640. doi:10.1109/TMI.2007.912817 PMID:18450536

Coughlan, J. (2007). Color targets: Fiducials to help visually impaired people find their way by camera phone. *EURASIP Journal on Image and Video Processing, 12*(1), 96–111.

Cromwell, L., Weibell, F. J., & Pfeiffer, E. A. (1980). *Biomedical instrumentation and measurements*. Prentice Hall.

Cui, Z., & Fan, Q. (2018). A "Nonconvex+Nonconvex" approach for image restoration with impulse noise removal. *Applied Mathematical Modelling, 62*, 254–271. doi:10.1016/j.apm.2018.05.035

Curtis, D., Shih, E., Waterman, J., Guttag, J., Bailey, J., Stair, T., . . . Ohno-Machado, L. (2008, March). Physiological signal monitoring in the waiting areas of an emergency room. In *Proceedings of the ICST 3rd international conference on Body area networks* (p. 5). ICST (Institute for Computer Sciences, Social-Informatics and Telecommunications Engineering). Available online on: http:// Minnie.tuhs .org/NetSec/Slides

Das, A. K., Hajra, S., & Mandal, M. K. (2018). RGB image encryption using microcontroller ATMEGA 32. *Microsystem Technologies, 5*(3980), 1–9. doi:10.100700542-018-3980-5

De Chazal, P., O'Dwyer, M., & Reilly, R. B. (2004). Automatic classification of heartbeats using ECG morphology and heartbeat interval features. *IEEE Transactions on Biomedical Engineering, 51*(7), 1196–1206. doi:10.1109/TBME.2004.827359 PMID:15248536

de Chazal, P., & Reilly, R. B. (2006). A patient-adapting heartbeat classifier using ECG morphology and heartbeat interval features. *IEEE Transactions on Biomedical Engineering, 53*(12), 2535–2543. doi:10.1109/TBME.2006.883802 PMID:17153211

De Lannoy, G., François, D., Delbeke, J., & Verleysen, M. (2012). Weighted conditional random fields for supervised interpatient heartbeat classification. *IEEE Transactions on Biomedical Engineering, 59*(1), 241–247. doi:10.1109/TBME.2011.2171037 PMID:21990327

de Oliveira, L. S. C., Andreão, R. V., & Sarcinelli-Filho, M. (2011). Premature ventricular beat classification using a dynamic Bayesian network. *Engineering in Medicine and Biology Society, EMBC, 2011 Annual International Conference of the IEEE*, 4984–4987 10.1109/IEMBS.2011.6091235

De, A., Sharma, D., Mata, S., & Devi, V. (2010). Masking based Segmentation of Diseased MRI Images. *International Conference on Information Science and Applications (ICISA)*, 1–7. 10.1109/ICISA.2010.5480274

Deutsch, D. (1985). Quantum Theory, the Church-Turing Principle and the Universal Quantum Computer. *Proceedings of the Royal Society A: Mathematical, Physical and Engineering Sciences, 400*(1818), 97–117. 10.1098/rspa.1985.0070

Devi, K. J. (2013). *A Sesure Image Steganography Using LSB Technique and Pseudo Random Encoding Technique*. National Institute of Technology-Rourkela Odisha.

Diffie, W., & Hellman, M. (1976). New directions in cryptography. *IEEE Transactions on Information Theory, 22*(6), 644–654. doi:10.1109/TIT.1976.1055638

Digital Signature Standard (DSS). (1994, May 19). Retrieved from FIPS PUB 186: csrc.nist.gov

Dimitriou, T., & Ioannis, K. (2008, October). Security issues in biomedical wireless sensor networks. In *Applied Sciences on Biomedical and Communication Technologies, 2008. ISABEL'08. First International Symposium on* (pp. 1-5). IEEE. 10.1109/ISABEL.2008.4712577

Dimitriou, N., & Delopoulos, A. (2013). Motion-based segmentation of objects using overlapping temporal windows. *Image and Vision Computing, 31*(9), 593–602. doi:10.1016/j.imavis.2013.06.005

Djerou, L., Khelil, N., Dehimi, H. E., & Batouche, M. (2009). Automatic Multilevel Thresholding Using Binary Particle Swarm Optimization for Image Segmentation. In *International Conference of Soft Computing and Pattern Recognition, 2009. SOCPAR '09*. Malacca: IEEE. 10.1109/SoCPaR.2009.25

Dmour, H. A., & Ani, A. A. (2016). Quality optimized medical image information hiding algorithm that employs edge detection and data coding. *Computer Methods and Programs in Biomedicine, 127*, 24–43. doi:10.1016/j.cmpb.2016.01.011 PMID:27000287

Donoho, D. L. (2006). Compressed sensing. *IEEE Transactions on Information Theory, 52*(4), 1289–1306. doi:10.1109/TIT.2006.871582

Dou, W., Ruan, S., Chen, Y., Bloyet, D., & Constans, J.-M. (2007). A framework of fuzzy information fusion for the segmentation of brain tumor tissues on MR images. *Image and Vision Computing, 25*(2), 164–171. doi:10.1016/j.imavis.2006.01.025

Dresher, R., & Irazoqui, P. (2007). A Compact Nanopower Low Output Impedance CMOS Operational Amplifier for Wireless Intraocular Pressure Recordings. In *29th Annual International Conference of the IEEE* (pp. 6055-6058). Engineering in Medicine and Biology Society. 10.1109/IEMBS.2007.4353729

Dunbar, B. (2002). *Steganographic A detailed look at*. Sans Institute.

Dunkels, A., Gr¨onvall, B., & Voigt, T. (2004). Contiki - a lightweight and flexible operating system for tiny networked sensors. In *First IEEE Workshop on Embedded Networked Sensors (Emnets-I)* (pp. 15-26). IEEE. 10.1109/LCN.2004.38

Ebrahimzadeh, A., & Khazaee, A. (2011). Higher order statistics for automated classification of ECG beats. *Electrical and Control Engineering (ICECE), 2011 International Conference on*, 5952–5955. 10.1109/ICECENG.2011.6057059

El Aziz, M. A., & Hassanien, A. E. (2016). Modified cuckoo search algorithm with rough sets for feature selection. *Neural Computing and Applications. Springer, 29*(4), 925–934. doi:10.100700521-016-2473-7

Eldar, Y. C., Kuppinger, P., & Bolcskei, H. (2010). Block-sparse signals: Uncertainty relations and efficient recovery. *IEEE Transactions on Signal Processing, 58*(6), 3042–3054. doi:10.1109/TSP.2010.2044837

ElGamal, T. (1985). A Public-Key Cryptosystem and a Signature Scheme Based on Discrete Logarithms. *IEEE Transactions on Information Theory, 31*(4), 469–472. doi:10.1109/TIT.1985.1057074

Elhaj, F. A., Salim, N., Harris, A. R., Swee, T. T., & Ahmed, T. (2016). Arrhythmia recognition and classification using combined linear and nonlinear features of ECG signals. *Computer Methods and Programs in Biomedicine, 127*, 52–63. doi:10.1016/j.cmpb.2015.12.024 PMID:27000289

El-latif, A. A. A., Abd-el-atty, B., & Talha, M. (2017). *Robust encryption of quantum medical images*. Academic Press.

Emory, F. A., & Lenert, L. A. (2005). MASCAL: RFID Tracking of Patients, Staff and Equipment to Enhance Hospital Response to Mass Casualty Events. In *The AMIA Annual Symposium* (pp. 261-265). AMIA.

Ephemeral Key. (2018, June 7). Retrieved from Wikipedia: https://en.wikipedia.org/wiki/Ephemeral_key

Eskofier, B., Lee, S., Baron, M., Simon, A., Martindale, C., Gaßner, H., & Klucken, J. (2017). An overview of smart shoes in the internet of health things: Gait and mobility assessment in health promotion and disease monitoring. *Applied Sciences, 7*(10), 986. doi:10.3390/app7100986

Eun, S., Jung, E., & Park, D. (2017). Effective Brain Contour Segmentation based on Active Contour Model. *Journal Of Next-Generation Convergence Information Services Technology, 6*(2), 75–88. doi:10.29056/jncist.2017.12.07

Feng, J. B., Lin, I. C., Tsai, C. S., & Chu, Y. P. (2006). Reversible watermarking: Current status and key issues. *International Journal of Network Security, 2*, 161–170.

Feng, W., Li, Y., Gao, S., Yan, Y., & Xue, J. (2016). A Novel Flame Edge Detection Algorithm via A Novel Active Contour Model. *International Journal Of Hybrid Information Technology, 9*(9), 275–282. doi:10.14257/ijhit.2016.9.9.26

Feynman, R. P. (1982). Simulating Physics With Computers By R P Feynman.pdf. *International Journal of Theoretical Physics, 21*(6–7), 467.

Filho, E. B. L., Rodrigues, N. M. M., Silva, E., Faria, S., Da Silva, E. A. B., & De Faria, S. M. M. (1923–1926). … De Carvalho, M. B. (2008). ECG signal compression based on dc equalization and complexity sorting. *IEEE Transactions on Biomedical Engineering, 55*(7), 1923–1926. doi:10.1109/TBME.2008.919880

Foucart, S., & Rauhut, H. (2013). *A mathematical introduction to compressive sensing.* Basel: Birkhäuser.

Francisco Ordonez, J., & Onate, L. (2016). Edge detection image using arm microcontroller. *Ingenius-. Revista de Ciencia y Tecnología, 16*, 30–35. doi:10.17163/ingenius.n16.2016.04

Fridrich, J. (1998). *Symmetric Ciphers Based on Two-Dimensional Chaotic Maps.* Academic Press.

Fu, C., Meng, W., Zhan, Y., Zhu, Z., Lau, F. C. M., Tse, C. K., & Ma, H. (2013). An efficient and secure medical image protection scheme based on chaotic maps. *Computers in Biology and Medicine, 43*(8), 1000–1010. doi:10.1016/j.compbiomed.2013.05.005 PMID:23816172

Fu, C., Zhang, G., Bian, O., Lei, W., & Ma, H. (2014). A Novel Medical Image Protection Scheme Using a 3-Dimensional Chaotic System. *PLoS One, 9*(12), e115773. doi:10.1371/journal.pone.0115773 PMID:25541941

Gao, H., Xu, W., Sun, J., & Tang, Y. (2010). Multilevel Thresholding for Image Segmentation Through an Improved Quantum-Behaved Particle Swarm Algorithm. *IEEE Transactions on Instrumentation and Measurement, 59*(4), 934–946. doi:10.1109/TIM.2009.2030931

Gao, R., Uchida, S., Shahab, A., Shafait, F., & Frinken, V. (2014). Visual Saliency Models for Text Detection in Real World. *PLoS One, 9*(12), e114539. doi:10.1371/journal.pone.0114539 PMID:25494196

Gao, Y., Kikinis, R., Bouix, S., Shenton, M., & Tannenbaum, A. (2012). A 3D interactive multi-object segmentation tool using local robust statistics-driven active contours. *Medical Image Analysis, 16*(6), 1216–1227. doi:10.1016/j.media.2012.06.002 PMID:22831773

Garthner. (2018, May). *Gartner Technical Research.* Retrieved from Internet of Things: http://www.gartner.com/technology/research/internet-of-things/

Gay, D., Levis, P., Von Behren, R., Welsh, M., Brewer, E., & Culler, D. (2014). The nesC language: A holistic approach to networked embedded systems. *ACM SIGPLAN Notices, 49*(4), 41–51. doi:10.1145/2641638.2641652

Georgiadis, P., Cavouras, D., Kalatzis, I., & Daskalakis, A. (2007). Non-linear Least Squares Features Transformation for Improving the Performance of Probabilistic Neural Networks in Classifying Human Brain Tumors on MRI. Computational Science and Its Applications – ICCSA 2007, 239–247. doi:10.1007/978-3-540-74484-9_21

Georgiadis, P., Cavouras, D., Kalatzis, I., Daskalakis, A., Kagadis, G. C., Sifaki, K., … Solomou, E. (2008). Improving brain tumor characterization on MRI by probabilistic neural networks and non-linear transformation of textural features. *Computer Methods and Programs in Biomedicine, 89*(1), 24–32. doi:10.1016/j.cmpb.2007.10.007 PMID:18053610

Ghebleh, M., & Kanso, A. (2014). A robust chaotic algorithm for digital image steganography. *Communications in Nonlinear Science and Numerical Simulation*, *19*(6), 1898–1907. doi:10.1016/j.cnsns.2013.10.014

Global Overview. (2018). Retrieved from https://public.dhe.ibm.com/common/ssi/ecm/55/en/55017055usen/2018-global-codb-report_06271811_55017055USEN.pdf

Gnawali, O., Fonseca, R., Jamieson, K., Moss, D., & Levis, P. (2009). Collection tree protocol. In *7th ACM conference on embedded networked sensor systems* (pp. 1-14). ACM.

Gobind v. State of Madhya Pradesh (July 27, 1992). India.

Gondal, A. H., & Khan, M. N. A. (2013). A review of fully automated techniques for brain tumor detection from MR images. *International Journal of Modern Education and Computer Science. Modern Education and Computer Science Press*, *5*(2), 55–61.

Gurtov, A., Komu, M., & Moskowitz, R. (2009). Host Identity Protocol (HIP): Identifier/locator split for host mobility and multihoming. *Internet Protocol Journal*, *12*(1), 27–32.

Halperin, D., Heydt-Benjamin, T. S., Fu, K., Kohno, T., & Maisel, W. H. (2008). Security and privacy for implantable medical devices. *IEEE Pervasive Computing*, *7*(1), 30–39. doi:10.1109/MPRV.2008.16

Hanjagi, A., Srihari, P., & Rayamane, A. (2007). A public health care information system using GIS and GPS: A case study of Shiggaon. *Springer: GIS for Health and the Environment*, *5*(1), 243–255.

Hansen, R. (2012, Jan.). *Gnu Privacy Guard*. Retrieved from GnuPG: https://www.gnupg.org/faq/gnupg-faq.html#compatible

Hayes, T. O. (2015, August 6). *American Action Forum*. Retrieved from https://www.americanactionforum.org/research/are-electronic-medical-records-worth-the-costs-of-implementation/

Hazewinkel & Michiel. (1994). Cyclic group. In *Encyclopedia of Mathematics*. Springer Science+Business Media B.V. / Kluwer Academic Publishers.

Healthcare Data Breach Statistics. (n.d.). Retrieved September 11, 2018, from https://www.hipaajournal.com/healthcare-data-breach-statistics/

Heer, T. (2007). LHIP lightweight authentication extension for HIP. *IETF*, *12*(3), 290–230.

He, H. (2016). Saliency and depth-based unsupervised object segmentation. *IET Image Processing*, *10*(11), 893–899. doi:10.1049/iet-ipr.2016.0031

Heidari, S., & Naseri, M. (2016). A Novel LSB Based Quantum Watermarking. *International Journal of Theoretical Physics*, *55*(10), 4205–4218. doi:10.100710773-016-3046-3

Helmy, M., El-Rabaie, E.-S. M., Eldokany, I. M., & El-Samie, F. E. A. (2017). 3-D Image Encryption Based on Rubik's Cube and RC6 Algorithm. *3D Research, 8*(4), 38.

Hemalatha, R., Radha, S., Raghuvarman, N., Soumya, B., & Vivekanandan, B. (2013). Energy Efficient Image Transmission over Bandwidth Scarce WSN using Compressed Sensing. *International Conference on IT and Intelligent Systems,* 57-61.

Hemanth, D. J., Vijila, C. K. S., Selvakumar, A. I., & Anitha, J. (2013). Distance metric-based time-efficient fuzzy algorithm for abnormal magnetic resonance brain image segmentation. *Neural Computing & Applications*, *22*(5), 1013–1022. doi:10.100700521-011-0792-2

Hidayatullah, H. M. (1984). Constitutional law of India. New Delhi: Bar Council of India Trust.

Hil, J., Szewczyk, R., Woo, A., Hollar, S., Culler, D., & Pister, K. (2000). System architecture directions for network sensors. *Operating Systems Review*, *34*(5), 93–104. doi:10.1145/384264.379006

Hodgetts, T., & Mackaway-Jones, K. (1995). *Major Incident Medical Management and Support, the Practical Approach*. BMJ Publishing Group.

Hongmei, T., Cuixia, W., Liying, H., & Xia, W. (2010). Image Segmentation Based on Improved PSO. In *International Conference on Computer and Communication Technologies in Agriculture Engineering Image*. Chengdue: IEEE.

Hong, W., & Chen, T. S. (2012). A novel data embedding method using adaptive pixel pair matching. *IEEE Transactions on Information Forensics and Security*, *7*(1), 176–184. doi:10.1109/TIFS.2011.2155062

Honsinger, C.W., Jones, P.W., Rabbani, M., & Stoffel, J.C. (2001). *Lossless recovery of an original image containing embedded data*. US Patent 6,278,791.

Horng, M. H. (2010). Multilevel minimum cross entropy threshold selection based on the honey bee mating optimization. *Expert Systems with Applications*, *37*(6), 4580–4592. doi:10.1016/j.eswa.2009.12.050

Horng, M.-H., & Liou, R.-J. (2011). Multilevel minimum cross entropy threshold selection based on the firefly algorithm. *Expert Systems with Applications*, *38*(12), 14805–14811. doi:10.1016/j.eswa.2011.05.069

Hossain, I., & Chellappan, K. (2014). Collaborative Compressed I-Cloud Medical Image Storage with Decompress Viewer. *Procedia Computer Science*, *42*, 114–121. doi:10.1016/j.procs.2014.11.041

Hossain, M., Islam, S. R., Ali, F., Kwak, K. S., & Hasan, R. (2018). An Internet of Things-based health prescription assistant and its security system design. *Future Generation Computer Systems*, *82*, 422–439. doi:10.1016/j.future.2017.11.020

Huang, H. F., Hu, G. S., & Zhu, L. (2012). Sparse representation-based heartbeat classification using independent component analysis. *Journal of Medical Systems*, *36*(3), 1235–1247. doi:10.100710916-010-9585-x PMID:20839036

Hua, Z., Yi, S., & Zhou, Y. (2018). Medical image encryption using high-speed scrambling and pixel adaptive diffusion. *Signal Processing*, *144*, 134–144. doi:10.1016/j.sigpro.2017.10.004

Hua, Z., Zhou, Y., Pun, C. M., & Chang, C. L. P. (2015). 2D Sine Logistic modulation map for image encryption. *Information Sciences*, *297*, 80–94. doi:10.1016/j.ins.2014.11.018

Hu, F., Jiang, M., Celentano, L., & Xiao, Y. (2008). Robust medical ad hoc sensor networks (MASN) with wavelet-based ECG data mining. *Ad Hoc Networks*, *6*(7), 986–1012. doi:10.1016/j.adhoc.2007.09.002

Hu, J., & Han, F. (2009). A pixel-based scrambling scheme for digital medical images protection. *Journal of Network and Computer Applications*, *32*(4), 788–794. doi:10.1016/j.jnca.2009.02.009

Hu, Y. H., Palreddy, S., & Tompkins, W. J. (1997). A patient-adaptable ECG beat classifier using a mixture of experts approach. *IEEE Transactions on Biomedical Engineering*, *44*(9), 891–900. doi:10.1109/10.623058 PMID:9282481

Ibaida, A. (2014). *Secure Steganography, Compression and Diagnoses of Electrocardiograms in Wireless Body Sensor Networks* (PhD Thesis). RMIT University.

Ibaida, A., & Khalil, I. (2013). Wavelet-based ECG steganography for protecting patient confidential information in point-of-care systems. *IEEE Transactions on Biomedical Engineering*, *60*(12), 3322–3330. doi:10.1109/TBME.2013.2264539 PMID:23708767

Ibaida, A., Khalil, I., & Al-Shammary, D. (2010) Embedding patients confidential data in ECG signal for healthcare information systems. *32nd Int. conf. of IEEE Buenos Aires, Argentina*, 3891-3894. 10.1109/IEMBS.2010.5627671

Imadali, S., Karanasiou, A., Petrescu, A., Sifniadis, I., Veque, V., & Angelidis, P. (2012). eHealth service support in IPv6 vehicular networks. In *IEEE Int. Conf. Wireless Mobile Comput., Netw. Commun. (WiMob)* (pp. 579-585). London: IEEE Digital eXplore. 10.1109/WiMOB.2012.6379134

Inan, O. T., Giovangrandi, L., & Kovacs, G. T. A. (2006). Robust neural-network-based classification of premature ventricular contractions using wavelet transform and timing interval features. *IEEE Transactions on Biomedical Engineering*, *53*(12), 2507–2515. doi:10.1109/TBME.2006.880879 PMID:17153208

Ince, T., Kiranyaz, S., Gabbouj, M., & Member, S. (2009b). *A Generic and Robust System for Automated Patient-Specific Classification of ECG Signals*. Academic Press.

Ince, T., Kiranyaz, S., & Gabbouj, M. (2009a). A generic and robust system for automated patient-specific classification of ECG signals. *IEEE Transactions on Biomedical Engineering*, *56*(5), 1415–1426. doi:10.1109/TBME.2009.2013934 PMID:19203885

Indian Express v. Union of India. AIR 1981 SC 365.

Ingenerf, J. (1999). Telemedicine and Terminology. *Different Needs of Context Information*, *3*(2), 92–100. PMID:10719490

Internet of Things. (2018, May). Retrieved from IEEE: http://iot.ieee.org/about.html

Intille, S. S. (2006). Using a live-in laboratory for ubiquitous computing research. In *International Conference on Pervasive Computing* (pp. 349-365). Berlin: Springer. 10.1007/11748625_22

Introduction to Internet of Things. (2016, March 17). Retrieved from https://www.slideshare.net/Blackvard/introduction-to-internet-of-things-iot

Ismail, S. M., Said, L. A., Rezk, A. A., Radwan, A. G., Madian, A. H., Abu-Elyazeed, M. F., & Soliman, A. M. (2017). Generalized fractional logistic map encryption system based on FPGA. *AEÜ. International Journal of Electronics and Communications*, *80*, 114–126. doi:10.1016/j.aeue.2017.05.047

Izham, M., Fukui, T., & Morinishi, K. (2014). Simulation of three-dimensional homogeneous isotropic turbulence using the moment-based lattice Boltzmann method and LES-lattice Boltzmann method. *Journal Of Fluid Science And Technology, 9*(4). doi:10.1299/jfst.2014jfst0064

Janab K. Abdul Rahim vs The Divisional Electrical AIR 1954 SC 1077 (December 16, 2002). AIR 1975 SC 148.

Janakiraman, S., Thenmozhi, K., Rayappan, J. B. B., & Amirtharajan, R. (2018). Lightweight chaotic image encryption algorithm for real-time embedded system: Implementation and analysis on 32-bit microcontroller. *Microprocessors and Microsystems*, *56*, 1–12. doi:10.1016/j.micpro.2017.10.013

Jara, A. J., Zamora, M. A., & Skarmeta, A. (2012). Knowledge acquisition and management architecture for mobile and personal health environments based on the Internet of Things. In *IEEE Int. Conf. Trust, Security Privacy Comput. Commun. (TrustCom)* (pp. 1811-1818). IEEE Digital eXplore. 10.1109/TrustCom.2012.194

Jero, S. E., Ramu, P., & Ramakrishnan, S. (2014). Discrete wavelet transform and singular value decomposition based ECG steganography for secured patient information transmission. *Journal of Medical Systems*, *38*(10), 132. doi:10.100710916-014-0132-z PMID:25187409

Jero, S. E., Ramu, P., & Ramakrishnan, S. (2015). ECG steganography using curvelet transform. *Biomedical Signal Processing and Control*, *22*, 161–169. doi:10.1016/j.bspc.2015.07.004

Jero, S. E., Ramu, P., & Ramakrishnan, S. (2015). Steganography in arrhythmic electrocardiogram signal. *Proceedings of the Annual International Conference of the IEEE Engineering in Medicine and Biology Society, EMBS, 2015-Novem*, 1409–1412. doi:10.1109/EMBC.2015.7318633

Jero, S. E., Ramu, P., & Ramakrishnan, S. (2016). Imperceptibility—Robustness trade-off studies for ECG steganography using continuous ant colony optimization. *Expert Systems with Applications*, *49*, 123–135. doi:10.1016/j.eswa.2015.12.010

Jiang, X., Zhang, L., Zhao, Q., & Albayrak, S. (2006). ECG arrhythmias recognition system based on independent component analysis feature extraction. TENCON 2006. 2006 IEEE Region 10 Conference, 1–4. doi:10.1109/TENCON.2006.343781

Jiang, H., Feng, R., & Gao, X. (2011). Level set based on signed pressure force function and its application in liver image segmentation. *Wuhan University Journal of Natural Sciences*, *16*(3), 265–270. doi:10.100711859-011-0748-5

Jiang, T., Yang, M., & Zhang, Y. (2015). Research and implementation of M2M smart home and security system. *Security and Communication Networks*, *8*(16), 2704–2711. doi:10.1002ec.569

Jiang, W., & Kong, S. G. (2007). Block-based neural networks for personalized ECG signal classification. *IEEE Transactions on Neural Networks*, *18*(6), 1750–1761. doi:10.1109/TNN.2007.900239 PMID:18051190

Jiang, Y., Liu, X., & Lian, S. (2016). Design and implementation of smart-home monitoring system with the Internet of Things technology. In *Wireless Communications, Networking and Applications* (pp. 473–484). New Delhi: Springer. doi:10.1007/978-81-322-2580-5_43

Jing, C., Wang, Y., & Hanxiao, W. (2012). A Coded Aperture Compressive Imaging Array and Its Visual Detection and Tracking Algorithms for Surveillance Systems. *Sensors (Basel)*, *12*(11), 14397–14415. doi:10.3390121114397 PMID:23202167

Ji, U., Bhardwaj, C., & Sood, M. (2017). Effectiveness of Reconstruction Methods in Compressive Sensing for Biomedical Images. *Journal of Global Pharma Technology*, *6*(9), 134–143.

Johnson, N. F., & Jajodia, S. (1998). Exploring steganography: Seeing the unseen. *Computers*, *31*(2), 26–34. doi:10.1109/MC.1998.4655281

Jones, J., Xie, X., & Essa, E. (2014). Combining region-based and imprecise boundary-based cues for interactive medical image segmentation. *International Journal for Numerical Methods in Biomedical Engineering*, *30*(12), 1649–1666. doi:10.1002/cnm.2693 PMID:25377853

Jung, W-H., & Lee, S-G. (2017). *An Arrhythmia Classification Method in Utilizing the Weighted KNN and the Fitness Rule*. Academic Press.

Justice K. S. Puttaswamy (Retd.) and Anr. vs Union Of India And Ors. (24 August 2017)

Kanan, H. R., & Nazeri, B. (2014). A novel image steganography scheme with high embedding capacity and tunable visual image quality based on a genetic algorithm. *Expert Systems with Applications*, *41*(14), 6123–6130. doi:10.1016/j.eswa.2014.04.022

Kanso, A., & Ghebleh, M. (2015). An efficient and robust image encryption scheme for medical applications. *Communications in Nonlinear Science and Numerical Simulation*, *24*(1–3), 98–116. doi:10.1016/j.cnsns.2014.12.005

Kanso, A., & Smaoui, N. (2009). Logistic chaotic maps for binary numbers generations. *Chaos, Solitons, and Fractals*, *40*(5), 2557–2568. doi:10.1016/j.chaos.2007.10.049

Kapur, J. N., Sahoo, P. K., & Wong, A. K. C. (1985). A new method for gray-level picture thresholding using the entropy of the histogram. *Computer Vision Graphics and Image Processing*, *29*(3), 273–285. doi:10.1016/0734-189X(85)90125-2

Karimifard, S., Ahmadian, A., Khoshnevisan, M., & Nambakhsh, M. S. (2006). Morphological heart arrhythmia detection using hermitian basis functions and kNN classifier. *Engineering in Medicine and Biology Society, 2006. EMBS'06. 28th Annual International Conference of the IEEE*, 1367–1370. 10.1109/IEMBS.2006.260182

Kashyap, R. (2019a). Security, Reliability, and Performance Assessment for Healthcare Biometrics. In D. Kisku, P. Gupta, & J. Sing (Eds.), Design and Implementation of Healthcare Biometric Systems (pp. 29-54). Hershey, PA: IGI Global. doi:10.4018/978-1-5225-7525-2.ch002

Kashyap, R. (2019b). Geospatial Big Data, Analytics and IoT: Challenges, Applications and Potential. In H. Das, R. Barik, H. Dubey & D. Sinha Roy (Eds.), Cloud Computing for Geospatial Big Data Analytics (pp. 191-213). Springer International Publishing.

Kashyap, R. (2018). Object boundary detection through robust active contour-based method with global information. *International Journal Of Image Mining, 3*(1), 22. doi:10.1504/IJIM.2018.093008

Kashyap, R. (2019c). Biometric Authentication Techniques and E-Learning. In A. Kumar (Ed.), *Biometric Authentication in Online Learning Environments* (pp. 236–265). Hershey, PA: IGI Global. doi:10.4018/978-1-5225-7724-9.ch010

Kashyap, R. (2019d). Machine Learning for Internet of Things. In I.-S. Comşa & R. Trestian (Eds.), *Next-Generation Wireless Networks Meet Advanced Machine Learning Applications* (pp. 57–83). Hershey, PA: IGI Global. doi:10.4018/978-1-5225-7458-3.ch003

Kashyap, R., & Gautam, P. (2015). Modified region based segmentation of medical images. In *International Conference on Communication Networks (ICCN)*. IEEE. 10.1109/ICCN.2015.41

Kashyap, R., & Gautam, P. (2017). Fast Medical Image Segmentation Using Energy-Based Method. *Biometrics, Concepts, Methodologies, Tools, and Applications, 3*(1), 1017–1042. doi:10.4018/978-1-5225-0983-7.ch040

Kashyap, R., & Piersson, A. D. (2018a). Impact of Big Data on Security. In G. Shrivastava, P. Kumar, B. Gupta, S. Bala, & N. Dey (Eds.), *Handbook of Research on Network Forensics and Analysis Techniques* (pp. 283–299). Hershey, PA: IGI Global. doi:10.4018/978-1-5225-4100-4.ch015

Kashyap, R., & Piersson, A. D. (2018b). Big Data Challenges and Solutions in the Medical Industries. In V. Tiwari, R. Thakur, B. Tiwari, & S. Gupta (Eds.), *Handbook of Research on Pattern Engineering System Development for Big Data Analytics* (pp. 1–24). Hershey, PA: IGI Global. doi:10.4018/978-1-5225-3870-7.ch001

Kashyap, R., & Tiwari, V. (2017). Energy-based active contour method for image segmentation. *International Journal of Electronic Healthcare, 9*(2–3), 210–225. doi:10.1504/IJEH.2017.083165

Kashyap, R., & Tiwari, V. (2018). Active contours using global models for medical image segmentation. *International Journal of Computational Systems Engineering, 4*(2/3), 195. doi:10.1504/IJCSYSE.2018.091404

Kass, R. E., & Clancy, C. E. (2005). *Basis and treatment of cardiac arrhythmias*. Springer Science & Business Media.

Kaur, T., Saini, B. S., & Gupta, S. (2016). Optimized Multi Threshold Brain Tumor Image Segmentation Using Two Dimensional Minimum Cross Entropy Based on Co-occurrence Matrix. In *Medical Imaging in Clinical Applications* (pp. 461–486). Springer International Publishing. doi:10.1007/978-3-319-33793-7_20

Kaur, T., Saini, B. S., & Gupta, S. (2018). A comparative study on Kapur's and Tsallis entropy for multilevel thresholding of MR images via particle swarm optimisation technique. *Int. J. Computing Systems in Engineering, 4*(2/3), 156–164. doi:10.1504/IJCSYSE.2018.091395

Kavitha, T., &Sridharan, D. (2010). Security vulnerabilities in wireless sensor networks: A survey. *Journal of information Assurance and Security, 5*(1), 31-44.

Keller, J. M., Gray, M. R., & Givens, J. A. (1985). A fuzzy k-nearest neighbor algorithm. *IEEE Transactions on Systems, Man, and Cybernetics, SMC-15*(4), 580–585. doi:10.1109/TSMC.1985.6313426

Kennedy, J., & Eberhart, R. (1995). Particle swarm optimization. In *Proceedings of ICNN'95 - International Conference on Neural Networks*. Perth, Australia: IEEE. 10.1109/ICNN.1995.488968

Keshavarz, A., Tabar, A. M., & Aghajan, H. (2006, October). Distributed vision-based reasoning for smart home care. *Proc. of ACM SenSys Workshop on DSC*.

Khadra, L., Al-Fahoum, A. S., & Binajjaj, S. (2005). A quantitative analysis approach for cardiac arrhythmia classification using higher order spectral techniques. *IEEE Transactions on Biomedical Engineering, 52*(11), 1840–1845. doi:10.1109/TBME.2005.856281 PMID:16285387

Khaing, A. S., & Naing, Z. M. (2011). Quantitative Investigation of Digital Filters in Electrocardiogram with Simulated Noises. *Int J Inf Electron Eng, 1*, 210.

Khalil, N., Abid, M. R., Benhaddou, D., & Gerndt, M. (2014, April). Wireless sensors networks for Internet of Things. In *2014 IEEE ninth international conference on Intelligent sensors, sensor networks and information processing (ISSNIP)* (pp. 1-6). IEEE. 10.1109/ISSNIP.2014.6827681

Khan, O. A., & Skinner, R. (2002). *Geographic Information Systems and Health Applications*. IGI Globa.

Kharak Singh vs The State Of U. P. & Others on (18 December, 1962)

Khazaee, A., & Ebrahimzadeh, A. (2010). Classification of electrocardiogram signals with support vector machines and genetic algorithms using power spectral features. *Biomedical Signal Processing and Control, 5*(4), 252–263. doi:10.1016/j.bspc.2010.07.006

Kittler, J., & Illingworth, J. (1986). Minimum error thresholding. *Pattern Recognition, 19*(1), 41–47. doi:10.1016/0031-3203(86)90030-0

Ko, J. L.-E., Dutton, R. P., Lim, J. H., Chen, Y., Musvaloiu-E, R., Terzis, A., ... Selavo, L. (2010). MEDiSN: Medical emergency detection in sensor networks. *ACM Transactions on Embedded Computing Systems, 10*(1), 89–101. doi:10.1145/1814539.1814550

Korurek, M., & Dogan, B. (2010). ECG beat classification using particle swarm optimization and radial basis function neural network. *Expert Systems with Applications, 37*(12), 7563–7569. doi:10.1016/j.eswa.2010.04.087

Koszat, S. S., Vlachos, M., Lucchese, C., & Herle, H. V. (2009). Embedding and Retrieving Private Metadata in Electrocardiograms. *Journal of Medical Systems, 33*(4), 241–259. doi:10.100710916-008-9185-1 PMID:19697691

Krumm, J. (2007). Inference attacks on location track. In *International Conference on Pervasive Computing* (pp. 127-143). Berlin: Springer. 10.1007/978-3-540-72037-9_8

Kumar, A., Jakhar, D. S., & Makkar, M. S. (2012). Comparative Analysis between DES and RSA Algorithm's. *International Journal of Advanced Research in Computer Science and Software Engineering, 2*(7), 386–391.

Kumar, P., & Lee, H. J. (2011). Security issues in healthcare applications using wireless medical sensor networks: A survey. *Sensors (Basel), 12*(1), 55–91. doi:10.3390120100055 PMID:22368458

Kurs, A., Karalis, A., Moffatt, R., Joannopoulos, J. D., Fisher, P., & Soljačić, M. (2007). Wireless power transfer via strongly coupled magnetic resonances. *Science, 317*(5834), 83-86.

Kutlu, Y., & Kuntalp, D. (2012). Feature extraction for ECG heartbeats using higher order statistics of WPD coefficients. *Computer Methods and Programs in Biomedicine, 105*(3), 257–267. doi:10.1016/j.cmpb.2011.10.002 PMID:22055998

Lagerholm, M., Peterson, C., Braccini, G., Edenbrandt, L., & Sornmo, L. (2000). Clustering ECG complexes using Hermite functions and self-organizing maps. *IEEE Transactions on Biomedical Engineering, 47*(7), 838–848. doi:10.1109/10.846677 PMID:10916254

Laiphrakpam, D. S., & Khumanthem, M. S. (2017). Medical image encryption based on improved ElGamal encryption technique. *Optik (Stuttgart), 147*, 88–102. doi:10.1016/j.ijleo.2017.08.028

Lakshminarayana, M., & Sarvagya, M. (2016). Algorithm to balance compression and signal quality using novel compressive sensing in medical images. In *Software Engineering Perspectives and Application in Intelligent Systems* (pp. 317–327). Cham: Springer. doi:10.1007/978-3-319-33622-0_29

Lankton, S., & Tannenbaum, A. (2008). Localizing Region-Based Active Contours. *IEEE Transactions on Image Processing, 17*(11), 2029–2039. doi:10.1109/TIP.2008.2004611 PMID:18854247

Laskar, S. A., & Hemachandran, K. (2013). Steganography based on random pixel selection for efficient data hiding. *International Journal of Computer Engineering and Technology, 4*(2), 31–44.

Latorre, J. I. (2005). *Image compression and entanglement.* Retrieved from http://arxiv.org/abs/quant-ph/0510031

Lee, H., & Buckley, K. M. (1999). ECG data compression using cut and align beats approach and 2-D transforms. *IEEE Transactions on Biomedical Engineering, 46*(5), 556–564. doi:10.1109/10.759056 PMID:10230134

Lee, S., Yoo, C. D., & Kalker, T. (2007). Reversible image watermarking based on integer-to-integer wavelet transform. *IEEE Transactions on Information Forensics and Security, 2*(3), 321–330. doi:10.1109/TIFS.2007.905146

Li Feng, X. (2014). Object Recognition Algorithm Utilizing Graph Cuts Based Image Segmentation. *Journal of Multimedia.* doi:10.4304/jmm.9.2.238-244

Li, X., Wang, L., Yan, Y., & Liu, P. (2016). An improvement color image encryption algorithm based on DNA operations and real and complex chaotic systems. *Optik - International Journal for Light and Electron Optics, 127*(5), 2558–2565.

Li, X., Zhao, Z., & Cheng, H. D. (1995). Fuzzy entropy threshold approach to breast cancer detection. *Information Sciences - Applications, 4*, 49–56.

Liang, D., & Ying, L. (2010, August). Compressed-sensing dynamic MR imaging with partially known support. In *Engineering in Medicine and Biology Society (EMBC), 2010 Annual International Conference of the IEEE* (pp. 2829-2832). IEEE. 10.1109/IEMBS.2010.5626077

Liao, L., Fox, D., & Kautz, H. (2005). BLocation-based activity recognition using relational Markov networks. *19th Int. In Joint Conf. Artif. Intell.*, 773-778.

Li, C., Zheng, C., & Tai, C. (1995). Detection of ECG characteristic points using wavelet transforms. *IEEE Transactions on Biomedical Engineering, 42*(1), 21–28. doi:10.1109/10.362922 PMID:7851927

Li, D., He, Q., Chunli, L., & Hongjie, Y. (2017). Local Binary Fitting Segmentation by Cooperative Quantum Particle Optimization. *TELKOMNIKA, 15*(1), 531. doi:10.12928/telkomnika.v15i1.3159

Li, H., Liang, H., Miao, C., Cao, L., Feng, X., Tang, C., & Li, E. (2016). Novel ECG Signal Classification Based on KICA Nonlinear Feature Extraction. *Circuits, Systems, and Signal Processing, 35*(4), 1187–1197. doi:10.100700034-015-0108-3

Liji, C. A., Indiradevi, K. P., & Anish, B. K. K. (2015) Integer wavelet transform for embedded lossy to lossless image compression. *International Conference on Emerging Trends in Engineering, Science and Technology, Procedia Technology, 24*, 1039–47.

Lima, J. B., Madeiro, F., & Sales, F. J. R. (2015). Encryption of medical images based on the cosine number transform. *Signal Processing Image Communication*, *35*, 1–8. doi:10.1016/j.image.2015.03.005

Linderman, M. D., Santhanam, G., Kemere, C. T., Gilja, V., O'Driscoll, S., Yu, B. M., ... Meng, T. (2008). Signal processing challenges for neural prostheses. *IEEE Signal Processing Magazine*, *25*(1), 18–28. doi:10.1109/MSP.2008.4408439

Lin, M., & Hua, Z. (2009). Improved PSO Algorithm with Adaptive Inertia Weight and Mutation. *World Congress on Computer Science and Information Engineering*, 622–625. 10.1109/CSIE.2009.428

Lin, Y. K. (2012). High capacity reversible data hiding scheme based upon discrete cosine transformation. *Journal of Systems and Software*, *85*(10), 2395–2404. doi:10.1016/j.jss.2012.05.032

Li, Q., Rajagopalan, C., & Clifford, G. D. (2014). A machine learning approach to multi-level ECG signal quality classification. *Computer Methods and Programs in Biomedicine*, *117*(3), 435–447. doi:10.1016/j.cmpb.2014.09.002 PMID:25306242

Liu, D. D., Liang, D., Liu, X., & Zhang, Y. T. (2012, August). Under-sampling trajectory design for compressed sensing MRI. In *Engineering in Medicine and Biology Society (EMBC), 2012 Annual International Conference of the IEEE* (pp. 73-76). IEEE.

Liu, T. Y., Lin, K. J., & Wu, H. C. (2017). ECG data encryption then compression using singular value decomposition. *IEEE Journal of Biomedical and Health Informatics*, *22*(3), 707–713. doi:10.1109/JBHI.2017.2698498 PMID:28463208

Liu, W., & Ruan, D. (2014). TU-F-BRF-05: Level Set Based Segmentation with a Dynamic Shape Prior. *Medical Physics*, *41*(6Part27), 471–472. doi:10.1118/1.4889323

Liu, Y., De Vos, M., Gligorijevic, I., Matic, V., Li, Y., & Van Huffel, S. (2013). Multi-structural signal recovery for biomedical compressive sensing. *IEEE Transactions on Biomedical Engineering*, *60*(10), 2794–2805. doi:10.1109/TBME.2013.2264772 PMID:23715599

Li, X., Jiang, D., Shi, Y., & Li, W. (2015). Segmentation of MR image using local and global region based geodesic model. *Biomedical Engineering Online*, *14*(1), 8. doi:10.1186/1475-925X-14-8 PMID:25971306

Li, Y., & Thai, M. T. (Eds.). (2008). *Wireless sensor networks and applications*. Springer Science & Business Media. doi:10.1007/978-0-387-49592-7

Llamedo, M., & Martinez, J. P. (2012). An automatic patient-adapted ECG heartbeat classifier allowing expert assistance. *IEEE Transactions on Biomedical Engineering*, *59*(8), 2312–2320. doi:10.1109/TBME.2012.2202662 PMID:22692868

Lopez-Nores, M., Pazos-Arias, J. J., Garcia-Duque, J., & Blanco-Fernandez, Y. (2008, January). Monitoring medicine intake in the networked home: The iCabiNET solution. In *Pervasive Computing Technologies for Healthcare, 2008. PervasiveHealth 2008. Second International Conference on* (pp. 116-117). IEEE.

Lu, S., Qiu, X., Shi, J., Li, N., Lu, Z.-H., Chen, P., ... Zhang, Y. (2017). A pathological brain detection system based on extreme learning machine optimized by bat algorithm. *CNS & Neurological Disorders-Drug Targets (Formerly Current Drug Targets-CNS & Neurological Disorders)*, *16*(1), 23–29.

Lu, C. H., & Fu, L. C. (2009). Robust location-aware activity recognition using wireless sensor network in an attentive home. *IEEE Transactions on Automation Science and Engineering*, *6*(4), 598–609. doi:10.1109/TASE.2009.2021981

Lu, C., Wu, Z., Liu, M., Chen, W., & Guo, J. (2013). A patient privacy protection scheme for medical information system. *Journal of Medical Systems*, *37*(6), 1–10. doi:10.100710916-013-9982-z PMID:24166018

Luo, Y., & Bradley-Schmieg, P. (2018). *China Issues New Personal Information Protection Standard.* Retrieved from www.insideprivacy.com/international/china/china-issues-new-personal-information-protection-standard/

M. P. Sharma And Others vs Satish Chandra. (15 March, 1954)

Madhukumar, N., & Baiju, P. S. (2015). Contourlet Transform Based MRI Image Compression using Compressed Sensing. *International Journal of Advanced Research in Electrical, Electronics and Instrumentation Engineering, 4*(7), 6434-6440.

Magaña-Espinoza, P., Aquino-Santos, R., Cárdenas-Benítez, N., Aguilar-Velasco, J., Buenrostro-Segura, C., Edwards-Block, A., & Medina-Cass, A. (2014). Wisph: A wireless sensor network-based home care monitoring system. *Sensors (Basel), 14*(4), 7096–7119. doi:10.3390140407096 PMID:24759112

Maglogiannis, C. D. (2012). Bringing IoT and cloud computing towards pervasive healthcare. In *Int. Conf. Innov. Mobile Internet Services Ubiquitous Comput. (IMIS),* (pp. 922-926). Academic Press.

Mahdavi, M., Fesanghary, M., & Damangir, E. (2007). An improved harmony search algorithm for solving optimization problems. *Applied Mathematics and Computation, 188*(2), 1567–1579. doi:10.1016/j.amc.2006.11.033

Ma, J., Nguyen, H., Mirza, F., & Neuland, O. (2017). Two way architecture between IoT sensors and cloud computing for remote health care monitoring applications. *Twenty-Fifth European Conference on Information Systems (ECIS),* 2834–2841.

Majumdar, A., Ward, R. K., & Aboulnasr, T. (2012). Compressed sensing based real-time dynamic MRI reconstruction. *IEEE Transactions on Medical Imaging, 31*(12), 2253–2266. doi:10.1109/TMI.2012.2215921 PMID:22949054

Manfredi, M., Grana, C., Cucchiara, R., & Smeulders, A. (2016). Segmentation models diversity for object proposals. *Computer Vision and Image Understanding.* doi:10.1016/j.cviu.2016.06.005

Manikandan, M. S., & Dandapat, S. (2007). Wavelet energy based diagnostic distortion measure for ECG. *Biomedical Signal Processing and Control, 2*(2), 80–96. doi:10.1016/j.bspc.2007.05.001

Manikandan, S., Ramar, K., Iruthayarajan, M. W., Srinivasagan, K. G. G., Willjuice Iruthayarajan, M., & Srinivasagan, K. G. G. (2014). Multilevel thresholding for segmentation of medical brain images using Real coded Genetic Algorithm. *Measurement, 47*(1), 558–568. doi:10.1016/j.measurement.2013.09.031

Marco, A., Casas, R., Falco, J., Gracia, H., Artigas, J. I., & Roy, A. (2008). Location-based services for elderly and disabled people. *Computer Communications, 31*(6), 1055–1066. doi:10.1016/j.comcom.2007.12.031

Mark, R., & Moody, G. (1997). Mit-bih arrhythmia database 1997.

Martínez-González, R. F., Díaz Méndez, J. A., Palacios-Luengas, L., López-Hernández, J., & Vázquez-Medina, R. (2016). A steganographic method using bernoulli's chaotic maps. *Computers & Electrical Engineering, 54,* 435–449. doi:10.1016/j.compeleceng.2015.12.005

Martis, R. J., Acharya, U. R., Ray, A. K., & Chakraborty, C. (2011). Application of higher order cumulants to ECG signals for the cardiac health diagnosis. *Engineering in medicine and biology society,* 1697–1700. doi:10.1109/IEMBS.2011.6090487

Martis, R. J., Acharya, U. R., Mandana, K. M., Ray, A. K., & Chakraborty, C. (2013). Cardiac decision making using higher order spectra. *Biomedical Signal Processing and Control, 8*(2), 193–203. doi:10.1016/j.bspc.2012.08.004

ME, M. S. S., Vijayakuymar, V. R., & Anuja, M. R. (2012). A survey on various compression methods for medical images. *International Journal of Intelligent Systems and Applications, 4*(3), 13.

Medical Informatics and Telemedicine. (n.d.). Retrieved from https://medicalinformatics.healthconferences.org/events-list/medical-informatics-and-biomedical-informatics

Medical Sample Images. (n.d.). Retrieved from http://www.barre.nom.fr/medical/samples/

Meingast, M., Roosta, T., & Sastry, S. (2006, August). Security and privacy issues with health are information technology. In *Engineering in Medicine and Biology Society, 2006. EMBS'06. 28th Annual International Conference of the IEEE* (pp. 5453-5458). IEEE. 10.1109/IEMBS.2006.260060

Melgani, F., Member, S., & Bazi, Y. (2008). Classification of Electrocardiogram Signals With Support Vector Machines and Particle Swarm Optimization. *IEEE Transactions on Information Technology in Biomedicine, 12*(5), 667–677. doi:10.1109/TITB.2008.923147 PMID:18779082

MIFA Shares Industry Wisdom on Medical Identity Theft and Fraud. (n.d.). Retrieved September 11, 2018, from https://www.hipaajournal.com/mifa-shares-industry-wisdom-on-medical-identity-theft-and-fraud-3657/

Minaie, A., Sanati-Mehrizy, A., Sanati-Mehrizy, P., &Sanati-Mehrizy, R. (2013). Application of wireless sensor networks in health care system. *Age, 23*(1).

Mishra, N. M., Parker, L., & Deshpande, S. (2017). Privacy and the Right to Information Act, 2005. *Indian Journal of Medical Ethics*. Retrieved from https://www.ncbi.nlm.nih.gov/pmc/articles/PMC5473905/

Mitra, U., Emken, B. A., Lee, S., Li, M., Rozgic, V., Thatte, G., & Levorato, M. (2012). KNOWME: A case study in wireless body area sensor network design. *IEEE Communications Magazine, 50*(5), 116–125. doi:10.1109/MCOM.2012.6194391

Mokji, M. M., & Abu Bakar, S. A. R. (2007). Adaptive thresholding based on co-occurrence matrix edge information. *Journal of Computers, 2*(8), 44–52. doi:10.4304/jcp.2.8.44-52

Morkel, T., Eloff, J. H. P., & Olivier, M. S. (2005). *An overview of image steganography*. ISSA.

Moskowitz, R. (2012). HIP Diet EXchange (DEX): Draft-moskowitz-hip-dex-00. *Standards Track, 19*(5), 120–135.

Mousa, A., & Hamad, A. (2006). Evaluation of the RC4 algorithm for data encryption. *IJCSA, 3*(2), 44–56.

Mousavi, S. M., Naghsh, A., & Abu-Bakar, S. (2014). Watermarking techniques used in medical images: A survey. *Journal of Digital Imaging, 27*(6), 714–729. doi:10.100710278-014-9700-5 PMID:24871349

Mr. X v. Hospital. AIR 2004 Del. 203 (India).

Ms. X vs Mr. Z. AIR 2002 Del 217 (India).

Mukhtar v. State of Maharashtra 2011 (2) ID 101 (SC).

Munn v. Illinois, 94 U.S. 113 (1876)

Nagesh, P., & Baoxin, L. (2009). A Compressive Sensing Approach for Expression-Invariant Face Recognition. *IEEE Conference on Computer Vision and Pattern Recognition*, 1518-1525. 10.1109/CVPR.2009.5206657

Nahar, P. C., & Kolte, M. T. (2014). An introduction to compressive sensing and its applications. *Int J Sci Res Publ, 4*(6).

Nakib, A., Roman, S., Oulhadj, H., & Siarry, P. (2007). Fast brain MRI segmentation based on two-dimensional survival exponential entropy and particle swarm optimization. *Proceedings of the 29th Annual International Conference of the IEEE EMBS*, 5563–6. 10.1109/IEMBS.2007.4353607

Nambakhsh, M. S., Ahmadian, A., & Zaidi, H. (2011). A contextual based double watermarking of PET images by patient ID and ECG signal. *Computer Methods and Programs in Biomedicine, 104*(3), 418–425. doi:10.1016/j.cmpb.2010.08.016 PMID:20934773

National Health Mission Report. (2018, August 14). Retrieved from http://nhm.gov.in/nrhm-components/rmnch-a/child-health-immunization/child-health/annual-report.html

Nausheen, N., Seal, A., Khanna, P., & Halder, S. (2018). A FPGA based implementation of Sobel edge detection. *Microprocessors and Microsystems*, *56*, 84–91. doi:10.1016/j.micpro.2017.10.011

Nayak, D. R., Patra, P. K., & Mahapatra, A. (2014). *A Survey on Two Dimensional Cellular Automata and Its Application in Image Processing*. arXiv Preprint ar Xiv:1407.7626

Ngoc, T. V. (2008). *Medical applications of wireless networks*. Washington, DC: Recent Advances in Wireless and Mobile Networking.

Nyberg, K., & Rueppel, R. A. (1996). Message recovery for signature schemes based on the discrete logarithm problem. *Designs, Codes and Cryptography*, *7*(1-2), 61–81. doi:10.1007/BF00125076

Office of Australian Information Commissioner. (n.d.). *Health Information and Medical Research*. Retrieved from https://www.oaic.gov.au/privacy-law/privacy-act/health-and-medical-research

Okamoto, T., & Uchiyama, S. (1998). A new public-key cryptosystem as secure as factoring. Advances in Cryptology — EUROCRYPT'98 Lecture Notes in Computer Science, 1403, 308–318.

Olivereau, Y. B. (2012). D-HIP: A distributed key exchange scheme for HIP-based Internet of Things. *IEEE Int'l Symp. on a World of Wireless, Mobile and Multimedia Networks (WoWMoM): IEEE Computer Society*, 1-7.

Osiri, X. DICOM Viewer | DICOM Image Library. (n.d.). Retrieved December 21, 2018, from http://www.osirix-viewer.com/resources/dicom-image-library/

Osowski, S., Hoai, L. T., & Markiewicz, T. (2004). Support vector machine-based expert system for reliable heartbeat recognition. *IEEE Transactions on Biomedical Engineering*, *51*(4), 582–589. doi:10.1109/TBME.2004.824138 PMID:15072212

Otsu, N. (1979). A threshold selection method from gray-level histograms. *IEEE Transactions on Systems, Man, and Cybernetics*, *SMC-9*(1), 62–66. doi:10.1109/TSMC.1979.4310076

P. Sharma v. Satish Chandra, District Magistrate Delhi on 30 August, 1954 SCC 494 (India).

Paillier, P. (1999). Public-Key Cryptosystems Based on Composite Degree Residuosity Classes. *EUROCRYPT*, 223–238.

Palumbo, F., Ullberg, J., Štimec, A., Furfari, F., Karlsson, L., & Coradeschi, S. (2014). Sensor network infrastructure for a home care monitoring system. *Sensors (Basel)*, *14*(3), 3833–3860. doi:10.3390140303833 PMID:24573309

Panda, R., Agrawal, S., & Bhuyan, S. (2013). Edge magnitude based multilevel thresholding using Cuckoo search technique. *Expert Systems with Applications*, *40*(18), 7617–7628. doi:10.1016/j.eswa.2013.07.060

Pandey, A., Saini, B. S., Singh, B., & Sood, N. (2016). A 2D electrocardiogram data compression method using a sample entropy-based complexity sorting approach. *Computers & Electrical Engineering*, *56*, 36–45. doi:10.1016/j.compeleceng.2016.10.012

Pandey, A., Saini, B. S., Singh, B., & Sood, N. (2016b). Analysis of electrocardiogram data compression techniques: A MATLAB-based approach. In *Computational Tools and Techniques for Biomedical Signal Processing* (Vol. 1, pp. 272–313). IGI Global. doi:10.4018/978-1-5225-0660-7.ch013

Pandey, A., Saini, B. S., Singh, B., & Sood, N. (2017). An integrated approach using chaotic map & sample value difference method for electrocardiogram steganography and OFDM based secured patient information transmission. *Journal of Medical Systems*, *41*(12), 187. doi:10.100710916-017-0830-4 PMID:29043502

Pandey, A., Saini, B. S., Singh, B., & Sood, N. (2018). Complexity sorting and coupled chaotic map based on 2D ECG data compression-then-encryption and its OFDM transmission with impair sample correction. *Multimedia Tools and Applications.* doi:10.100711042-018-6681-2

Pandey, A., Singh, B., Saini, B. S., & Sood, N. (2016). A joint application of optimal threshold based discrete cosine transform and ASCII encoding for ECG data compression with its inherent encryption. *Australasian Physical & Engineering Sciences in Medicine, 39*(4), 833–855. doi:10.100713246-016-0476-4 PMID:27613706

Pandey, A., Singh, B., Saini, B. S., & Sood, N. (2016b). Nonlinear complexity sorting approach for 2D ECG data compression. In *Computational Tools and Techniques for Biomedical Signal Processing* (Vol. 1, pp. 1–21). IGI Global. doi:10.4018/978-1-5225-0660-7.ch001

Pang, Z., Chen, Q., & Zheng, L. (2009, November). A pervasive and preventive healthcare solution for medication non-compliance and daily monitoring. In *Applied Sciences in Biomedical and Communication Technologies, 2009. ISABEL 2009. 2nd International Symposium on* (pp. 1-6). IEEE. 10.1109/ISABEL.2009.5373681

Pan, J., & Tompkins, W. J. (1985). A real-time QRS detection algorithm. *IEEE Transactions on Biomedical Engineering, BME-32*(3), 230–236. doi:10.1109/TBME.1985.325532 PMID:3997178

Paoli, C. (2014). 6 Security Tools To Protect Enterprise Data. *Redmond Magazine.* Retrieved November 19, 2018, from https://redmondmag.com/articles/2014/11/01/security-tools.aspx

Parisot, S., Wells, W., Chemouny, S., Duffau, H., & Paragios, N. (2014). 'Concurrent tumor segmentation and registration with uncertainty-based sparse non-uniform graphs', *Medical Image Analysis. Elsevier B., 18*(4), 647–659. PMID:24717540

Park, J. Y., & Wakin, M. B. (2009, May). A multiscale framework for compressive sensing of video. In *Picture Coding Symposium, 2009. PCS 2009* (pp. 1-4). IEEE. 10.1109/PCS.2009.5167440

Pathan, A. S. K., Lee, H. W., & Hong, C. S. (2006, February). Security in wireless sensor networks: issues and challenges. In *Advanced Communication Technology, 2006. ICACT 2006. The 8th International Conference* (Vol. 2, pp. 6-pp). IEEE. 10.1109/ICACT.2006.206151

Patrick, K. (2007). *A tool for geospatial analysis of physical activity: Physical activity location measurement system (palms).* San Diego, CA: NIHGEI project at the University of California.

Pattichis, C. S., Kyriacou, E., Voskarides, S., Pattichis, M. S., Istepanian, R., & Schizas, C. N. (2002). Wireless telemedicine systems: An overview. *IEEE Antennas & Propagation Magazine, 44*(2), 143–153. doi:10.1109/MAP.2002.1003651

Peng, Y., Zhu, Y., & Wang, Y. (2016). A fast medical image segmentation method based on the initial contour forecast segmentation model. *International Journal Of Computing Science And Mathematics, 7*(3), 212. doi:10.1504/IJCSM.2016.077863

Peres, A. (1985). Reversible logic and Quantum Computers. *Physical Review A., 32*(6), 3266–3276. doi:10.1103/PhysRevA.32.3266 PMID:9896493

Phadikar, A. (2013). Multibit quantization index modulation: A high-rate robust data-hiding method. *Journal of King Saud University-Computer and Information Sciences, 25*(2), 163–171. doi:10.1016/j.jksuci.2012.11.005

Polastre, J., Szewczyk, R., & Culler, D. (2005). Telos: Enabling Ultra-Low Power Wireless Research. *4th International Conference on Information Processing in Sensor Networks: Special track on Platform Tools and Design Methods for Network Embedded Sensors (IPSN/SPOTS),* 57-62.

Ponemon Organization. (2015, May 7). Retrieved from Ponemon Institute: https://www.ponemon.org/news-2/66

Poornachandra, S. (2008). Wavelet-based denoising using subband dependent threshold for ECG signals. *Digit Signal Process A Rev J., 18*, 49–55. doi:10.1016/j.dsp.2007.09.006

Pragnya, K. R., Harshini, G. S., &Chaitanya, J. K. (2013). Wireless home monitoring for senior citizens using ZigBee network. *Advance in Electronic and Electric Engineering.*

Prasad, G. K., & Sahambi, J. S. (2003). Classification of ECG arrhythmias using multi-resolution analysis and neural networks. *TENCON 2003. Conference on Convergent Technologies for the Asia-Pacific Region*, 227–231. 10.1109/TENCON.2003.1273320

Praveenkumar, P., Amirtharajan, R., Thenmozhi, K., & Balaguru Rayappan, J. B. (2015). Medical Data Sheet in Safe Havens - A Tri-layer Cryptic Solution. *Computers in Biology and Medicine, 62*(C), 264–276. doi:10.1016/j.compbiomed.2015.04.031 PMID:25966921

Qasim, A. F., Meziane, F., & Aspin, R. (2018). Digital watermarking: Applicability for developing trust in medical imaging workflows state of the art review. *Computer Science Review, 27*, 45–60. doi:10.1016/j.cosrev.2017.11.003

Qin, C., Zhang, G., Zhou, Y., Tao, W., & Cao, Z. (2014). Integration of the saliency-based seed extraction and random walks for image segmentation. *Neurocomputing, 129*, 378–391. doi:10.1016/j.neucom.2013.09.021

Qu, X., Cuo, X., Guo, D., Hu, C., & Chen, Z. (2010). Compress sensing MRI with combined sparisifying transforms and smoothed l0 norm minimization. *International Conference of IEEE*, 626-629.

Radcliffe, J. (2011). *Hacking medical devices for fun and insulin.* Retrieved from Breaking the human scada system: http://media.blackhat.com/bh-us-11/Radcliffe/BH US 11 Radcliffe_Hacking Medical Devices WP.pdf

Raeiatibanadkooki, M., Quchani, S. R., KhalilZade, M. M., & Bahaadinbeigy, K. (2016). Compression and encryption of ECG signal using wavelet and chaotically huffman code in telemedicine application. *Journal of Medical Systems, 40*(3), 1–8. doi:10.100710916-016-0433-5 PMID:26779641

Raghunathan, S., Ward, M., Roy, K., & Irazoqui, P. (2009). A lowpower implantable event-based seizure detection algorithm. In *4th International IEEE/EMBS Conference* (pp. 151-154). IEEE.

Rajagopal, K. (2018, January 9). *Right to privacy verdict: A timeline of SC hearings.* Retrieved from https://www.the-hindubusinessline.com/news/national/right-to-privacy-verdict-a-timeline-of-sc-hearings/article9829124.ece

Rajagopalan, S., Dhamodaran, B., Ramji, A., Francis, C., Venkatraman, S., & Amirtharajan, R. (2017). Confusion and diffusion on FPGA- On chip solution for medical image security. In *Computer Communication and Informatics (ICCCI), 2017 International Conference on* (pp. 1–6). Academic Press.

Rajagopalan, S., Rethinam, S., Arumugham, S., Upadhyay, H. N., Rayappan, J. B. B., & Amirtharajan, R. (2018). Networked hardware assisted key image and chaotic attractors for secure RGB image communication. *Multimedia Tools and Applications*, 1–34.

Rajagopalan, S., Sivaraman, R., Upadhyay, H. N., Rayappan, J. B. B., & Amirtharajan, R. (2018). ON-Chip Peripherals are ON for Chaos--an Image fused Encryption. *Microprocessors and Microsystems, 61*, 257–278. doi:10.1016/j.micpro.2018.06.011

Raja, K. B., Venugopal, K. R., & Patnaik, L. M. (2004). *A Secure Stegonographic Algorithm using LSB, DCT and Image Compression on Raw Images. Technical Report.* Department of Computer Science and Engineering.

Rajaraman, V. (2016). IEEE standard for floating point numbers. *Resonance, 21*(1), 11–30. doi:10.100712045-016-0292-x

Raj, S., Chand, G. S. S. P., & Ray, K. C. (2015a). Arm-based arrhythmia beat monitoring system. *Microprocessors and Microsystems*, *39*(7), 504–511. doi:10.1016/j.micpro.2015.07.013

Raj, S., Maurya, K., & Ray, K. C. (2015b). A knowledge-based real time embedded platform for arrhythmia beat classification. *Biomedical Engineering Letters*, *5*(4), 271–280. doi:10.100713534-015-0196-9

Ramalingam, B., Amirtharajan, R., & Rayappan, J. B. B. (2016). Multiplexed stego path on reconfigurable hardware: A novel random approach. *Computers & Electrical Engineering*, *55*, 153–163. doi:10.1016/j.compeleceng.2016.02.010

Ramalingam, B., Rengarajan, A., & Rayappan, J. B. B. (2017). Hybrid image crypto system for secure image communication– A VLSI approach. *Microprocessors and Microsystems*, *50*, 1–13. doi:10.1016/j.micpro.2017.02.003

Rangayyan, R. M. (2002). *Biomedical Signal Analysis: A Case-Study Approach*. John Wiley and Sons, Inc. doi:10.1002/9780470544204

Ravichandran, D., Praveenkumar, P., Rayappan, J. B. B., & Amirtharajan, R. (2016). Chaos based crossover and mutation for securing DICOM image. *Computers in Biology and Medicine*, *72*, 170–18. doi:10.1016/j.compbiomed.2016.03.020 PMID:27046666

Ravichandran, D., Praveenkumar, P., Rayappan, J. B. B., & Amirtharajan, R. (2017). DNA Chaos Blend to Secure Medical Privacy. *IEEE Transactions on Nanobioscience*, *16*(8), 850–858. doi:10.1109/TNB.2017.2780881 PMID:29364129

Ravichandran, D., Rajagopalan, S., Upadhyay, H. N., Rayappan, J. B. B., & Amirtharajan, R. (2018). Encrypted Biography of Biomedical Image-a Pentalayer Cryptosystem on FPGA. *Journal of Signal Processing Systems for Signal, Image, and Video Technology*, 1–27.

Ravishankar, S., & Bresler, Y. (2011, August). Adaptive sampling design for compressed sensing MRI. In *Engineering in Medicine and Biology Society, EMBC, 2011 Annual International Conference of the IEEE* (pp. 3751-3755). IEEE. 10.1109/IEMBS.2011.6090639

Ray, K. C., & Sharma, P. (2016). Efficient methodology for electrocardiogram beat classification. *IET Signal Processing*, *10*(7), 825–832. doi:10.1049/iet-spr.2015.0274

Raymond, D. R., & Midkiff, S. F. (2008). Denial-of-service in wireless sensor networks: Attacks and defenses. *IEEE Pervasive Computing*, *7*(1), 74–81. doi:10.1109/MPRV.2008.6

Reza, S., & Iftekharuddin, K. M. (2013). Multi-class Abnormal Brain Tissue Segmentation Using Texture Features. In *MICCAI Challenge on Multimodal Brain Tumor Segmentation* (pp. 38–42). Nagoya, Japan: IEEE.

Rivest, R., Shamir, A., & Adleman, L. (1978). A Method for Obtaining Digital Signatures and Public-Key Cryptosystems. *Communications of the ACM*, *21*(2), 120–126. doi:10.1145/359340.359342

Rodriguez, J., Goni, A., & Illarramendi, A. (2005). Real-time classification of ECGs on a PDA. *IEEE Transactions on Information Technology in Biomedicine*, *9*(1), 23–34. doi:10.1109/TITB.2004.838369 PMID:15787004

Rubio, O., Alesanco, A., & García, J. (2013). Secure information embedding into 1D biomedical signals based on SPIHT. *Journal of Biomedical Informatics*, *46*(4), 653–664. doi:10.1016/j.jbi.2013.05.002 PMID:23707304

S.P. Gupta v. Union of India (2003) 1 SCC 500 (India).

Saini, I., Singh, D., & Khosla, A. (2013). QRS detection using K-Nearest Neighbor algorithm (KNN) and evaluation on standard ECG databases. *Journal of Advanced Research*, *4*(4), 331–344. doi:10.1016/j.jare.2012.05.007 PMID:25685438

Salman, N., Ghafour, B., & Hadi, G. (2015). *Medical Image Segmentation Based on Edge Detection Techniques*. Advances in Image and Video Processing; doi:10.14738/aivp.32.1006

Samira Kohli vs Dr. Prabha Manchanda & Anr (January 16, 2018)

Sang, J., Wang, S., & Niu, X. (2016). Quantum realization of the nearest-neighbor interpolation method for FRQI and NEQR. *Quantum Information Processing*, *15*(1), 37–64. doi:10.100711128-015-1135-5

Sarkar, P. (2000). A brief history of cellular automata. *ACM Computing Surveys*, *32*(1), 80–107. doi:10.1145/349194.349202

Sarkar, S., Sen, N., Kundu, A., Das, S., & Chaudhuri, S. S. (2012). A differential evolutionary multilevel segmentation of near infra-red images using renyi's entropy. *International Conference on Frontiers of Intelligent Computing: Theory and Applications*, 699–706.

Sarma, H. K. D., & Kar, A. (2006, October). Security threats in wireless sensor networks. In *Carnahan Conferences Security Technology, Proceedings 2006 40th Annual IEEE International* (pp. 243-251). IEEE.

Sathya, P. D., & Kayalvizhi, R. (2010). Optimum multilevel image thresholding based on tsallis entropy method with bacterial foraging algorithm. *International Journal of Computer Science Issues*, *7*(5), 336–343.

Satyan, S. (2013). *The Use of Compressive Sensing in Video* (Doctoral dissertation).

Saxena, M. (2007). *Security in wireless sensor networks-a layer based classification*. Department of Computer Science, Purdue University.

Sayadi, O., Shamsollahi, M. B., & Clifford, G. D. (2010). Robust detection of premature ventricular contractions using a wave-based Bayesian framework. *IEEE Transactions on Biomedical Engineering*, *57*(2), 353–362. doi:10.1109/TBME.2009.2031243 PMID:19758851

Schade UMeinecke C. (2013). Spatial competition on the master-saliency map. *Frontiers in Psychology*. doi:10.3389/fpsyg.2013.00394 PMID:23847568

Seera, M., Lim, C. P., Liew, W. S., Lim, E., & Loo, C. K. (2015). Classification of Electrocardiogram and Auscultatory blood pressure signals using machine learning models. *Expert Systems with Applications*, *42*(7), 3643–3652. doi:10.1016/j.eswa.2014.12.023

Selvam, P., Balachandran, S., Iyer, S. P., & Jayabal, R. (2017). Hybrid transform based reversible watermarking technique for medical images in telemedicine applications. *Optik-International Journal for Light and Electron Optics*, *145*, 655–671. doi:10.1016/j.ijleo.2017.07.060

Sen, P., & Darabi, S. (2011). Compressive Rendering: A Rendering Application of Compressed Sensing. *IEEE Transactions on Visualization and Computer Graphics*, *17*(4), 487–499. doi:10.1109/TVCG.2010.46 PMID:21311092

Sevak, M. M., Thakkar, F. N., Kher, R. K., & Modi, C. K. (2012, May). CT image compression using compressive sensing and wavelet transform. In *Communication Systems and Network Technologies (CSNT), 2012 International Conference on* (pp. 138-142). IEEE. 10.1109/CSNT.2012.39

Shahamabadi, M. S., Ali, B. B., Varahram, P., & Jara, A. (2013). A network mobility solution based on 6LoWPAN hospital wireless sensor network (NEMO-HWSN). In *7th Int. Conf. Innov. Mobile Internet Services Ubiquitous Comput. (IMIS)* (pp. 433-438). IMIS. 10.1109/IMIS.2013.157

Shaikh, R. A., Lee, S., Song, Y. J., & Zhung, Y. (2006, June). Securing distributed wireless sensor networks: Issues and guidelines. In *Sensor Networks, Ubiquitous, and Trustworthy Computing, 2006. IEEE International Conference on* (Vol. 2, pp. 226-231). IEEE.

Shelke, F. M., Dongre, A. A., & Soni, P. D. (2014). Comparison of different techniques for Steganography in images. *International Journal of Application or Innovation in Engineering & Management*, *3*(2), 171–176.

Shi, G., & Ming, Y. (2016). Wireless Communications. *Networking and Applications*, 1269-1278.

Shi, E., & Perrig, A. (2004). Designing secure sensor networks. *IEEE Wireless Communications*, *11*(6), 38–43. doi:10.1109/MWC.2004.1368895

Shiqian, M., Wotao, Y., Yin, Z., & Chakraborty, A. (2008). An Efficient Algorithm for Compressed MR Imaging using Total Variation and Wavelets. *IEEE Conference on Computer Vision and Pattern Recognition*, 1-8. 10.1109/CVPR.2008.4587391

Shiu, H. J., Lin, B. S., Chien, H. H., Chiang, P. Y., & Lei, C. L. (2017). Preserving privacy of online digital physiological signals using blind and reversible steganography. *Computer Methods and Programs in Biomedicine*, *151*, 159–170. doi:10.1016/j.cmpb.2017.08.015 PMID:28946998

Shi, Y., & Eberhart, R. (1998). A modified particle swarm optimizer. In *IEEE World Congress on Computational Intelligence*. Anchorage, AK: IEEE.

Shi, Y., Yi, Y., Yan, H., Dai, J., Zhang, M., & Kong, J. (2014). Region contrast and supervised locality-preserving projection-based saliency detection. *The Visual Computer*, *31*(9), 1191–1205. doi:10.100700371-014-1005-7

Shrividya, G., & Bharathi, S. H. (2018, February). A study of Optimum Sampling Pattern for Reconstruction of MR Images using Compressive Sensing. In *2018 Second International Conference on Advances in Electronics, Computers and Communications* (pp. 1-6). IEEE. 10.1109/ICAECC.2018.8479422

Shuang, Y., & Zhou, Y. (2017). Binary-block embedding for reversible data hiding in encrypted images. *Signal Processing, 133*, 40–51. doi:10.1007/SpringerReference_24796

Shukla, R., Gupta, R. K., & Kashyap, R. (2019). A multiphase pre-copy strategy for the virtual machine migration in cloud. In S. Satapathy, V. Bhateja, & S. Das (Eds.), *Smart Intelligent Computing and Applications. Smart Innovation, Systems and Technologies* (Vol. 104). Singapore: Springer. doi:10.1007/978-981-13-1921-1_43

Silva, B. M. C., Rodrigues, J. J. P. C., Canelo, F., Lopes, I. M. C., & Lloret, J. (2014). Towards a cooperative security system for mobile-health applications. *Electronic Commerce Research*, (1). doi:10.100710660-014-9171-2

Singh, P. P., & Garg, R. D. (2014). Classification of high resolution satellite images using spatial constraints-based fuzzy clustering. *Journal of Applied Remote Sensing*, *8*(1).

Singh, B. N., & Tiwari, A. K. (2006). Optimal selection of wavelet basis function applied to ECG signal denoising. *Digital Signal Processing*, *16*(3), 275–287. doi:10.1016/j.dsp.2005.12.003

Singh, G. (2013). A study of encryption algorithms (RSA, DES, 3DES and AES) for information security. *International Journal of Computers and Applications*, *67*(19).

Singh, M. G., Singla, M. A., & Sandha, M. K. (2011). Cryptography algorithm comparison for security enhancement in wireless intrusion detection system. *International Journal of Multidisciplinary Research*, *1*(4), 143–151.

Singh, M., Verma, A., & Sharma, N. (2017). Bat optimization based neuron model of stochastic resonance for the enhancement of MR images. *Biocybernetics and Biomedical Engineering*, *37*(1), 124–134. doi:10.1016/j.bbe.2016.10.006

Singh, Y. S., Devi, B. P., & Singh, K. M. (2013). A review of different techniques on digital image watermarking scheme. *International Journal of Engine Research*, *2*(3), 193–199.

Slimane, Z. E. H., & Naït-Ali, A. (2010). QRS complex detection using empirical mode decomposition. *Digital Signal Processing*, *20*(4), 1221–1228. doi:10.1016/j.dsp.2009.10.017

Society, B. (1996). *IEEE Standard for Medical Device Communications — Overview and Framework*. IEEE.

Song, S., Zhang, J., Liao, X., Du, J., & Wen, Q. (2011). A novel secure communication protocol combining steganography and cryptography. *Procedia Engineering, 15*, 2767–2772. doi:10.1016/j.proeng.2011.08.521

Song, X. H., Wang, S., Liu, S., Abd El-Latif, A. A., & Niu, X. M. (2013). A dynamic watermarking scheme for quantum images using quantum wavelet transform. *Quantum Information Processing, 12*(12), 3689–3706. doi:10.100711128-013-0629-2

Srinivas, N., & Biswas, A. (2012). *Protecting Patient Information in India: Data Privacy Law and its Challenges.* Retrieved from www.docs.manupatra.in/newsline/articles/Upload/B3C7F081-838F-489F-9F77-AF1E209C26F8.pdf

Srinivasan, V., Stankovic, J., & Whitehouse, K. (2008). Protecting your daily in-home activity information from a wireless snooping attack. In *10th international conference on Ubiquitous computing* (pp. 202-211). ACM.

Staal, F. J. T., Van Der Luijt, R. B., Baert, M. R. M., Van Drunen, J., Van Bakel, H., Peters, E., & ... . (2002). A novel germline mutation of PTEN associated with brain tumours of multiple lineages. *British Journal of Cancer, 86*(10), 1586–1591. PMID:12085208

Stankovic, J. A., Cao, Q., Doan, T., Fang, L., He, Z., Kiran, R., . . . Wood, A. (2005, June). Wireless sensor networks for in-home healthcare: Potential and challenges. In High confidence medical device software and systems (HCMDSS) workshop (Vol. 2005). Academic Press.

Stroulia, E., Chodos, D., Boers, N. M., Huang, J., Gburzynski, P., & Nikolaidis, I. (2009, May). Software engineering for health education and care delivery systems: The Smart Condo project. In *Software Engineering in Health Care, 2009. SEHC'09. ICSE Workshop on* (pp. 20-28). IEEE.

Subhedar, M. S., & Mankar, V. H. (2014). Current status and key issues in image steganography: A survey. *Computer Science Review, 13-14*, 95–113. doi:10.1016/j.cosrev.2014.09.001

Sudeepa, K. B., Raju, K., Ranjan Kumar, H. S., & Aithal, G. (2016). A New Approach for Video Steganography Based on Randomization and Parallelization. *Physics Procedia, 78*, 483–490. doi:10.1016/j.procs.2016.02.092

Sunil Batra v. Delhi Administration, (1997) SC 568 (India).

Surjit Singh Thind vs Kanwaljit Kaur. AIR 2003 P&H 353 (India).

T., H. (2007). *LHIP lightweight authentication extension for HIP.* Draft-heer-hip-lhip-00, IETF.

Tabar, A. M., Keshavarz, A., & Aghajan, H. (2006, October). Smart home care network using sensor fusion and distributed vision-based reasoning. In *Proceedings of the 4th ACM international workshop on Video surveillance and sensor networks* (pp. 145-154). ACM. 10.1145/1178782.1178804

Tang, K., Yuan, X., Sun, T., Yang, J., & Gao, S. (2011). An improved scheme for minimum cross entropy threshold selection based on genetic algorithm. *Knowledge-Based Systems. Elsevier B, 24*(8), 1131–1138.

Thirumuruganathan, S. (2010). *A detailed introduction to K-nearest neighbor (KNN) algorithm.* Academic Press.

Tiwari, S., Gupta, R. K., & Kashyap, R. (2019). To enhance web response time using agglomerative clustering technique for web navigation recommendation. In H. Behera, J. Nayak, B. Naik, & A. Abraham (Eds.), *Computational Intelligence in Data Mining. Advances in Intelligent Systems and Computing* (Vol. 711). Singapore: Springer. doi:10.1007/978-981-10-8055-5_59

Toffoli, T. (1980). *Reversible computing.* Berlin: Springer. doi:10.21236/ADA082021

Tran, T. D., Duc, T. T., & Bui, T. T. (2010, November). Combination compress sensing and digital wireless transmission for the MRI signal. In *Micro-NanoMechatronics and Human Science (MHS), 2010 International Symposium* (pp. 273-276). IEEE.

Tremoulheac, B., Dikaios, N., Atkinson, D., & Arridge, S. R. (2014). Dynamic MR Image Reconstruction–Separation From Undersampled (k, t)-Space via Low-Rank Plus Sparse Prior. *IEEE Transactions on Medical Imaging, 33*(8), 1689–1701. doi:10.1109/TMI.2014.2321190 PMID:24802294

Trinder, J., Kleiman, J., Carrington, M., Smith, S., Breen, S., Tan, N., & Kim, Y. (2001). Autonomic activity during human sleep as a function of time and sleep stage. *Journal of Sleep Resolution, 10*(4), 253–264. doi:10.1046/j.1365-2869.2001.00263.x PMID:11903855

Tropp, J. A. (2004). Greed is good: Algorithmic results for sparse approximation. *IEEE Transactions on Information Theory, 50*(10), 2231–2242. doi:10.1109/TIT.2004.834793

Tropp, J. A., Gilbert, A. C., & Strauss, M. J. (2006). Algorithms for simultaneous sparse approximation. Part I: Greedy pursuit. *Signal Processing, 86*(3), 572–588. doi:10.1016/j.sigpro.2005.05.030

Tsallis, C. (1988). Possible generalization of boltzmann- gibbs statistics. *Journal of Statistical Physics, 52*(1), 479–487. doi:10.1007/BF01016429

Urien., P. (2013, Oct). *HIP support for RFIDs.* draft-irtf-hiprg-rfid-07.txt.

Utyuzh, O., Wilk, G., & Wodarczyk, Z. (2007). Numerical symmetrization of state of identical particles. *Brazilian Journal of Physics, 37*(2c). doi:10.1590/S0103-97332007000500007

Van de Weijer, J., Gevers, T., & Bagdanov, A. (2006). Boosting color saliency in image feature detection. *IEEE Transactions on Pattern Analysis and Machine Intelligence, 28*(1), 150–156. doi:10.1109/TPAMI.2006.3 PMID:16402628

Venegas-Andraca, S. E., & Bose, S. (2003). *Storing, processing, and retrieving an image using quantum mechanics.* Academic Press.

Venegas-Andraca, S. E., & Ball, J. L. (2010). Processing images in entangled quantum systems. *Quantum Information Processing, 9*(1), 1–11. doi:10.100711128-009-0123-z

Wang, Y., Attebury, G., & Ramamurthy, B. (2006). *A survey of security issues in wireless sensor networks.* Academic Press.

Wang, G., Bresler, Y., & Ntziachristos, V. (2011). Guest editorial compressive sensing for biomedical imaging. *IEEE Transactions on Medical Imaging, 30*(5), 1013–1016. doi:10.1109/TMI.2011.2145070 PMID:21692237

Wang, K., Lu, Z. M., & Hu, Y. J. (2013). A high capacity lossless data hiding scheme for JPEG images. *Journal of Systems and Software, 86*(7), 1965–1975. doi:10.1016/j.jss.2013.03.083

Wang, M., Wang, X., Zhang, Y., & Gao, Z. (2018). A novel chaotic encryption scheme based on image segmentation and multiple diffusion models. *Optics & Laser Technology, 108*, 558–573. doi:10.1016/j.optlastec.2018.07.052

Wang, S., Yang, B., & Niu, X. (2010). A secure steganography method based on genetic algorithm. *Journal of Information Hiding and Multimedia Signal Processing, 1*(1), 28–35. www.physionet.org/cgi-bin/atm/ATM

Wang, X., & Liu, C. (2017). A novel and effective image encryption algorithm based on chaos and DNA encoding. *Multimedia Tools and Applications, 76*(5), 6229–6245. doi:10.100711042-016-3311-8

Wang, X.-Y., Zhang, Y.-Q., & Bao, X.-M. (2015). A novel chaotic image encryption scheme using DNA sequence operations. *Optics and Lasers in Engineering, 73*, 53–61. doi:10.1016/j.optlaseng.2015.03.022

Waoo, N., Kashyap, R., & Jaiswal, A. (2010). DNA Nano array analysis using hierarchical quality threshold clustering. In *The 2nd IEEE International Conference on Information Management and Engineering*. IEEE. 10.1109/ICIME.2010.5477579

Warren, S., & Jovanov, E. (2006, January). The need for rules of engagement applied to wireless body area networks. *Proc. of the IEEE consumer communications and networking conference, CCNC*. 10.1109/CCNC.2006.1593184

Wen, W., He, C., Li, M., & Zhan, Y. (2012). Adaptively Active Contours Based on Variable ExponentLp(|∇I|)Norm for Image Segmentation. *Mathematical Problems in Engineering, 2012*, 1–20. doi:10.1155/2012/490879

Wiegand, T., Sullivan, G. J., Bjontegaard, G., & Luthra, A. (2003). Overview of the H. 264/AVC video coding standard. *IEEE Transactions on Circuits and Systems for Video Technology, 13*(7), 560–576. doi:10.1109/TCSVT.2003.815165

Wilson, C. B. (1999). Sensors in Medicine. *The Western Journal of Medicine, 11*(5), 322–335. PMID:18751196

Wood, A. D., Fang, L., Stankovic, J. A., & He, T. (2006). SIGF: a family of configurable, secure routing protocols for wireless sensor networks. In *4th ACM workshop on Security of ad hoc and sensor networks* (pp. 35-48). ACM. 10.1145/1180345.1180351

Wood, A. D., Stankovic, J. A., Virone, G., Selavo, L., He, Z., Cao, Q., ... Stoleru, R. (2008). Context-aware wireless sensor networks for assisted living and residential monitoring. *IEEE Network, 22*(4), 26–33. doi:10.1109/MNET.2008.4579768

Wright, J., Yang, A. Y., Ganesh, A., Sastry, S. S., & Ma, Y. (2009). Robust Face Recognition via Sparse Representation. *IEEE Transactions on Pattern Analysis and Machine Intelligence, 31*(2), 210–227. doi:10.1109/TPAMI.2008.79 PMID:19110489

Wu, W., Au, L., Jordan, B., Stathopoulos, T., Batalin, M., & Kaiser, W. (2008). The smartcane system: an assistive device for geriatrics. In ICST (Institute for Computer Sciences, Social-Informatics and Telecommunications Engineering) 3rd international (pp. 1-4). BodyNets '08.

Wu, Y., Member, S., Noonan, J. P., & Member, L. (2011, April). NPCR and UACI Randomness Tests for Image Encryption. *Cyber Journals: Multidisciplinary Journals in Science and Technology, Journal of Selected Areas in Telecommunications*, 31–38.

Xie, S., Guan, C., Huang, W., & Lu, Z. (2015). Frame-based compressive sensing MR image reconstruction with balanced regularization. In *Engineering in Medicine and Biology Society (EMBC), 2015 37th Annual International Conference* (pp. 7031-7034). IEEE.

Xu, M., & Zhang, H. (2014). Saliency detection with color contrast based on boundary information and neighbors. *The Visual Computer, 31*, 355–364. doi:10.100700371-014-0930-9

Yachana, K. N., & Sood, S. K. (2017). A trustworthy system for secure access to patient centric sensitive information. *Telematics and Informatics*. doi:10.1016/j.tele.2017.09.008

Yager, P., Edwards, T., Fu, E., Helton, K., Nelson, K., Tam, M. R., & Weigl, B. H. (2006). Microfluidic diagnostic technologies for global public health. *Nature, 442*(7101), 412–418. doi:10.1038/nature05064 PMID:16871209

Yan, H., Xu, Y., Gidlund, M., & Nohr, R. (2008, August). An experimental study on home-wireless passive positioning. In *Sensor Technologies and Applications, 2008. SENSORCOMM'08. Second International Conference on* (pp. 223-228). IEEE.

Yang, C. Y., & Wang, W. F. (2016). Effective electrocardiogram steganography based on coefficient alignment. *Journal of Medical Systems, 40*(3), 66. doi:10.100710916-015-0426-9 PMID:26711443

Yang, H., Sun, X., & Sun, G. (2009). A high-capacity image data hiding scheme using adaptive LSB substitution. *Wuxiandian Gongcheng, 18*(4), 509–516.

Yang, H., Wong, K.-W., Liao, X., Zhang, W., & Wei, P. (2010). A fast image encryption and authentication scheme based on chaotic maps. *Communications in Nonlinear Science and Numerical Simulation, 15*(11), 3507–3517. doi:10.1016/j.cnsns.2010.01.004

Yang, S., & Shen, H. (2013). Heartbeat classification using discrete wavelet transform and kernel principal component analysis. In *TENCON Spring Conference, 2013* (pp. 34–38). IEEE. doi:10.1109/TENCONSpring.2013.6584412

Yang, X. S. (2010). A new metaheuristic bat-inspired algorithm. In *Nature inspired cooperative strategies for optimization* (pp. 65–74). Springer. doi:10.1007/978-3-642-12538-6_6

Ye, C., Kumar, B. V. K. V., & Coimbra, M. T. (2012). Heartbeat classification using morphological and dynamic features of ECG signals. *Biomed Eng IEEE Trans, 59*(10), 2930–2941. doi:10.1109/TBME.2012.2213253 PMID:22907960

Yeh, J.-P., & Wu, K.-L. (2008). A simple method to synchronize chaotic systems and its application to secure communications. *Mathematical and Computer Modelling, 47*(9), 894–902. doi:10.1016/j.mcm.2007.06.021

Yin, P.-Y. (2007). Multilevel minimum cross entropy threshold selection based on particle swarm optimization. *Applied Mathematics and Computation, 184*(2), 503–513. doi:10.1016/j.amc.2006.06.057

Yin, S., Zhao, X., Wang, W., & Gong, M. (2014). Efficient multilevel image segmentation through fuzzy entropy maximization and graph cut optimization. *Pattern Recognition, 47*(9), 2894–2907. doi:10.1016/j.patcog.2014.03.009

Yoon, J. W., & Kim, H. (2010). An image encryption scheme with a pseudorandom permutation based on chaotic maps. *Communications in Nonlinear Science and Numerical Simulation, 15*(12), 3998–4006. doi:10.1016/j.cnsns.2010.01.041

Yu, C., Zhang, W., & Wang, C. (2015). A Saliency Detection Method Based on Global Contrast. International Journal of Signal Processing. *Image Processing and Pattern Recognition, 8*(7), 111–122. doi:10.14257/ijsip.2015.8.7.11

Zacharaki, E. I., Wang, S., Chawla, S., & Soo, D. (2009). Classification of brain tumor type and grade using MRI texture and shape in a machine learning scheme. *Magnetic Resonance in Medicine, 62*(6), 1609–1618. doi:10.1002/mrm.22147 PMID:19859947

Zhang, Q., Zhang, J., & Sei-ichiro, K. (2016). Adaptive sampling and wavelet tree based compressive sensing for MRI reconstruction. In *Image Processing (ICIP), 2016 IEEE International Conference,* (pp. 2524-2528). IEEE.

Zhang, X., & Wen, J. (2012, September). Compressive video sensing using non-linear mapping. In *Image Processing (ICIP), 2012 19th IEEE International Conference on* (pp. 885-888). IEEE. 10.1109/ICIP.2012.6467002

Zhang, J., Ma, W., Ma, L., & He, Z. (2013). Fault diagnosis model based on fuzzy support vector machine combined with weighted fuzzy clustering. *Transactions of Tianjin University, 19*(3), 174–181. doi:10.100712209-013-1927-6

Zhang, S., Gao, T., & Gao, L. (2014). A Novel Encryption Frame for Medical Image with Watermark Based on Hyperchaotic System. *Mathematical Problems in Engineering, 2014,* 1–11. doi:10.1155/2014/917147

Zhang, S., Gao, T., & Gao, L. (2014). A novel encryption frame for medical image with watermark based on hyperchaotic system. *Mathematical Problems in Engineering, 2014.* doi:10.1155/2014/240749

Zhang, X., Wen, J., Han, Y., & Villasenor, J. (2011, February). An improved compressive sensing reconstruction algorithm using linear/non-linear mapping. In *Information Theory and Applications Workshop (ITA), 2011* (pp. 1-7). IEEE. 10.1109/ITA.2011.5743577

Zhang, Y., Lu, K., Gao, Y., & Xu, K. (2013). A novel quantum representation for log-polar images. *Quantum Information Processing*, *12*(9), 3103–3126. doi:10.100711128-013-0587-8

Zhang, Y., & Wu, L. (2011). Optimal Multi-Level Thresholding Based on Maximum Tsallis Entropy via an Artificial Bee Colony Approach. *Entropy (Basel, Switzerland)*, *13*(4), 841–859. doi:10.3390/e13040841

Zhang, Z., Dong, J., Luo, X., Choi, K.-S., & Wu, X. (2014). Heartbeat classification using disease-specific feature selection. *Computers in Biology and Medicine*, *46*, 79–89. doi:10.1016/j.compbiomed.2013.11.019 PMID:24529208

Zhao, C., Ma, S., Zhang, J., Xiong, R., & Gao, W. (2017). Video compressive sensing reconstruction via reweighted residual sparsity. *IEEE Transactions on Circuits and Systems for Video Technology*, *27*(6), 1182–1195. doi:10.1109/TCSVT.2016.2527181

Zhao, F., Liang, H., Wu, X., & Ding, D. (2017). Region-based Active Contour Segmentation Model with Local Discriminant Criterion. *International Journal Of Security And Its Applications*, *11*(7), 73–86. doi:10.14257/ijsia.2017.11.7.06

Zhou, X., & Tang, X. (2011, August). Research and implementation of RSA algorithm for encryption and decryption. *Strategic Technology (IFOST), 2011 6th International Forum on*, *2*, 1118–1121.

Zhou, Y., Bao, L., & Chen, C. L. P. (2014). A new 1D chaotic system for image encryption. *Signal Processing*, *97*, 172–182. doi:10.1016/j.sigpro.2013.10.034

Zhuang, M., Dierckx, R., & Zaidi, H. (2016). Generic and robust method for automatic segmentation of PET images using an active contour model. *Medical Physics*, *43*(8Part1), 4483–4494. doi:10.1118/1.4954844 PMID:27487865

Zia, T., & Zomaya, A. (2006, October). Security issues in wireless sensor networks. In Null (p. 40). IEEE. doi:10.1109/ICSNC.2006.66

Zimmermann, P. (2010, June). *Where to Get PGP*. Retrieved from Phil Zimmermann & Associates LLC: https://philzimmermann.com/EN/findpgp/

About the Contributors

Butta Singh received his Bachelor's degree in Electronics and Communication Engineering from Guru Nanak Dev Engineering College, Ludhiana, Punjab, India in 2002, Master's degree in Instrumentation and Control Engineering from Sant Longowal Institute of Engineering and Technology, Longowal, Sangrur, Punjab, India in 2005 and Ph.D. in Engineering from National Institute of Technology, Jalandhar, Punjab, India. He is serving as Assistant Professor in the Department of Electronics and Communication Engineering, Guru Nanak Dev University, Regional Campus, Jalandhar, Punjab, India. His professional research interests are in signal processing, in particular, applied to biomedical applications. He has published over 50 research articles in internationally reputed journals and conference proceedings.

* * *

Rengarajan Amirtharajan received his B.E. degree from P.S.G. College of Technology, Bharathiyar University, Coimbatore, India in 1997. He received M.Tech. and PhD degrees from SASTRA Deemed University, Thanjavur, India in 2007 and 2012, respectively. He is currently working as an Associate Professor in the School of EEE, SASTRA Deemed University. His research interests include image security, information hiding and information security. He has patented a novel embedding scheme which has been issued by USPTO during March 2015. He has also published more than 150 research articles in National & International journals.

Charu Bhardwaj is a Ph.D. Research Scholar and teaching assistant in the Department of Electronics and Communication Engineering, JUIT Waknaghat, Solan. Her research area is Digital Signal Processing, Digital Image Processing and Biomedical Image Processing. The Author has published articles in 4th IEEE Conference on "Computing for Sustainable Global Development" (INDIACOM 2017) and Journal of Global Pharma Technology. As a Research Associate, she is currently working in JUIT and giving her constant efforts to make the research work a success.

Dinesh Bhatia received his Ph.D. in the field of bio-rehabilitation engineering from Motilal Nehru National Institute of Technology (MNNIT), Allahabad. His specific interests lie in the development of bio-rehabilitative devices, and the study of EMG signals. He is currently an Associate Professor and Head of Department of the Biomedical Engineering, North Easrtern Hill University, Shillong, India. He was the recipient of the BOYSCAST Fellowship and INAE Fellowships and was also the International Young Biomedical Scientist.

Savita Gupta is currently working as a Professor in the Department of Computer Science and Engineering, University Institute of Engineering and Technology, Panjab University, Chandigarh. She completed her PhD degree from the PTU, Jalandhar in 2007 in the field of ultrasound image processing. Her research interests include wavelet-based image processing, network security, image compression and denoising.

Shruti Jain has received PhD degree from Jaypee University of Information Technology, Waknaghat, Solan. She has a teaching experience of around 13 years and before joining JUIT, she worked as Assistant Professor in Haryana Engineering College, Jagadhari, Ambala College of Engineering, Ambala. She has specialization in Biomedical Signal Processing, Computer- Aided design of FPGA and VLSI circuits, combinatorial optimization. She has published more than 50 papers in reputed journals and 30 papers in International conferences. She is a senior member of IEEE, life member of Biomedical Engineering Society of India and member of IAENG. She is currently working as Associate Professor in the Department of Electronics and Communication Engineering, JUIT Waknaghat.

Siva Janakiraman received his B.E. Degree from Bharathidasan University, Tiruchirapalli, India in 2003. He received M.Tech. Degree in Embedded Systems and Ph.D. Degree from SASTRA Deemed University, Thanjavur, India in 2007 and 2017 respectively. He is currently working as Senior Assistant Professor in the School of EEE, SASTRA Deemed University. His research interests include embedded system and information security. He has also published more than 25 research articles in peer- reviewed international journals.

Ramgopal Kashyap's areas of interest are image processing, pattern recognition, and machine learning. He has published many research papers in international journals and conferences like Springer, Inderscience, Elsevier, ACM, and IGI-Global indexed by Science Citation Index (SCI) and Scopus (Elsevier) and many book chapters. He has Reviewed Research Papers in the Science Citation Index Expanded, Springer Journals and Editorial Board Member and conferences programme committee member of the IEEE, Springer international conferences and journals held in countries: Czech Republic, Switzerland, UAE, Australia, Hungary, Poland, Taiwan, Denmark, India, USA, UK, Austria, and Turkey. He has written many book chapters published by IGI Global, USA.

Taranjit Kaur received her BTech and MTech in Electronics and Communication Engineering from the Guru Nanak Dev Engineering College, Ludhiana in 2010 and 2012. She did her PhD from Dr. B.R. Ambedkar National Institute of Technology, Jalandhar, Punjab in the area of medical image processing in year 2017. Currently, she is a post doctoral fellow in the Department of Electrical Engineering, Indian Institute of Technology, Delhi (IIT Delhi). Prior to the joining at IIT Delhi she has also worked as an Assistant Professor at Guru Nanak Dev Engineering College, Ludhiana.Her research interest include application of the optimization techniques for the medical image analysis.

Padmapriya Praveenkumar received her B.E (ECE) from Angala Amman college of Engineering and Technology and M.E (Communication system) from Jayaram college of Engineering and Technology. Currently she is working as an Senior Assistant Professor in the Department of ECE in SASTRA Deemed University, Thanjavur. She has a teaching experience of 15 years and she has published 45 Research articles in National & International journals. Her research area includes image encryption, Quantum medical image encryption, Wireless communication and Steganography.

SanthiyaDevi R. completed her B.Tech and M.Tech from SASTRA Deemed university. She is currently pursuing her Ph.D. in SASTRA Deemed University. Her area of interest includes Image Encryption and Quantum Medical Image Encryption.

Surendra Rahamatkar areas of interest are pattern recognition, and machine learning. He has published many research papers in international journals and conferences like Springer, Inderscience, Elsevier, ACM, and IGI-Global indexed by Science Citation Index (SCI) and Scopus (Elsevier) and many book chapters. He has Reviewed Research Papers in the Science Citation Index Expanded, Springer Journals.

Sundararaman Rajagopalan completed his B.Tech. in Electronics & Instrumentation Engg., M.Tech. in Advanced Communication Systems and Ph.D. in the domain of hardware steganography in the years 2005, 2007 and 2015 respectively from SASTRA University, Thanjavur, India. He is currently working as Senior Asst. Professor in the Dept. of ECE, SASTRA University. He has recently completed a DRDO, Govt. of India funded project in the domain of Random Key Generation. He was also a Co-Principal Investigator in a DRDO, Govt. of India funded project on steganography. Also, he was a WIPRO ULK faculty resource guide team Contributor for FPGA based experiments with Unified Technology Learning Platform (UTLP). He was also a faculty guide for IBM Remote Mentoring Projects for the years 2011 and 2012. He has published 30 research articles in national and international journals.

Barjinder Singh Saini was born in Jalandhar, India. He received his B.Tech and M.Tech degrees in Electronics & Communication Engineering. He then obtained his Ph.D. degree in Engineering on ''Signal Processing of Heart Rate Variability'' from Dr. B. R. Ambedkar National Institute of Technology, Jalandhar. His areas of interest are medical image processing, digital signal processing and embedded systems.

Indu Saini received her B. Tech degree in Electronics and Communication Engineering from Guru Nanak Dev University, India, in 1994 and then obtained her M. Tech (by Research) and PhD degree in Electronics & Communication Engineering from Dr B. R. Ambedkar National Institute of Technology Jalandhar, where she is also serving as Assistant Professor in Electronics & Communication Engineering Department since 2002. Her professional research interests are Very Large Scale Integration (VLSI) design, Biomedical Signal/Image Processing, and Machine Learning Algorithms.

Neetika Soni received her M.Tech Degree from Punjab Technical University, Punjab India in year 2008 and currently pursuing her PhD in Biomedical Signal Processing. She is working as an Assistant Professor in Department of Electronics and Communication Engineering, GNDU, RC, Jalandhar, Punjab since 2004. Her areas of interest includes Biomedical Signal Processing and Embedded System Design.

Meenakshi Sood is a Senior Assistant Professor in the Department of Electronics and Communication Engineering at Jaypee University of Information Technology, Waknaghat, H.P, India and received her Ph.D in Biomedical Signal Processing. She is Gold Medalist and has been awarded Academic Award for her performance in Master of Engineering (Hons.) from Panjab Univeristy, Chandigarh. Her research areas interests are Image and Signal processing, Antenna Design, Metamaterials and Soft Computing. She has published more than 25 papers in reputed journals and 30 papers in International conferences. She is a senior member of IEEE and giving her continuous guidance and efforts as Department Coordinator at JUIT. She has published course material of "Digital Electronics and Microprocessors " for ICDOEL, H.P University. She had been selected as GSE member of Rotary International and visited USA in Exchange Program.

Neetu Sood works as assistant professor in the Department of Electronics and Communication Engineering at Dr B R Ambedkar National Institute of Technology, Jalandhar in India since 2007. Her research interest includes wireless communication system design, OFDM based systems, channel modelling & its simulations, Biomedical signal processing and plant signalling.

Ankita Tiwari received his B.Tech degree in the field of Electronics and Communication Engineering from Dr. APJ Abdul Kalam Technical University (AKTU) and M.Tech degree in the field of Embedded System and Technology from Amity University Uttar Pradesh. Her specific interest lies in the Biomedical Signal Processing, Artificial Neural Networks, Intelligent Biomedical Devices and Embedded Systems.

Raghuvendra Pratap Tripathi received his B.Tech and M.Tech degree in the field of Electronics and Communication Engineering from Amity University Uttar Pradesh. His specific interests lie in the Biomedical Signal Processing, Artificial Neural Networks, Intelligent Biomedical Devices and Embedded Systems. He is currently working as a Junior Research Fellow in Department of the Biomedical Engineering, North Eastern Hill University, Shillong, India.

Index

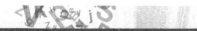
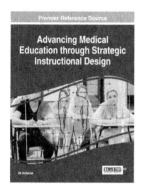
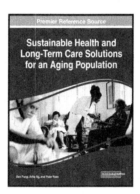
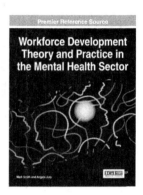
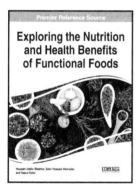
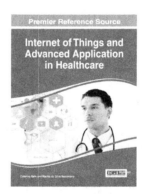
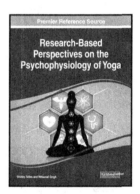
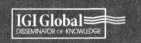

Ensure Quality Research is Introduced to the Academic Community

Become an IGI Global Reviewer for Authored Book Projects

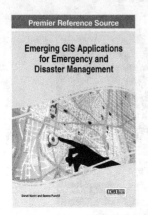

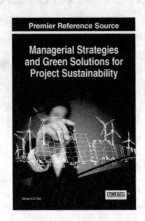

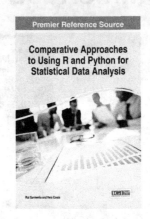

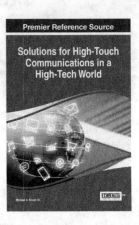

The overall success of an authored book project is dependent on quality and timely reviews.

In this competitive age of scholarly publishing, constructive and timely feedback significantly expedites the turnaround time of manuscripts from submission to acceptance, allowing the publication and discovery of forward-thinking research at a much more expeditious rate. Several IGI Global authored book projects are currently seeking highly qualified experts in the field to fill vacancies on their respective editorial review boards:

Applications may be sent to:
development@igi-global.com

Applicants must have a doctorate (or an equivalent degree) as well as publishing and reviewing experience. Reviewers are asked to write reviews in a timely, collegial, and constructive manner. All reviewers will begin their role on an ad-hoc basis for a period of one year, and upon successful completion of this term can be considered for full editorial review board status, with the potential for a subsequent promotion to Associate Editor.

If you have a colleague that may be interested in this opportunity, we encourage you to share this information with them.

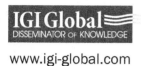

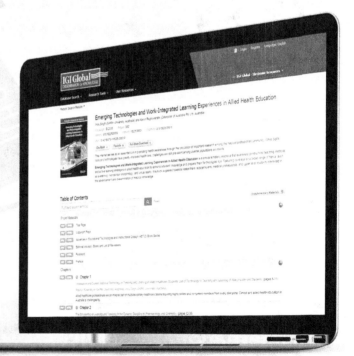

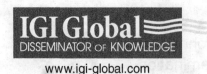
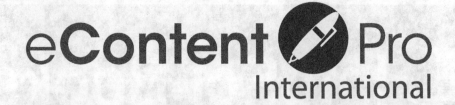

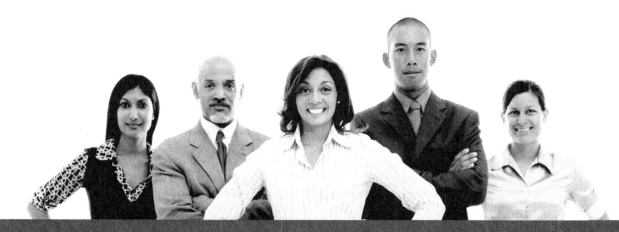

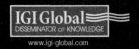
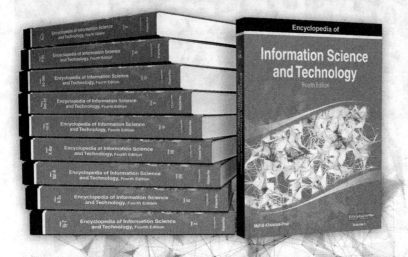

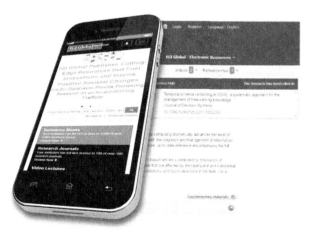
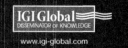

Printed in the United States
By Bookmasters